Allergy Methods and Protocols

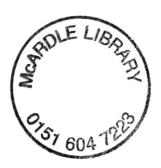

METHODS IN MOLECULAR MEDICINE

John M. Walker, SERIES EDITOR

METHODS IN MOLECULAR MEDICINE

Allergy Methods and Protocols

Edited by

Meinir G. Jones

Department of Occupational and Environmental Medicine
Imperial College
London, United Kingdom

and

Penny Lympany

St. George's University of London
London, United Kingdom

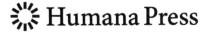
Humana Press

Production Editor: Christina Thomas

Cover Design: Mark Buckley and Andrew F. Walls

Cover Illustration: From Ch. 24 Fig. 1.A. mast cells identified around the crypts in human colonic tissue, using an immunohistochemical procedure specific for tryptase.

For additional copies, pricing for bulk purchases, and/or information about other Humana titles, contact Humana at the above address or at any of the following numbers: Tel.: 973-256-1699; Fax: 973-256-8341; E-mail: orders@humanapr.com; or visit our Website: www.humanapress.com

Printed in the United States of America. 10 9 8 7 6 5 4 3 2 1
eISBN: 978-1-59745-366-0

Library of Congress Control Number: 2007932488

Preface

Allergy is a major problem in the 'Westernized' countries, and its prevalence continues to rise. It is therefore important to try and understand the reasons for the increase in allergy. Research in recent years has focused on the causes and mechanisms of allergy. In parallel, there is also an impetus to try to understand mechanisms of natural tolerance and immunotherapy where allergy is being dampened. This volume *Allergy Methods and Protocols* in the *Methods in Molecular Medicine* series aims to assist the researcher to gain an insight into the molecular mechanisms involved in allergy by featuring an array of protocols. These cover a range of disciplines including allergy, immunology, cell biology and histology and include methods to investigate the cellular response to allergens, cytokine profile, MHC restriction, T regulatory cells. The book is intended to be a useful bench tool for anyone embarking or continuing with their research in allergy. Techniques discussed include; B and T cell epitope mapping, characterisation of allergens, conjugation of haptens, preparation of monoclonal antibodies, collection and sampling of airborne allergens, IgG antibodies and facilitated antigen blocking assays, identification and purification of mast cells and *in situ* hybridisation. We thank all the authors who have shared their protocols with us and made this book possible.

Meinir G. Jones

Contents

Contributors

ALLAN B. BECKER • *Department of Immunology, University of Manitoba, Winnipeg, Canada*

MELANIE BLANCHARD • *Department of Immunology, University of Manitoba, Winnipeg, Canada*

MICHAEL BUCKLEY • *Immunopharmacology Group, Southampton General Hospital, Southampton*

DARREN CAMPBELL • *Department of Immunology, University of Manitoba, Winnipeg, Canada*

KEVIN COOMBS • *Department of Immunology, University of Manitoba, Winnipeg, Canada*

OLIVER CROMWELL • *Allergopharma Joachim Ganzer, Reinbek, Germany*

SANDRA DE LUCCA • *Department of Medicine, University of Sydney, Australia*

STEN DREBORG • *Lerum, Sweden*

RENÉE DOUVILLE • *Department of Immunology, University of Manitoba, Winnipeg, Canada*

JAMES N. FRANCIS • *Department of Allergy and Clinical Immunology, National Heart and Lung Institute, Imperial College, South Kensington, London*

SUSAN GORDON • *Institute of Occupational Medicine, Research Park North, Riccarton, Dinburgh, Scotland*

GITTE NORDSKOV HANSEN • *ALK-Abello, Denmark*

KENT T. HAYGLASS • *Department of Immunology, University of Manitoba, Winnipeg, Canada*

SHAOHENG HE • *Immunopharmacology Group, Southampton General Hospital, Southampton*

HAYLEY JEAL • *Department of Occupational and Environmental Medicine, National Heart and Lung Institute, Imperial College School of Medicine, London, UK*

ERIKA JENSEN-JAROLIM • *Medical University of Vienna, Vienna, Austria*

MEINIR JONES • *Department of Occupational and Environmental Medicine, National Heart and Lung Institute, Imperial College School of Medicine, London, UK*

HELGA KAHLERT • *Allergopharma Joachim Ganzer KG, Germany*

MERYL KAROL • *Department of Environmental and Occupational Health, University of Pittsburgh, Pittsburgh, PA*

MARK LARCHE • *Department of Allergy and Clinical Immunology, Imperial College London, National Heart and Lung Institute, London, UK*
JØRGEN NEDERGAARD LARSEN • *ALK-Abello, Horsholm, Denmark*
PER H. LARSSON • *Mabtech AB, Nacka Strand, Sweden*
RANULFO LEMUS • *Department of Environmental and Occupational Health, University of Pittsburgh, Pittsburgh, PA*
YURIY LISSITSYN • *Department of Immunology, University of Manitoba, Winnipeg, Canada*
ALAN R. MCEUEN • *Immunopharmacology Group, Southampton General Hospital, Southampton, UK*
PETER NICKERSON • *Department of Immunology, University of Manitoba, Winnipeg, Canada*
ALISTAIR NOBLE • *Department of Asthma, Allergy and Respiratory Science, King's College London, London, UK*
KAYHAN T. NOURI-ARIA • *Department of Allergy and Clinical Immunology, National Heart and Lung Institute, Imperial College, South Kensington, London, UK*
TIM O'MEARA • *Department of Medicine, University of Sydney, Australia*
LEANNE POULOS • *Department of Medicine, University of Sydney, Australia*
MAGDALENA RAHL • *ALLERGON AB, Ängelholm, Sweden*
MONIKA RAULF-HEIMSOTH • *Institut der Ruhr-Universität Bochum, Bereich Allergologie/Immunologie, Germany*
ANNE RENSTRÖM • *Lung-och allergiforskning, Karolinska Institutet, Stockholm, Sweden*
ISABELLA SCHÖLL • *Centre of Physiology and Pathophysiology, Medical University of Vienna, Vienna, Austria*
F ESTELLE SIMONS • *Department of Immunology, University of Manitoba, Winnipeg, Canada*
WILLIAM P. STEFURA • *Department of Immunology, University of Manitoba, Winnipeg, Canada*
MONIQUE J. STINSON • *Department of Immunology, University of Manitoba, Winnipeg, Canada*
SUN-SANG J. SUNG • *Division of Rheumatology, University of Virginia Health Sciences Center, Charlottesville, VA*
EUAN TOVEY • *Department of Medicine, University of Sydney, Australia*
ADRIENNE VERHOEF • *Department of Allergy and Clinical Immunology, National Heart and Lung Institute, Imperial College School of Medicine, South Kensington, London, UK*
TUOMAS VIRTANEN • *Department of Clinical Microbiology, University of Kuopio, Kuopio, Finland*

BEEJAL VYAS • *Department of Asthma, Allergy and Respiratory Science, King's College London, London, UK*
ANDREW F. WALLS • *Immunopharmacology Group, Southampton General Hospital, Southampton, UK*
THOMAS ZEILER • *Department of Clinical Microbiology, University of Kuopio, Kuopio, Finland*

1

Understanding of the Molecular Mechanisms of Allergy

Meinir Jones

Abstract

The prevalence of allergic disease has dramatically increased over the past 30 years in Westernised countries. It is unlikely that the rapid increase in the prevalence of allergic disease is the result of genetic changes, which highlights the importance of environmental factors in the development of allergic disease. The 'hygiene hypothesis' was put forward in 1989 and focused attention on the notion that exposure to microbes and their products in early life can modify the risk for development of allergic disease. Infections were thought to polarize the immunological response towards a Th2-mediated immune responses causing allergic disease. However it is likely that the Th1/Th2 imbalance is too simplistic to explain the increased prevalence of allergic disease. Current research is focusing on understanding the role of T regulatory cells in inducing a state of tolerance and the resulting modified Th2 response observed in natural and induced tolerance.

Key Words: Allergic disease; hygiene hypothesis; immunoregulation; immunotolerance.

1. Introduction

The term 'allergy' was introduced in 1906 by von Pirquet *(1)*, who recognized that in both protective immunity and hypersensitivity reactions, antigens had induced changes in reactivity. Allergy is now used to describe a hypersensitivity reaction initiated by immunologic mechanism *(2)*. Allergic diseases include allergic rhinitis, allergic conjunctivitis, asthma, atopic eczema, and food allergy. IgE-mediated diseases are often referred to as atopy (from the Greek atopos, meaning out of place). The definition of atopy is a personal or familial tendency to produce IgE antibodies in response to low doses of allergens, usually proteins, and to develop typical symptoms such as asthma, rhinoconjunctivitis, or eczema/dermatitis *(3)*.

Atopic individuals have a genetic predisposition to produce IgE antibodies against common environmental allergens. Atopic disorders are thought to be

From: *Methods in Molecular Medicine: Allergy Methods and Protocols*
Edited by: M. G. Jones and P. Lympany © Humana Press Inc., Totowa, NJ

because of complex interactions between genetic and environmental factors. The prevalence of allergic disease has dramatically increased over the past 30 yr *(4–7)*, especially in Westernized countries. It is unlikely that the rapid increase in the prevalence of allergic disease is the result of genetic changes, which highlights the importance of environmental factors in the development of allergic disease. The increased prevalence of allergy in Westernized countries highlights the potential influence of improved hygiene and better infection control on the development of allergy. An interesting observation was made after the reunification of Germany: before reunification, allergic rhinitis and asthma were less common in East Germany compared with West Germany *(8)*. However, since reunification, the prevalence of atopy and hay fever, but not asthma, has increased among children who spent their early childhood in East Germany *(9)*. Interestingly, exposure to farm animals remains a protective factor in the development of allergy *(10)*, which is similar to that observed with hay fever at the turn of the century. These observations suggest that our Westernized lifestyle accounts for the increase in prevalence. Interestingly, hay fever was first reported back in the early nineteenth century and was thought to be essentially the disease of the upper social class and urban dwellers *(3)*. The rural working population was considered to have become tolerant through high-dose exposure in the fields.

2. Hygiene Hypothesis

The 'hygiene' hypothesis was put forward in 1989 *(11)*, and focused attention on the notion that exposure to microbes and their products in early life can modify the risk for development of allergic disorders. It is thought that helminth infection, mycobacteria, Hepatitis A, endotoxin, and early life infections create a milieu which protects against the development of allergic reactions. The distinction of Th1 and Th2 cells in mice (1989) *(12)* and humans (1994) *(13)* provided a plausible immunological mechanism for the hygiene hypothesis. Th1 cells are responsible for cell-mediated immune responses against intracellular pathogens whereas Th2 cells direct immune responses against intestinal helminths *(12)*. Th1 cells cause autoimmune diseases, while Th2 cells cause allergic diseases and asthma. Th1 and Th2 cells crossregulate each other, thus it was proposed that in allergic disease there were too many Th2 cells and not enough Th1 cells. Exposure to microbial products leads to a polarization toward the Th1 cells potentially suppressing the Th2 immune response involved in IgE-mediated allergy. Thus lack of exposure to microbes in early childhood may lead to a predominantly Th2 immune response causing allergic disease.

In parallel with an increase in prevalence of allergy in the last 30 yr, there has been a similar increase in autoimmune diseases such as Type 1 diabetes, multiple sclerosis, inflammatory bowel disease, and systemic lupus erythe-matosus *(14,15)*. An increase in the incidence of autoimmune diseases, plus the relative absence of autoimmunity in developing countries where chronic infections are endemic, has led to the theory that infection may actually inhibit the development of autoimmunity *(14)*. In view of increased prevalence of both Th1 autoimmune diseases and Th2 allergic disease in recent years, it is likely that the Th1/Th2 imbalance is too simplistic. It is more likely that there are other control mechanisms of T-cell regulation, which controls harmful T-cell responses.

3. Family Size and Allergy

One of the most robust findings in allergy which has stood the test of time is the epidemiological observation of the inverse association of allergic disease with family size, which was reported with hay fever, skin prick positivity, and specific IgE *(16,17)*. Other factors found to be protective against sensitization are exposure to farm animals or domestic pets, day care attendance, and large family size *(10)*. The protective influence of large family size has been inter-preted as evidence in support of the hygiene hypothesis. However, this does not preclude other mechanisms related to birth order *(18)*.

It is possible that pregnancy may influence the atopic status of both the mother and the fetus. Pregnancy is an immunological challenge to the mother and it is possible that the immunoregulation, which takes place to avoid fetal rejection, may also influence the allergic response in both the mother and the fetus *(19)*. There is some evidence in support of this hypothesis. Mothers of higher parity have lower levels of total IgE, as do their newborn children *(20)*. They report higher rates of remission from allergic rhinitis *(21)* and lower rates of allergic conjunctivitis *(22)*. Cord blood mononuclear cell responses to house dust mite are reduced in higher birth order children *(23)* although this may be explained by maternal age.

In a cross-sectional study, it was observed that multiparous mothers are less often atopic, although this did not hold true for the fathers *(24,25)*. In a prospec-tive study, over a period of 7 yr, it was observed that the loss of maternal atopy and hay fever are associated with a higher number of intervening pregnancies *(26)*. Expansion of regulatory T cells has been demonstrated in both mice *(27)* and humans *(28)*. In mice, the cells were alloantigen-independent although capable of suppressing an aggressive response against the fetus. Their deletion led to a failure of gestation because of immunological fetal rejection. This effect was true only for allogeneic pregnancies, the outcome of syngeneic pregnancies being unaffected. In humans, T regulatory cells increase during early pregnancy, peaking during the second trimester and declining postpartum although remaining higher than prepregnancy *(28)*. The cells are capable of suppressing an allogeneic response. Allergic mothers and their neonates were found to have a stronger lymphoproliferation to alloantigen than nonallergic mothers and their neonates *(29)*, suggesting the possibility of greater immunoregulation in nonallergic than in allergic mothers. It is not known whether the degree of regulation varies with a mother's parity and whether it is transferred to her children.

4. Indoor Allergens

Atopic individuals are, by definition, sensitized to the common environmental allergens. The major allergens of the Westernized countries are Der p 1 and Der p 2 from the house dust mite (*Dermatophagoides pteronyssinus*); Fel d 1 from the cat (*Felis domesticus*); tree allergens including Bet v 1 from the birch tree (*Betula verrucosa*); and many grasses such as Phl p 1 and Phl p 5 from timothy (*Phleum pratense*) and the ragweed allergens Amb a 1, 2, 3, 5, and 6 from short ragweed (*Ambrosia aretmisiifolia*) *(1)*. Another allergen which has become common over the last 25 yr is the glycypahgus dust mite *Blomia tropicalis*, in heavily populated tropical regions *(3)*. This allergen was uncommon; however, it is now estimated that 1 billion individuals are currently sensitized.

At present, there is a drive to target immunotherapy selectively to immunodominant allergens *(3)*. It is currently unknown whether the immunodominant allergens have intrinsic adjuvant properties that contribute to their potency. It will be intriguing to see whether removing or neutralizing the host response to immunodominant allergens will silence the allergy or redirect the immune response toward different specificities. The main allergens represent a diverse group of proteins; several are proteases which are thought to be important in the development of allergy. Currently, there is much interest in the lipid-binding property of immunodominant allergens *(30)*.

Much focus has been given to understanding the mechanisms of the development of sensitization in recent years. It was proposed that exposure to indoor allergens early in life would increase the risk of allergic sensitization. If this were the case, then it would follow that avoidance of allergen early in life would decrease the risk of allergic sensitization. Exposure–response studies with allergen and sensitization have demonstrated an apparent dose–response relationship with a bell-shaped curve, suggestive of a tolerance mechanism at high exposures. A bell-shaped curve was described with cat *(31,32)* and house dust mite *(32)* allergens. Allergen avoidance trial demonstrated that reducing house dust mite concentration did not reduce but increased sensitization rates to house dust mite *(33)*. Cat ownership has been associated with a reduced prevalence of sensitization *(34–36)* and physician-diagnosed asthma *(34)*.

Immunologically, it is known that low-dose antigen exposure favors Th2 priming whereas high-dose priming leads to a Th1 type of response *(3)*.

5. Endotoxin

Animal exposures at home or at work may also result in high exposures to microbial and associated products including endotoxin. Conceivably, this coexposure may confer protection, manifest as an attenuation of the immune response to allergen at high doses. Regulatory T cells selectively express toll-like receptors which are activated by endotoxin. Exposure of CD4+CD25+ cells to the Toll-like receptor-4 ligand lipopolysaccharide induces upregulation of several activation markers and enhances their survival/proliferation *(37)*.

The host response to environmental endotoxin appears to depend, in part, on the time and dose of exposure. Low dose of endotoxin induces a Th2 response whereas high-level endotoxin favors a Th1 response. In an experimental model of allergy, exposure of rats to endotoxin during early sensitization protects against their development of ovalbumin-specific IgE; coexposure of endotoxin with allergen results in dose-dependent inhibition of acute and late phase allergic inflammation and bronchial hyperresponsiveness. Exposures to endotoxin after allergen challenge further exacerbate the allergic response *(38)*. Adult pig farmers have an inverse relationship between endotoxin and sensitization to common allergens, and the overall prevalence of atopic sensitization in this population is low *(39)*.

In contrast, other studies suggest that endotoxin is not protective. Homes of cat owners did not have higher endotoxin levels than homes without cats *(40,41)*. Similarly in a study of laboratory animal workers, there was no significant relationship between rat-related symptoms and endotoxin levels *(42)*. These results argue that the effects of cat and rat ownership cannot be explained by increased exposure to endotoxin.

6. Cellular Response to Allergens

Cellular response of T cells in peripheral blood is often present in both healthy and sensitized individuals *(43)*. The epitopes recognized within allergens is also found to be similar between healthy and allergic individuals *(44–48)*. The cytokine profile from the in vitro T cell culture is predominantly Th2 in the allergic individual. Th2 cytokines IL-4 and IL-13 stimulate the production of IgE; IL-5 and IL-9 are involved in the development of eosinophils; IL-4 and IL-9 promote the development of mast cells; IL-9 and IL-13 promote airway hyperresponsiveness, and IL-4, IL-9, and IL-13 promote the overproduction of mucus *(1)*.

7. Modified Th2 Response

High-dose attenuation of risk of sensitization with cat allergen exposure is associated with high-titer IgG and IgG_4 antibodies *(31)*. This response was described as a modified Th2 response because both IgE and IgG$_4$ require Th2 cytokine IL-4 for their production. The modified Th2 response is suggestive of clinical tolerance because the shift from specific IgE to IgG$_4$ resulted in a decrease in both sensitization and asthma *(49)*.

We have recently established a modified Th2 response in laboratory animal workers. Within our cohort and cross-sectional studies on laboratory animal allergy, we observed increasing risks of sensitization and work-related symptoms with increasing exposures to rats, except at highest exposure level where risks of both outcomes were lower *(50,51)*. We established a significantly increased ratio of IgG$_4$:IgE in the most heavily exposed workers *(50)*. There was an almost twofold reduction in those who produced both specific IgG$_4$ and IgE as compared to those producing specific IgE only. The attenuation at high exposures and the increased ratio of IgG$_4$:IgE in laboratory animal workers are suggestive of a natural form of immunotherapy.

The enteric mucosal immune system plays an extremely efficient and pivotal role in the development of tolerance. Repeated exposure to allergen through the gastrointestinal tract during life leads to the development of tolerance, even in highly atopic individuals *(52)*. It is proposed that exposure to aeroallergens through this route may promote the local (IgA) immune responses, which promote persistent systemic tolerance, preventing the emergence of pathogenic Th2-responsive memory T cells. The information regarding the role of IgA in mediating tolerance to allergens is at present very limited. Immunotherapy studies have shown increases in the levels of TGF-β following treatment *(53)*. TGF-β plays a suppressor role in mucosal allergens such as house dust mite or birch pollen and this cytokine is known to induce IgA, which works as a non-inflammatory immunoglobulin isotype *(53)*. Levels of IgA antibodies have been shown to be upregulated following venom immunotherapy *(54)*.

8. Natural Killer Cells

Mouse models of allergic asthma indicate that natural killer T cells are required for the development of allergen-induced airway hyperreactivity *(55)*. Natural killer T cells have a unique property of responding to glycolipid antigens, rather than peptide antigens presented by the nonpolymorphic class I MHC-like protein CD1d, expressed on antigen-presenting cells. Invariant natural killer T cells rapidly produce large quantities of both Th1 and Th2 cytokines, which enhance the function of dendritic cells, natural killer cells, and B cells, as well as the conventional CD4+ and CD8+ T cells *(56)*. The rapid production of cytokines by invariant natural killer T cells is a manifestation of innate-like immunity and provides these T cells with the capacity to link innate and adaptive immune responses and critically regulate adaptive immunity and a host of inflammatory diseases *(56)*. Recently, it was observed that CD4+ invariant natural killer T cells are abundant in the lungs of patients with chronic asthma but are virtually absent from the lungs of controls and patients with sarcoidosis *(56)*. These natural killer cells express an invariant T-cell receptor that recognizes glycolipid antigens, which appear to be highly conserved in both man and mice. It will be important to identify glycolipid allergens from our major allergens to determine their role in both allergy and asthma.

9. Immunoregulation

The peripheral immune response has evolved several mechanisms to maintain a state of tolerance to innocuous antigens, which involve clonal deletion, anergy, and active suppression mediated by regulatory cells. Several subsets of regulatory T cells (Tr) with distinct phenotypes and distinct mechanisms of action have now been identified *(57)*. Recent studies suggest that naturally occurring T regulatory cells and antigen-induced IL-10 producing T regulatory cells have a physiological role in protecting against human allergic disease *(58)*. A rare mutation in the gene encoding FOXP3 results in a disease called immune-dysregulation, polyendocrinopathy, and enteropathy, X-linked (IPEX). Individuals with IPEX syndrome suffer from a range of autoimmune endocrine pathologies as well as allergic symptoms including severe eczema, increased serum IgE levels, eosinophilia, and food allergies *(58)*. Within allergy, there is evidence that CD4+CD25+ T cells producing IL-10 are important in regulating a nonallergic response. Healthy beekeepers show a substantial increase in IL-10 producing CD4+CD25+ T cells and monocytes, suggesting that these regulatory T cells induce tolerance to bee stings *(59)*.

Recent interest has focused on the role of T regulatory cells in allergic disease and immunotherapy. Seasonal atopic patients were found to have a diminished suppressive effect of T regulatory cells compared with nonatopic controls and this was more pronounced during the hay fever season *(60)*. The degree of allergen exposure is likely to alter the suppressive effect of T regulatory cells in allergic patients. On high grass pollen exposure, regulatory cells from nonatopic donors retained both the ability to inhibit proliferation and cytokine production whilst allergic donors failed to inhibit proliferation. At high allergen doses of wasp venom, T regulatory cells from both allergic and healthy controls lose their regulatory function, whereas nonallergic donors retained their regulatory function at low allergen doses *(61)*. A study investigating regulatory differences before and after cat peptide immunotherapy demonstrated that antigen-specific proliferative responses of memory T cells were reduced after peptide immunotherapy compared with preimmunotherapy samples *(62)*. The CD4 cells isolated after peptide immunotherapy suppressed the proliferative response of baseline CD4-negative cells in the coculture experiments, suggesting that peptide immunotherapy induces a population of CD4 T cells with suppressive/regulatory activity.

Grass pollen immunotherapy is associated with an increase in T regulatory cells with IL-10+CD4+CD25+ phenotype *(63)*. Similarly bee venom immunotherapy demonstrated a significant increase in levels of IL-10 after therapy *(64)*. In a study of cat peptide immunotherapy, they were able to demonstrate reduced antigen-specific proliferative responses in memory T cells following treatment. IL-10 is a potent suppressor of both total and allergen-specific IgE, whereas it simultaneously increases IgG_4 production *(65)*. Specific IL-10 secreting T reg cells consistently represent the dominant subsets against common environmental allergens in healthy individuals, in contrast to the high frequency of allergen-specific IL-4 secreting T cells in allergic individuals *(66)*.

In a recent pilot study, in which we investigated the role of CD4+CD25+ T cells in laboratory animal allergy, CD4+CD25– cells proliferated to a significantly greater degree than either PBMCs ($p < 0.01$) or CD25+ cells ($p < 0.001$) in all individuals (Hayley Jeal, personal communication). Inhibition of proliferation to rat by CD4+CD25+ T cells did not differ between cases and controls. IL-5 suppression was increased in controls than cases although not significantly. Results from this pilot study indicate that the ability of CD4+CD25+ T regulatory cells to suppress proliferation in rat-sensitized individuals compared with controls does not differ, but failure of these cells to suppress IL-5 production in cases could contribute to the development of their allergic disease.

10. Genetics

HLA class II antigens are involved in the presentation of epitopes of foreign proteins at the antigen-presenting cell surface and are important in the development of a hypersensitivity response. Epitope mapping of the major cat allergen, Fel d 1, has revealed several T-cell epitopes *(67)*. One of these T-cell epitopes located in the carboxy terminus of chain 2 of Fel d is associated with HLA-DRB1*0701 with preferential IL-10 induction. Production of IL-10 was enhanced in PBMC from DR-7 positive modified responders compared to their DR-7 negative counterparts. Expression of HLA-DR7, coupled with high-dose exposure to cat allergen, could favor optimal induction of T regulatory cells in parallel with Th1 cells. When this occurs during the initiation phase of the immune response, it may result in imprinting of the regulatory mechanism necessary to prevent expansion of Th2 cells. A second immunodominant region within the chain induced IL-5 and a strong T cell proliferation in allergic and modified Th2 responders but not in control subjects *(67)*. Thus the ratio between TR1 and Th2 cells may determine the development of a healthy or allergic immune response. The generation of allergen-specific T reg cells and increased production of suppressive cytokines IL-10 and TGF-β are essentially early events in allergen-specific immunotherapy *(65,66)*.

Several studies have demonstrated HLA associations with low molecular weight chemical sensitizers *(68–71)*. It is likely to be more difficult to establish a HLA association with larger allergen as multiple T-cell epitopes are likely to be presented by different HLA molecules, diluting any single HLA association. We have established in laboratory animal allergy that HLA-DR7 was associated with sensitization to rat allergen and respiratory symptoms at work whereas HLA-DR3 was protective against sensitization *(72)*. The major rat allergen, Rat n 1, is a relatively low molecular weight protein with just five identical T-cell epitopes.

11. Intradermal Exposure

The high-dose attenuation of risk of sensitization and symptoms demonstrated with laboratory animal allergens is similar to both natural tolerance seen with beekeepers that have been frequently stung by bees and the induced tolerance by subcutaneous injection of natural allergen in immunotherapy. One common theme with bee keepers, laboratory animal workers, and cat owners, who develop tolerance at high exposures, is that they are at high risk of being bitten and scratched. We suggest the intradermal exposure to the allergens is responsible for the induced tolerance. In support of our hypothesis is the observation that repeated inhalation of cat peptides as an experimental method of immunotherapy was not—in contrast to an intradermal method—associated with the induction of hyporesponsiveness ('tolerance') in the skin or the lung. Other groups of workers at risk of developing occupational asthma, for example bakers and detergent workers, do not develop attenuation at high exposure—these workers are less likely to have an intradermal exposure.

12. Immunotherapy

Specific allergen injection immunotherapy is an effective treatment for IgE-mediated allergic diseases, which may confer long-term benefit for at least 3 yr after discontinuation *(73)*. Immunotherapy is generally administered by either subcutaneous injection or sublingual administration of allergen.

The mechanisms associated with immunotherapy are thought to involve both humoral and cellular responses. Following immunotherapy, there is a modest reduction in allergen-specific IgE and increases in allergen-specific IgG antibodies, particularly the IgG_4 subclass. Effector cells are reduced at the site of allergic inflammation, including a reduction in the numbers of mast cells, eosinophils, basophils, and the release in mediator secretion. There is thought to be an immune deviation toward a Th1-type response or the induction of T regulatory cells producing IL-10 and transforming growth factor beta.

Ratios of IgE to IgG_4 have been found to change during specific immunotherapy *(59)*. Specific serum levels of both IgE and IgG_4 increase during the early phase of therapy, but the increase in specific IgG_4 is more pronounced and the ratio of specific IgG_4:IgE is increased 10 to 100-fold, suggesting a protective role for IgG_4 *(59)*. IL-10 is a potent suppressor of both total and allergen-specific IgE, whereas it simultaneously increases IgG_4 production *(65)*.

Successful immunotherapy is associated with increases in allergen-specific IgG_1 and IgG_4 antibody concentrations that correlate with the clinical outcome *(74–77)*. It is not known whether allergen-specific IgG or IgG_4 antibodies associated with the modified Th2 response exhibit functional activity. It is possible that IgG antibodies may play a protective role by blocking leukocyte histamine release, inhibiting signal transduction and mediator release through the high-affinity IgE receptor (FcεR1) and IgG (FcγRIIB) receptors *(78–81)*, and blocking allergen-induced IgE-dependent histamine release by basophils *(82)*. IgG antibodies may exert their effect by competitive inhibition of allergen– IgE complexes, which prevents complexes binding to the low-affinity IgE receptor, CD23, and subsequent antigen presentation. Others have suggested that not only quantitative changes occur with the IgG antibody but also the spectrum of the specificity of the IgG is altered *(83)*. One grass pollen immunotherapy study demonstrated a blunting of seasonal increases in serum allergen-specific IgG and IgG_4. Further examination showed the postimmunotherapy serum to exhibit inhibitory activity, which coeluted with IgG_4 and blocked IgE-facilitated binding of allergen–IgE complexes to B cells. Increases in IgG and the IgG blocking activity correlated with the patients' overall assessment of improvement *(76)*.

References

1. Kay, A. B. (2001) Allergy and allergic diseases. *N. Engl. J. Med.* **344,** 30–37.
2. Johansson, S. G. O., Hourihane, J. O. B., Bousquet, J., et al. (2001) A revised nomenclature for allergy. *Allergy* **56,** 813–824.
3. Holt, P. G. and Thomas, W. R. (2005) Sensitization to airborne environmental allergens: unresolved issues. *Nat. Immunol.* **6,** 957–960.
4. The International Study of Asthma and Allergies in Childhood (ISAAC) Steering Committee (1998) Worldwide variation in prevalence of asthma, allergic rhinoconjuctivitis, and atopic eczema: ISAAC. *Lancet* **351,** 1225–1232.
5. Aberg, N., Hesselmar, B., Aberg, B., and Eriksson, B. (1995) Increase of asthma, allergic rhinitis and eczema in Swedish schoolchildren between 1979 and 1991. *Clin. Exp. Allergy* **25,** 815–819.
6. Celedon, J. C., Soto-Quiros, M. E., Hanson, L. A., and Weiss, S. T. (2002) The relationship among markers of allergy, asthma, allergic rhinitis, and eczema in Costa Rica. *Pediatr. Allergy Immunol.* **13,** 91–97.
7. Ninan, T. K. and Russell, G. (1992) Respiratory symptoms and atopy in Aberdeen school-children: evidence from two surveys 25 years apart. *BMJ* **304,** 873–875.
8. von Mutius, E., Martinez, F. D., Fritzch, C., Nicolai, T., Roell, G., and Thiemann, H. H. (1994) Prevalence of asthma and atopy in two areas of East and West Germany. *Am. J. Respir. Crit. Care Med.* **149,** 358–364.
9. von Mutius, E., Weiland, S. K., Fritasch, C., Duhme, H., and Keil, U. (1998) Increasing prevalence of hay fever and atopy among children in Leipzig, East Germany. *Lancet* **351,** 862–866.

10. Upham, J. W. and Holt, P. G. (2005) Environment and development of atopy. *Curr. Opin. Allergy Clin. Immunol.* **5,** 67–172.
11. Strachan, D. P. (1989) Hay fever, hygiene and household size. *BMJ* **299,** 1259–1260.
12. Mosmann, T. R. and Coffman, R. L. (1989) Th1 and Th2 cells: differential patterns of lymphokine secretion lead to different functional properties. *Annu. Rev. Immunol.* **7,** 145–173.
13. Romagnani, S. (1994) Lymphokine production by human T cells in disease states. *Annu. Rev. Immunol.* **12,** 27–257.
14. Cooke, A., Zaccone, P., Raine, T., Phillips, J. M., and Dunne, D. W. (2004) Infection and autoimmunity: are we winning the war, only to lose the peace? *Trends Parasitol.* **20,** 316–321.
15. Bach, J. F. (2002) The effect of infections on susceptibility to autoimmune and allergic diseases. *N. Engl. J. Med.* **347,** 911–920.
16. Strachan, D. P. (1997) Allergy and family size, a riddle worth solving. *Clin. Exp. Allergy* **27,** 235–236.
17. Karmaus, W. and Botezan, C. (2002) Does a higher number of siblings protect against the development of allergy and asthma? A review. *J. Epidemiol. Commun. Health* **56,** 209–217.
18. Cullinan, P. (2006) Childhood allergies, birth order and family size. *Thorax* **61,** 3–5.
19. Sacks, G., Sargent, I., and Redman, C. (1999) An innate view of human pregnancy. *Immunol. Today* **20,** 114–118.
20. Karmaus, W., Arshad, S. H., Sadeghnejad, A., and Twiselton, R. (2004) Does maternal immunoglobulin E decrease with increasing order of live offspring? Investigation into maternal immune tolerance. *Clin. Exp. Allergy* **34,** 853–859.
21. Westergaard, T., Begtrup, K., Rostgaard, K., Krause, T. G., Benn, C. S., and Melbye, M. (2003) Reproductive history and allergic rhinitis among 31145 Danish women. *Clin. Exp. Allergy* **33,** 301–305.
22. Forastiere, F., Sunyer, J., Farchi, S., et al. (2005) Number of offspring and maternal allergy. *Allergy* **60,** 510–514.
23. Devereux, G., Barker, R. N., and Seaton, A. (2002) Antenatal determinants of neonatal immune responses to allergens. *Clin. Exp. Allergy* **32,** 43–50.
24. Sunyer, J., Anto, J. M., Harris, J., et al. (2001) Maternal atopy and parity. *Clin. Exp. Allergy* **31,** 1352–1355.
25. Karmaus, W. and Eneli, I. (2003) Maternal atopy and the number of offspring, is there an association? *Pediatr. Allergy Immunol.* **14,** 470–474.
26. Harris, J. M., White, C., Moffat, S., Mills, P., Newman Taylor, A. J., and Cullinan, P. (2004) New pregnancies and loss of allergy. *Clin. Exp. Allergy* **34,** 369–372.
27. Aluvihare, V. R., Kallikourdis, M., and Betz, A. G. (2004) Regulatory T cells mediate maternal tolerance to the fetus. *Nature Immunol.* **5,** 266–271.
28. Somerset, D. A., Zheng, Y., Kilby, M. D., Sansom, D. M., and Drayson, M. T. (2004) Normal human pregnancy is associated with an elevation in the immune suppressive CD25+CD4+ regulatory T-cell subset. *Immunology* **112,** 38–43.

29. Prescott, S. L., Taylor, A., Roper, J., et al. (2005) Maternal reactivity to fetal alloantigens is related to newborn immune responses and subsequent allergic disease. *Clin. Exp. Allergy* **35**, 417–425.
30. Thomas, W., Hales, B., and Smith, W. (2005) Genetically engineered vaccines. *Curr. Allergy Asthma Rep.* **5**, 388–393.
31. Platts-Mills, T., Vaughan, J., Squillace, S., Woodfolk, J., and Sporik, R. (2001) Sensitisation, asthma, and a modified Th2 response in children exposed to cat allergen, a population-based cross-sectional study. *Lancet* **357**, 752–756.
32. Cullinan, P., MacNeill, S. J., Harris, J., et al. (2004) Early allergen exposure, skin prick responses, and atopic wheeze at age 5 in English children, a cohort study. *Thorax* **59**, 855–861.
33. Woodcock, A., Lowe, L. A., Murray, C. S., et al. (2004) National Asthma Campaign Manchester Asthma and Allergy Study Group. Early life environmental control, effect on symptoms, sensitization, and lung function at age 3 years. *Am. J. Respir. Crit. Care Med.* **170**, 433–439.
34. Perzanowski, M. S., Ronmark, E., Platts-Mills, T. A., and Lundback, B. (2002) Effect of cat and dog ownership on sensitization and development of asthma among pre-teenage children. *Am. J. Respir. Crit. Care Med.* **166**, 696–702.
35. Ownby, D. R., Johnson, C. C., and Peterson, E. L. (2002) Exposure to dogs and cats in the first year of life and risk of allergic sensitization at 6 to 7 years of age. *JAMA* **288**, 963–972.
36. Custovic, A., Simpson, B. M., Simpson, A., et al. (2003) National Asthma Campaign Manchester Asthma and Allergy Study Group. Current mite, cat, and dog allergen exposure, pet ownership, and sensitization to inhalant allergens in adults. *J. Allergy Clin. Immunol.* **111**, 402–407.
37. Caramalho, I., Lopes-Carvalho, T., Ostler, D., Zelenay, S., Haury, M., and Demengeot, J. (2003) Regulatory T cells selectively express Toll-like receptors and are activated by lipopolysaccharide. *J. Exp. Med.* **197**, 403–411.
38. Tulic, M. K., Holt, P. G., and Sly, P. D. (2002) Modification of acute and late-phase allergic responses to ovalbumin with lipopolysaccharide. *Int. Arch. Allergy Immunol.* **129**, 119–128.
39. Portengen, L., Preller, L., Tielen, M., Doekes, G., and Heederik, D. (2005) Endotoxin exposure and atopic sensitization in adult pig farmers. *J. Allergy Clin. Immunol.* **115**, 797–802.
40. Lau, S., Illi, S., Platts-Mills, T. A., et al. (2005) Multicentre Allergy Study Group. Longitudinal study on the relationship between cat allergen and endotoxin exposure, sensitization, cat-specific IgG and development of asthma in childhood—report of the German Multicentre Allergy Study (MAS 90). *Allergy* **60**, 766–773.
41. Platts-Mills, J. A., Custis, N. J., Woodfolk, J. A., and Platts-Mills, T. A. (2005) Airborne endotoxin in homes with domestic animals, implications for cat-specific tolerance. *J. Allergy Clin. Immunol.* **116**, 384–389.
42. Lieutier-Colas, F., Meyer, P., Pons, F., et al. (2002) Prevalence of symptoms, sensitization to rats, and airborne exposure to major rat allergen (Rat n 1) and to endotoxin in rat-exposed workers, a cross-sectional study. *Clin. Exp. Allergy* **32**, 1424–1429.

43. Jeal, H., Draper, A., Harris, J., Newman Taylor, A., Cullinan, P., and Jones, M. (2004) Determination of the T cell epitopes of the lipocalin allergen, Rat n 1. *Clin. Exp. Allergy* **34,** 1919–1925.
44. Ebner, C., Schenk, S., Najafian, N., et al. (1995) Nonallergic individuals recognize the same T cell epitopes of Bet v 1, the major birch pollen allergen, as atopic patients. *J. Immunol.* **154,** 1932–1940.
45. O'Hehir, R. E., Verhoef, A., Panagiotopoulou, E., et al. (1993) Analysis of human T cell responses to the group II allergen of Dermatophagoides species, localization of major antigenic sites. *J. Allergy Clin. Immunol.* **92,** 105–113.
46. Verhoef, A., Higgins, J. A., Thorpe, C. J., et al. (1993) Clonal analysis of the atopic immune response to the group 2 allergen of Dermatophagoides spp, identification of HLA-DR and –DQ restricted T cell epitopes. *Int. Immunol.* **5,** 1589–1597.
47. Van Neerven, R. J., Van de Pol, M. M., Van Milligen, F. J., Jansen, H. M., Aalberse, R. C., and Kapsenberg, M. L. (1994) Characterisation of cat ander-specific T lymphocytes from atopic patients. *J. Immunol.* **152,** 4203–4210.
48. Carballido, J. M., Carballido-Perrig, N., Kagi, M. K., et al. (1993) T cell epitope specificity in human allergic and nonallergic subjects to bee venom phospholipase A2. *J. Immunol.* **150,** 3582–3591.
49. Hesselmar, B., Aberg, B., Eriksson, B., Bjorksten, B., and Aberg, N. (2003) High-dose exposure to cat is associated with clinical tolerance—a modified Th2 immune response? *Clin. Exp. Allergy* **33,** 1681–1685.
50. Jeal, H., Draper, A., Harris, J., Newman Taylor, A. J., Cullinan, P., and Jones, M. (2006) Modified Th2 responses at high dose exposures to allergen using an occupational model. *Am. J. Respir. Crit. Care Med.* Apr 7 [eprint ahead of publication].
51. Cullinan, P., Cook, A., Gordon, S., et al. (1999) Allergen exposure, atopy and smoking as determinants of allergy to rats in a cohort of laboratory employees. *Eur. Respir. J.* **13,** 1139–1143.
52. Holt, P. G. (1994) A potential vaccine strategy for asthma and allied atopic diseases during early childhood. *Lancet* **344,** 456–458.
53. Jutel, M., Akdis, M., Budak, F., et al. (2003) IL-10 and TGF-Beta cooperate in the regulatory cell response to mucosal allergens in normal immunity and specific immunotherapy. *Eur. J. Immunol.* **33,** 1205–1214.
54. Jutel, M., Akdis, M., Blaser, K., and Akdis, C. A. (2005) Are regulatory T cells the target of venom immunotherapy? *Curr. Opin. Allergy Clin. Immunol.* **116,** 608–613.
55. Dombrowicz, D. (2005) Exploiting the innate immune system to control allergic asthma. *Eur. J. Immunol.* **35,** 2786–2788.
56. Akbari, O., Faul, J. L., Hoyte, E. G., et al. (2006) CD4+ invariant T-cell-receptor+ natural killer T cells in bronchial asthma. *N. Engl. J. Med.* **354,** 1117–1129.
57. Akbari, O., DeKruyff, R. H., and Umetsu, D. T. (2001) Pulmonary dendritic cells producing IL-10 mediate tolerance induced by respiratory exposure to antigen. *Nat. Immunol.* **2,** 725–731.
58. Hawrylowicz, C. M. (2005) Regulatory T cells and IL-10 in allergic inflammation. *J. Exp. Med.* **202,** 1459–1463.

59. Akdis, C. A. and Blaser, K. (1999) IL-10 induced anergy in peripheral T cell and reactivation by microenvironmental ctokines, two key steps in specific immunotherapy. *FASEB J.* **13**, 603–619.

60. Ling, E. M. and Robinson, D. S. (2004) Relation of CD4+CD25+ regulatory T-cell suppression of allergen-driven T-cell activation to atopic status and expression of allergic disease. *Lancet* **363**, 608–615.

61. Bellinghausen, I., Konig, B., Bottcher, I., Knop, J., and Saloga, J. (2005) Regulatory activity of human CD4+CD25+ T cells depends on allergen concentration, type of allergen and atopy status of the donor. *Immunology* **116**, 103–111.

62. Verhoef, A., Alexander, C., Kay, A. B., and Larche, M. (2005) T cell epitope immunotherapy induces a CD4+ T cell population with regulatory activity. *PLoS Med.* Mar **2(3)**, e78. Epub Mar 29.

63. Francis, J. N., Till, S. J., and Durham, S. R. (2003) Induction of IL-10+CD4+CD25+ T cells by grass pollen immunotherapy. *J. Allergy Clin. Immunol.* **111**, 1255–1261.

64. Tarzi, M., Klunker, S., Texier, C., et al. (2006) Induction of interleukin-10 and suppressor of cytokine signalling-3 gene expression following peptide immunotherapy. *Clin. Exp. Allergy* **36**, 465–474.

65. Akdis, C. A., Blesken, T., Akdis, M., Wuthrich, B., and Blaser, K. (1998) Role of interleukin 10 in specific immunotherapy. *J. Clin. Investig.* **102**, 98–106.

66. Akdis, M., Blaser, K., and Akdis, C. A. (2005) T regulatory cells in allergy, novel concepts in the pathogenesis, prevention, and treatment of allergic diseases. *J. Allergy Clin. Immunol.* **116**, 961–968.

67. Woodfolk, J. A. (2005) High-dose allergen exposure leads to tolerance. *Clin. Rev. Allergy Immunol.* **28**, 43–58.

68. Jones, M. G., Nielsen, J., Welch, J., et al. (2004) Association of HLA-DQ5 and HLA-DR1 with sensitization to organic acid anhydrides. *Clin. Exp. Allergy* **34**, 812–816.

69. Map, C. E., Balboni, A., Baricordi, R., and Fabbri, L. M. (1997) Human leukocyte antigen associations in occupational asthma induced by isocyanantes. *Am. J. Respir. Crit. Care Med.* **156**, S139–S143.

70. Newman Taylor, A. J., Cullinan, P., Lympany, P. A., Harris, J. M., Dowdeswell, R. J., and du Bois, R. M. (1999) Interaction of HLA phenotype and exposure intensity in sensitization to complex platinum salts. *Am. J. Respir. Crit. Care Med.* **160**, 435–438.

71. Young, R. P., Barker, R. D., Pile, K. D., Cookson, W. O., and Newman Taylor, A. J. (1995) The association of HLA-DR3 with specific IgE to inhaled acid anhydrides. *Am. J. Respir. Crit. Care Med.* **151**, 219–221.

72. Jeal, H., Draper, A., Jones, M., et al. (2003) HLA associations with occupational sensitisation to rat lipocalin allergens, a model for other animal allergies? *J. Allergy Clin. Immunol.* **111**, 759.

73. Francis, J. and Larche, M. (2005) Peptide-based vaccination, where do we stand? *Curr. Opin. Allergy Clin. Immunol.* **5**, 537–543.

74. Gehlhar, K., Schlaak, M., Becker, W., and Bufe, A. (1999) Monitoring allergen immunotherapy of pollen-allergic patients, the ratio of allergen-specific IgG4 to IgG1 correlates with clinical outcome. *Clin. Exp. Allergy*, **29**, 497–506.

75. Jutel, M., Akdis, M., Budak, F., Aebischer-Casaulta, C., Wrzyszcz, M., and Blaser, K. (2003) IL-10 and TGF-beta cooperate in the regulatory T cell response to mucosal allergens in normal immunity and specific immunotherapy. *Eur. J. Immunol.* **33**, 1205–1214.

76. Nouri-Aria, K. T., Wachholz, P. A., Francis, J. N., et al. (2004) Grass pollen immunotherapy induces mucosal and peripheral IL-10 responses and blocking IgG activity. *J. Immunol.* **172**, 3252–3259.

77. Djurup, R. and Osterballe, O. (1984) IgG subclass antibody response in grass pollen-allergic patients undergoing specific immunotherapy. Prognostic value of serum IgG subclass antibody levels early in immunotherapy. *Allergy* **39**, 433–441.

78. Golden, D. B., Meyers, D. A., Kagey-Sobotka, A., Valentine, M. D., and Lichtenstein, L. M. (1982) Clinical relevance of the venom-specific immunoglobulin G antibody level during immunotherapy. *J. Allergy Clin. Immunol.* **69**, 489–493.

79. Daeron, M., Malbec, O., Latour, S., Arock, M., and Fridman, W. H. (1995) Regulation of high affinity IgE receptor-mediated mast cell activation by murine low-affinity IgG receptors. *J. Clin. Investig.* **95**, 577–585.

80. Daeron, M. (1997) Negative regulation of mast cell activation by receptors for IgG. *Int. Arch. Allergy Immunol.* **113**, 138–141.

81. Zhu, D., Kepley, C. L., Zhang, M., Zhang, K., and Saxon, A. (2002) A novel human immunoglobulin Fc gamma Fc epsilon bifunctional fusion protein inhibits Fc epsilon R1-mediated degranulation. *Nature Med.* **8**, 518–521.

82. Ball, T., Sperr, W. R., Valent, P., et al. (1999) Induction of antibody responses to new B cell epitopes indicates vaccination character of allergen immunotherapy. *Eur. J. Immunol.* **29**, 2026–2036.

83. Wachholz, P. A. and Durham. S. R. (2003) Induction of 'blocking' IgG antibodies during immunotherapy. *Clin. Exp. Allergy* **33**, 1171–1174.

2

T Cell — Primary Culture from Peripheral Blood

Monika Raulf-Heimsoth

Abstract

Peripheral blood mononuclear cells (PBMC) can be used to assess cell-mediated immunity in general or, via antigen-specific stimulation, to detect previous exposure to a variety of antigens/allergens and to monitor the response to immunotherapies. Peripheral blood is the most common source of mononuclear cells for in vitro cultures, although mononuclear cells can be obtained from other sources involved in the allergic reaction. PBMC from individuals previously exposed to an antigen proliferate in vitro when stimulated with the specific antigen. Proliferation is measured by the incorporation of (^{3}H)-thymidine into newly synthesized DNA. This parameter is often used as an end point of lymphocyte stimulation induced by antigen or antigen fragments (e.g., synthetic peptides), mitogens, or anti-CD3/anti-CD28 combinations.

The aim of this chapter is to describe the culture of T cells obtained from peripheral blood and the collection of cell supernatants for cytokine measurement.

Key Words: Peripheral blood mononuclear cells; T-cell culture; proliferation; cytokines.

1. Introduction

The investigation of the human immune system is a key element in understanding allergic reactions. Peripheral blood mononuclear cells (PBMC) can be used to assess cell-mediated immunity in general or, via antigen-specific stimulation, to detect previous exposure to a variety of antigens/allergens and to monitor the response to immunotherapies.

Peripheral blood is the most common source of mononuclear cells (lymphocytes and monocytes; PBMC) for in vitro cultures, although mononuclear cells can be obtained from other sources involved in the allergic reaction (lung, skin, etc.). PBMC from individuals previously exposed to an antigen proliferate in vitro when stimulated with the specific antigen. Proliferation is measured by the incorporation of (^{3}H)-thymidine into newly synthesized DNA. This parameter

From: Methods in Molecular Medicine: Allergy Methods and Protocols
Edited by: M. G. Jones and P. Lympany © Humana Press Inc., Totowa, NJ

is often used as an end point of lymphocyte stimulation induced by antigen or antigen fragments (e.g., synthetic peptides), mitogens, or anti-CD3/anti-CD28 combinations.

Measurable amounts of cytokines can be detected in such cultures. In some cases, an enhanced expression of cytokine receptors and activation markers can be detected on lymphocyte surfaces by flow cytometry.

In addition to basic nutrients, in vitro cultures of PBMC require a serum supplement, usually of human or fetal calf origin.

It is frequently difficult to perform studies on PBMC the same day they are obtained. However, it is feasible to freeze and thaw the separated PBMC without significant function loss.

2. Materials

2.1. General Comments on Sterile Working and Biosafety Practice

All solutions and equipment coming into contact with cells must be sterile and a proper sterile technique should be used accordingly. Usually a lamina flow hood filtering the air to remove airborne bacteria and fungi is necessary. Immunological studies of the human immune system pose special safety problems associated with the risk of infection with human disease agents. Invariably, blood samples should be treated as though they are a potential source of hepatitis or HIV infection and appropriate personal protective equipment should be used, i.e., wearing laboratory suits, latex gloves, and eye protectors. Disinfection of all equipment after use is recommended (e.g., with alcohol or Barrycidal).

Work in the laboratory environment is closely regulated by legislation; usually reinforced and exemplified by institutional and local codes of practice. Many of the requirements for "good laboratory practice" rely on common sense or are based on a thorough knowledge of the likely risks and their avoidance (e.g., hazardous procedures or chemicals). Eating, drinking, smoking, or application of cosmetics in laboratory areas should be prohibited. A large number of commonly used laboratory chemicals are potentially carcinogenic or mutagenic, for example, phorbol esters (PMA) or propidium iodide, and handling them with care is necessary *(1,2)*.

In addition, there are defined legal requirements for the handling of radioisotopes (*see* (³H)-thymidine labeling). The work area should be especially designed for their use. The design of apparatus and experimental procedures should minimize the handling of radioactive material and avoid exposure to radiation. Appropriate shielding and distance reduces the radioactive dose received.

2.2. Culture Media, Supplements, Reagents, and Equipment

Many different culture media are available. RPMI 1640 was specifically designed for the culture of human cells. It is a double-buffering system containing bicarbonate (24 mM) and HEPES (50 mM) (*N*-2-hydroxyethyl-piperazine *N*-2-ethanesulphonic acid) buffered by CO_2 in the air, as this approximates physiological conditions in closed culture conditions (5% CO_2 in air in a gassed incubator). Although 20 mM HEPES alone can control the pH of the culture medium within physiological limits, cells grow better in the presence of CO_2 and HCO_3^-. Oxygen tension is also important for the growth of cells. In static cultures, the depth of the medium should be greater than about 5 mM. Most cells grow well at pH 7.4. At this pH phenol red, the most commonly used indicator, is salmon. It is orange at pH 7.0, yellow at pH 6.5, and blue ("livid") under alkaline conditions.

For the prevention of bacterial contamination in cell cultures, an antibiotic cocktail of penicillin (100 U/mL) and streptomycin sulfate (100 µg/mL) or gentamycin (30 µg/mL; more stable but more expensive) is recommended. Protection from yeast contamination is possible by adding fungicone (amphotericin B) up to a final concentration of 10 µg/mL.

The growth of cells in cultures requires a complex mixture of nutrients and other essential components. Theoretically, it should consist of a totally defined set of media additives that result in vigorous cell growth without causing extraneous cell stimulation. Such media additives have been devised but they are usually not as satisfactory as fetal calf serum (FCS), an easily obtained and relatively cheap material that normally contains all components necessary for the growth of human cells (heat inactivation for 30 min at 56°C reduces the number of viral and other adventitious contaminants and inactivate complements; filter-sterilized [0.45-µm filter]).

Alternatively, cell cultures can grow in serum-free medium (e.g., Ultraculture; Yssel's medium which is based on a modification of Iscove's modified Dulbeccos's medium) *(3)*. In some cases, stimulation experiments will performed in serum-free ultra culture medium (Bioproducts, Heidelberg, Germanzy) supplemented with 2 mM GlutaMAX™ 1 (Life Style Technology), antibiotic/antimycotic solution (Sigma, Deisenhofen, Germany) and 20 mM β-mercaptoethanol (2-ME; Life Style Technology) *(4)*.

In some experiments involving the culture of human lymphocytes, it is preferable to replace FCS with human AB serum because FCS can be mitogenic for human cells. Because the capacity of human AB serum to support lymphocyte cultures can vary, the screening of various batches is recommended. In addition, human AB serum should be heated inactivated for 30 min at 56°C.

Nonessential amino acids may be required for some applications. Glutamine is a nonessential amino acid that serves not only as a primary respiratory fuel, but also as a necessary substrate for nucleotide synthesis in rapidly proliferating cells such as lymphocytes. Glutamine can be produced in sufficient quantities under stable conditions, but it becomes a limiting substrate during metabolic stress. Optimal lymphocyte functions have been demonstrated when the glutamine concentration is set around 0.6–2.0 mM *(5,6)*.

Although the precise mode(s) of action of 2-ME has not been defined, it must be included in the media (final concentration 50 μM) used for procedures with primary cultures. 2-ME (50 mM in PBS diluted solution; stored at 4°C) must be added to media immediately before use because its activity rapidly declines if diluted.

A variety of ingredients and reagents are supplemented to the media shortly before use; they are typically made in large batches at 100× or 200× concentrations and stored in small aliquots of convenient size until use at −20°C and prewarmed at 37°C before use.

It is possible to purchase sterile media in solution. Alternatively, packaged, premixed powders can be purchased and reconstituted in 10 to 20-L batches, which must then be filter-sterilized (0.45-μM filter). The media can be stored at 4°C (*see* manufacturer's recommendations).

1. Complete RPMI (*R*oswell *P*ark *M*emorial *I*nstitute) medium (500 mL) containing: 439.5 mL RPMI 1640 cell culture medium with GlutaMAX™ I-supplement and 25 mM HEPES (Gibco, BRL; Life Technologies GmbH Paisley; UK), 5 mL penicillin/streptomycin (10,000 U/mL penicillin and 10,000 μg/mL streptomycin; Gibco, BRL), 5 mL sodium pyruvate MEM (100 mM; Gibco, BRL), 0.5 mL 2-ME (1000×, Gibco, BRL), 50 mL FCS (Biochrom, Berlin), or human AB-serum (both heat-inactivated).
2. Hanks balanced salt solution (HBSS) without calcium and magnesium: D-glucose (1.0 g/L), KCl (0.4 g/L), KH_2PO_4 (0.06 g/L), NaCl (8.0 g/L), $NaHCO_3$ (0.35 g/L), Na_2HPO_4 (0.048 g/L).
3. PBS (phosphate-buffered saline; Dulbecco's) (10×): 80 g NaCl, 23 g $Na_2H\,PO_4\cdot2$ H_2O, 2 g $KH_2\,PO_4$, 2 g KCl. Make up to 1000 mL with H_2O. For the ready-to-use PBS (1×), mix 100 mL PBS (10×) with 800 mL H_2O; adjust to desired pH (7.2–7.4) with NaOH. Make up to 1000 mL with H_2O.

For cell cultures and experiments, special equipment and utensils are necessary including CO_2-humidified incubator, biosafety cabinet (laminar flow hood; Kendro Laboratory Products), autoclave, centrifuges (e.g., Beckman Instruments, Munich), multiwell harvester or cell harvester (PHD, Cambridge Technologies or 1450 Microbeta Trilux, Perkin Elmer Wallac GmbH, Freiburg).

1. *Thymidine*: (^{3}H)-labeled thymidine-methyl is added to each cell-containing well for determination of the proliferation response. Purchased from Dupont, NEN Division, Dreieich, Germany.
2. *Ficoll-Paque* (or Ficoll-Paque plus; Amersham Biosciences Europe GmbH, Freiburg, Germany or Pharmacia LKB, Uppsala, Sweden) for in vitro isolation of lymphocytes; should be stored between 4 and 25°C and protected from direct light. Cold storage will increase the shelf life. Ficoll-Paque plus provides a sterile,

ready-to-use Ficoll-sodium diatrizoate solution (contains nonionic saccharose polymer, sodium-diatrizoate, and ethylenediamintetraacetylacid di-sodium) of the appropriate density, viscosity, and osmotic pressure for use in a simple and rapid lymphocyte isolation procedure.

3. *PBS, BSA, EDTA* buffers used for the pan T-cell isolation kit. PBS with 0.5% bovine serum albumin (BSA) and 2 mM EDTA; should be degassed by applying vacuum or sonification.

4. *Eosin B* for microscopy (Merck Eurolab, Darmstadt, Germany). Prepare the 1% eosin stock solution by dissolving 100 mg eosin in 10 mL complete medium and sterile filtration; storage at +4°C for 1 mo is possible; dilute the stock solution 1:10 with complete medium for use.

5. *Freezing Medium*: A mixture prepared of 440 mL RPMI 1640 with Glutamax I, 5 mL penicillin/streptomycin, 5 mL sodium pyruvate, 100 mL FCS medium, and 50 mL dimethyl sulfoxide (DMSO). Aliquoted in 50 mL and stored at −20°C.

6. *PHA* (phytohemagglutinin; lectin from *Phaseolus vulgaris*; Sigma, Deisenhofen, Germany): 5 mg lyophylisate should be dissolved in 1 mL sterile HBSS (allowed to stand for 10 min for complete dissolution); carefully mixed, aliquoted in 10 µL portion (50 µg) and store at −20°C.

7. Hapten-antibody cocktail of antibodies for pan T-cell isolation kit: a cocktail of CD11b, CD16, CD19, CD36, and CD56 antibodies is used for the depletion of non-T cells. These antibodies are hapten-conjugated.

8. Reagents for polyclonal cell stimulation: use combinations of PMA (1 ng/mL) and calcium ionophore A23187 (500 ng/mL), both from "Sigma Chemicals"; PMA and soluble anti-CD3 mAb (1 µg/mL) (anti-CD3 were purchased from Ortho Pharmaceuticals); anti-CD28 mAb (1 µg/mL) and coated anti-CD3 mAb to plates.

3. Methods

3.1. Obtaining Peripheral Blood

Blood should be taken by trained staff in designated areas, and biosafety practices must be followed. Collect blood in heparinized tubes (20 mL heparinized blood for $2–3 \times 10^7$ cells).

3.2. Preparation of Human Mononuclear Cell Population (PBMC)

The use of human peripheral blood as a source of lymphoid cells is facilitated by Ficoll-Hypaque density gradient centrifugation *(7)*. This simple and rapid method of purifying PBMC takes advantage of the density differences between mononuclear cells and other blood materials. Mononuclear cells and platelets collect on top of the Ficoll-Hypaque layer because they have a lower density: in contrast, erythrocytes and granulocytes (neutrophils and eosinophils) have a higher density than Ficoll-Hypaque and collect at the bottom of the gradient. Platelets are separated from the mononuclear cells by subsequent washing.

Removal of immature cells (contaminants of cord blood and peripheral blood from infants) requires additional steps. All procedure steps have to be done under sterile conditions using a laminar flow cabinet.

1. Transfer the fresh heparinized blood into a 15- or 50-mL conical centrifuge tube, add an equal volume of HBSS (room temperature) or PBS and mix it well. (Using blood from a leukophoresis donor, blood dilution with buffer of 1:3 or 1:4 [blood:buffer] is recommended.) (Alternatively, instead of 50-mL conical centrifuge tubes use LeucoSep tubes [Greiner, Frickenhausen, Germany] which have a special permeable disk membrane in the lower part of the tube).
2. Place Ficoll-Paque Plus solution (Pharmacia LKB, Uppsala, Sweden; density 1.077 g/L) in a 15- or 50-mL conical centrifuge tube. Use 3 mL Ficoll-Paque solution per 10 mL blood/buffer mixture.
3. Slowly layer the blood/buffer mixture over the Ficoll-Paque solution by placing the tip of the pipette containing the blood/buffer mixture at the surface of the Ficoll-Paque solution. (Alternatively, slowly layer the Ficoll-Paque solution underneath the blood/buffer mixture by placing the tip of the pipette containing the Ficoll-Paque solution at the bottom of the tube).
4. Centrifuge the capped tube 30 min at 900g (room temperature) using no brake.
5. Use a sterile pipette and remove the upper layer containing the plasma and most of the platelets. Change the pipette and transfer the next layer containing the mononuclear cells (lymphocytes, monocytes, and basophils) to another centrifuge tube.
6. Wash the PBMC by adding excess HBSS (more than three times the volume of the cell layer) and centrifuge them for 10 min at 400g at room temperature. Discard the supernatant into an appropriate disinfectant solution, resuspend the cell pellet carefully in HBSS (step by step; first in a small volume, mixing gently, adding HBSS to a final volume of 10 mL into the tube), and repeat the washing procedure once again.
7. Resuspend the PBMC in complete RPMI medium. Count cells and determine viability (*see* **Section 3.4.**).

3.3. Isolation of T Cells (Immunomagnetic Purification of T Cells)

For some research applications, isolation of purified T cells is necessary (e.g., studies on signal transduction, regulation of T-cell cytokine expression, induction of T-cell anergy). We used the magnetic activated cell sorter (MACS®) T-cell isolation kit for indirect isolation of untouched CD3$^+$ T cells from human peripheral blood mononuclear cells (MACS®, Miltenyi Biotech, Bergisch-Gladbach, Germany). This T-cell isolation kit is based on an indirect magnetic labeling system with depletion of B cells, monocytes, NK cells, dendritic cells, erythroid cells, platelets, and basophils. For this purpose, a cocktail of CD11b, CD16, CD19, CD36, and CD56 antibodies is useful for the depletion of non-T cells. The T cells are isolated following the manufacturer's instructions.

In brief, a MACS® column type LS⁺/VS⁺ is used. It is a prerequisite to isolate PBMC cells without any clumps as the cells pass through a 30-mm nylon mesh or filter.

1. Count the isolated PBMC cells (*see* **Section 3.4.**) and wash them with PBS with 2 mM EDTA and 0.5% BSA (*see* **Note 1**) by centrifugation of the cell suspension for 10 min at 400g at room temperature.
2. Remove supernatant completely and resuspend cell pellet in PBS with 2 mM EDTA and 0.5% BSA to a total volume of 80 µL/1×10^7 total cells.
3. Add 20 µL haptene antibody cocktail to 1×10^7 total cells, mix well, and incubate for 10 min at 6–12°C.
4. Wash the cells carefully with PBS with 2 mM EDTA and 0.5% BSA by adding 10–20 times the labeling volume.
5. Centrifuge for 10 min at 400g at room temperature and remove the supernatant.
6. Repeat the washing step. Resuspend the cells carefully in 80 µL of PBS with 2 mM EDTA and 0.5% BSA for 1×10^7 total cells.
7. Add 20 µL MACS® anti-haptene microbeads to 1×10^7 total cells, to label the cells magnetically.
8. Mix the cell suspension well and incubate them for 15 min at 6–12°C.
9. Wash the cells carefully with PBS with 2 mM EDTA and 0.5% BSA by adding 10–20 times volume (approx. 15 mL) and centrifuging at 400g for 10 min.
10. Place the column in the magnetic field of an appropriate MACS® separator.
11. Prepare the LS⁺/VS⁺ column by washing with 3 mL PBS with 2 mM EDTA and 0.5% BSA.
12. Apply cell suspension onto the column; the unlabeled cells will not be retained on the column and will come out in the effluent.
13. Collect the effluent as negative fraction, representing the enriched T-cell fraction.
14. Rinse with 3–4 mL of PBS with 2 mM EDTA and 0.5% BSA and collect the effluent (enriched T-cell fraction).
15. Remove the column from the separator and elute outside of the magnetic field all positive non-T cells.
16. Check the purity of the untouched T cells by staining an aliquot of the T-cell fraction with the fluorochrome conjugate antibody against T cells (e.g., CD3-PE) and analyze by flow cytometry. To determine if any remaining non-T cells in the T-cell fraction are leukocytes or rather erythroid cells, counterstain an aliquot of the cell fractions with an antibody against CD45 coupled to another fluorochrome (e.g., CD45-FITC). In this case, T cells are double positive staining.

3.4. Determination of Cell Count and Cell Viability

Cells can be counted using Coulter counter or a hemocytometer. A Coulter counter is an electronic particle counter. It is based on the principle that particles (cells suspended in an electrolyte) passing through an aperture in which an electronic current is flowing will alter the electrical resistance of the electrolyte and give rise to changes in the current flow and voltage. A hemocytometer (improved by Neubauer ruling; Brand, Wertheim, Germany) is a special type of microscope slide (cell counting chamber), which is divided into squares of a defined area over which a defined volume of cell suspension is distributed. Counting the number of cells in a defined volume can give us the number of cells per milliliter in a cell suspension. The hemocytometer can be used to count all cells or determine the number of viable cells in a culture. Viability is determined by either trypan blue or eosin dye exclusion test (*see* **Note 2**). Determination of cell viability is recommended when using thawed PBMC.

The following procedure can be used for the determination of viable cells with eosin dye exclusion test.

1. Centrifuge the cell suspension (10 min at $400g$ at room temperature), remove the supernatant completely, and resuspend in a defined volume (e.g., 1 mL) in complete medium RPMI. The cells need to be well mixed and uniformly suspended in the suspension.
2. Ensuring that both are clean and free from any grease, place coverslip on hemocytometer.
3. Gently mix 50 µL cell suspension with 450 µL eosin ready-to-use solution in a small plastic tube.
4. Dip a 0.1- or 1-mL pipette into the cell–eosin suspension to form a small drop on the end of the pipette and transfer gently to the surface of the slide at periphery of the coverslip.
5. Place hemocytometer on the stage of the microscope and focus on the cells.
6. Count the number of viable cells (unstained, in contrast to the red dead cells) at each of the four corner squares (the total volume of each corner square is 0.1 mm^3) (*see* **Note 3**). Cells falling across the top and left border lines of a square are considered to be in that square, whereas those that lie on the bottom and right borders are excluded. Count any clumps of cells as one cell.
7. Calculate the viable number of cells per milliliter of cell suspension as follows:viable cell number/mL = (total number of cells in four corner squares/4) $\times 10^5$—the factor 10^5 includes the cell dilution of 1:10 in eosin.

3.5. Cryopreservation of Cells (Freezing and Thawing of Cells)

Freshly isolated PBMC or cell lines should be used for culturing and stimulation experiments. However, they can be stored in culture medium at 4°C for at least 2 d prior to use or frozen as soon as possible. Cell concentrations up to 10^7 cells/mL can be successfully frozen in special cryovial tubes (sterile; volume 1.8 mL; Nunc, Roskilde, Denmark). A stepwise freezing process is recommended (1–2°C/min for the first 30°C). DMSO (or alternatively, glycerol) as an additive in the culture medium (cryoprotection solution) avoids the development of ice crystals during the freezing process. DMSO must be handled with care (avoid skin contact), and avoid the accumulation of toxic peroxide in the DMSO solution by using a fresh bottle every 3 mo.

1. Prepare freezing medium with DMSO (RPMI with GlutaMAX™ with 20% FCS, 10% DMSO, 1% penicillin/streptomycin, 1% sodium pyruvate) and store at −20°C (add DMSO to medium and not vice versa).
2. Centrifuge the PBMC at 500g (room temperature) using a 50-mL conical centrifuge tube, discard the supernatant, and save the cell pellet. Place the cells in the tube in an ice bath.
3. Add the precooled freezing medium (+4°C) to the cell pellet to achieve a final cell concentration of $2×10^6$ cells/mL and resuspend cells gently (avoid cell sedimentation).
4. Transfer 1 mL of the resuspended cells to each labeled cryovial (use an indelible marker). Cap the vial and immediately place it for 1 h in a freezer storage box in −20°C freezer. Then, place the cryovials overnight into a −70°C freezer. For long-term storage (several years for human freshly isolated PBMC), transfer cells to a liquid nitrogen container (−196°C).
5. Thawing the frozen PBMC begins with precooling the cells (+4°C). Retrieve the cryovial containing the cells from the "liquid nitrogen freezing container".
6. Take the cryovial to the laminar flow and disinfect the outside of the vial with alcohol (70%).
7. Swirl cryovial gently in glove-protected and disinfected hands until PBMC are thawed or alternatively thaw vial quickly in 37°C water bath.
8. Open the cryovial gently and transfer the cells into a sterile 15-mL Falcon tube containing 12 mL of the precooled media. (Alternatively, resuspend the cells gently using a sterile 1-mL pipette, transfer them into a sterile 15-mL Falcon tube, and add dropwise 9 mL complete RPMI media with gentle shaking over a time period of about 2–3 min).
9. Cap the tube, centrifuge for 5 min at 500g at room temperature, and discard the supernatant (under sterile conditions in the laminar flow), resuspend the cells in complete RPMI, and repeat the washing procedure as above twice. Examine the cell viability and determine cell count. The cells are ready for use at this stage and should be transferred to tissue culture plates or flasks.
10. In some cases, it is necessary to remove the dead cells. For this purpose, centrifuge the cells (10 min at 400g at room temperature), resuspend in 2 mL sterile PBS, and by using a 2-mL pipette, place 2 mL of FCS under the cell suspension and centrifuge the suspension for 5 min at 500g and remove the supernatant. Wash the cells once with complete RPMI and determine the number of viable cells.

3.6. Culturing and Stimulation of PBMC

A number of agents can specifically or nonspecifically induce T-cell activation resulting in cytokine production, cytokine receptor expression, and ultimately proliferation of the activated T cells. Some agents are capable of nonspecific activation of unprimed T cells in culture. Calcium ionophore and phorbol ester stimulation can directly crosslink the T-cell receptor (TCR) on a large percentage of responder cells. Lectins, such as PHA, indirectly crosslink the TCR; accessory cells are necessary with concentrations of 1–5 μg/mL.

The use of anti-CD3 or anti-TCR antibodies in soluble forms (rather than plate bound) also requires accessory cells. When using super antigens, such as staphylococcus enterotoxin, accessory cells must express the appropriate MHC class II molecules.

For antigen-specific stimulation of PBMC, peripheral blood cells from donors previously exposed to antigen can be used successfully. In the case of tetanus toxoid, donors should ideally have received a booster injection about 1 mo to 1 yr prior to the use of their PBMCs. To study PBMC reaction induced by allergens, peripheral blood from atopic donors can be stimulated specifically with allergens, which induced the IgE response in this subject (for example, house dust mite allergen [Der p 1] or grass pollen [Phl p 1–5], latex allergen [e.g., Hev b 1–10] and so on). Patients should be tested for allergen-specific serum IgE levels. Although there is not always a positive correlation between RAST score and success rate in the induction of allergen-specific PBMC response, in some cases (e.g., for the generation of Th2 clones) donors with a RAST class > 3 should be chosen preferentially.

The antigen concentration used for T-cell proliferation assay needs to be optimized. It is common for Th2 responses to be induced preferentially with low allergen concentrations, whereas Th1 responses are more frequently induced by higher allergen concentration. The sensitization is not important for stimulation of PBMCs, as cells from nonallergic but exposed subjects also demonstrate proliferation response in the presence of allergen (8). This is not surprising, as cells from nonallergic but exposed subjects recognize the antigen and show strong IgG binding to the antigen, and immunocompetent cells are stimulated in this polyclonal system. The observation that nonallergic subjects show a proliferative response to allergen is in accordance with the observation of other authors, although there is some controversy regarding whether the proliferation of PBMC from allergic and nonallergic subjects is similar or lower for the latter (3,8).

3.7. Measurement of Proliferative Responses of Cultured Lymphocytes (Mitogen- and Antigen-Induced)

Although proliferation is not a specific effector function of T lymphocytes, in contrast to helper function for B lymphocytes or cytotoxicity, proliferation assays are reliable, simple and easy to perform, and have been widely used to assess the overall immunocompetence of the T cells.

1. For the proliferation assay, PBMC were "seeded" at a concentration of 2×10^4 cells/well in a 96-well culture plate (U-bottom; total volume 200 µL) in triplicate or increased number of replicates (hexaplicates) and stimulated with the antigen (*see* **Note 3**). Appropriate dilutions of various antigens (10–0.01 µg/mL) in complete

medium were then added in 0.1-mL aliquots. As a positive control, stimulation with the mitogen PHA (5 µg/mL) is used. Cells incubated with no antigen provide a medium control, to give a baseline level of T-cell proliferation.

In the case of mitogen-specific stimulation, an incubation time of 3 d is performed. In the case of allergens, 5 or 6 d is a good time, although this needs to be optimized for each allergen. For (^{3}H)-thymidine incorporation with allergens we performed a 5-d incubation in a humidified atmosphere at 37°C and 5% CO_2 (*see* **Notes 4–8**).

2. For the final 12 h of incubation, 37.4 kBq (1 µCi) of (^{3}H)-thymidine-methyl (Dupont, NEN Division, Dreieich, Germany) was added to each well (20 µL) and the incorporated radioactivity was assessed.

3. A semiautomated cell harvesting apparatus is used to lyse the cells with water and precipitate the tritium-labeled DNA onto glass fiber filters. The dried filter pads were counted by liquid scintillation spectroscopy.

4. Results were calculated as stimulation indices (SI-value). The SI-value is the ratio of the mean counts per minute obtained in three (or more) similar cultures with allergen or antigen to that obtained in the antigen-free culture (the medium control).

5. In the case of allergen-specific stimulation, it is important to set a cutoff point for determination of a positive response. An SI-value of 1.0 indicates that there is no antigen-specific response. An SI-value of 2 or 3 is often considered as a positive stimulation index.

3.8. Measurement of Receptors and Activation Markers on Lymphocyte Surfaces by Flow Cytometry

T-cell activation can be determined by measuring activation markers expressed on the cell surface of stimulated cells. For example, markers like CD25 (IL-2 receptor) and/or CD71 (transferrin receptor) are expressed on proliferated cells. The expression of these special markers is time-dependent, e.g., CD69 is an early proliferation marker. In addition, expression of TCRs or intracellular cytokines for further characterization of T cells can also be determined in PBMC cultures by flow cytometry.

1. Using sterile technique, 2×10^6 PBMC/mL are incubated in a 24-well culture plate in the presence or absence of antigen/allergen at different concentrations and for different times at 37°C in 5% CO_2.

2. After incubation, the cells are harvested and transferred to tubes and centrifuged for 10 min at 500g. Discard the supernatant.

3. Resuspend the cells in medium and count. Adjust cell count to 2×10^6/mL.

4. Pipette 50 µL PBMC cell suspension in a polypropylene tube and incubate with 8–10 µL of the chosen fluorochrome-labeled antibody to determine its expression.

5. Incubate in the dark for 30 min at 4°C.

6. Add 2 mL PBS and centrifuge the labeled cell suspension for 5 min at 500g. Discard the supernatant.

7. Repeat the washing step. Add 250 µL PBS with 0.2% paraformaldehyde to fix the cells.
8. Measure activation and cell surface marker expression by flow cytometry.

3.9. Collecting Supernatants for Further Cytokine Determination

The concentrations of soluble cytokines (like IL-4, IL-5, IL-10, IL-13, and interferon-gamma [IFNγ]) in culture supernatants could be measured with commercially available sandwich ELISAs (technique using combinations of unlabeled and biotin-coupled mAb of different epitopes of each cytokine).

1. Incubate 10^6 PBMCs/mL in the presence or absence of antigen/allergen in either 24 (final volume 1 mL), 48 (500 µL), or 96-well (200 µL) plate.
2. For polyclonal stimulation, use combinations of PMA (1 ng/mL) and calcium ionophore A23187 (500 ng/mL), both from "Sigma Chemicals"; PMA and soluble anti-CD3 mAb (1 µg/mL); anti-CD28 mAb (1 µg/mL and coated anti-CD3 mAb) to coat plates with anti-CD3 mAb, incubate a 96-well flat bottom plate with 10 µg/mL anti-CD3 mAb diluted in PBS and washed twice with 100 µL of RPMI.
3. Incubate the cells at 37°C, 5% CO_2 for 16 h/24 h (for IL-4 and IL-2) and 48 h or longer for IFNγ, IL-5, IL-13, etc., and harvest the supernatant which can be frozen (–20°C or better –70°C) prior to cytokine analysis.
4. Determine cytokine production levels by specific cytokine ELISAs. Be sure that the supernatant is cell-free (supernatant should be used after centrifugation).

4. Notes

1. Buffer is degassed by vacuum pump or sonication. Excess gas in buffer can form bubbles in the matrix of the column during separation, which may lead to clogging of the column and decrease the quality of separation.
2. Dye exclusion test is based on the principle that nonelectrolyte dyes penetrate into dead cells, whereas live cells with intact plasma membranes do not allow the entry of such substances. Exclusion dyes will eventually penetrate live cells, so quantification should be performed within 30 min of adding dye to cell suspension. Antigen preparations can lead to nonspecific activation of T cells, e.g., casein which if contaminated with lipopolysaccharide (LPS) can result in unspecific T-cell stimulation *(9)*. LPS can be removed from the protein fractions by polymyxin B coupled to a solid phase as described *(10)*.
3. As an alternative to (^{3}H)-thymidine incorporation, cell growing (proliferation) can be monitored using nonradioactive methods. Proliferation can be determined by photometric method using MTT (3-[4,5 dimethythiazol-2-yl]-2,5-diphenyl tetrazolium bromide) or else by flow cytometry using a combination of ethidium bromide and brom desoxyuridin (BrdU).
4. The level of (^{3}H)-thymidine incorporation should not be regarded only as a reflection of cellular proliferation: some nondividing cells will synthesize DNA, and "cold" thymidine released by disintegrating cells will compete with incorporation of labeled thymidine. Therefore, measurements of DNA synthesis should be

accompanied by counting viable cells over the length of the culture period if a true estimate of cellular proliferation is to be obtained. Of course, cell death of non-activated cells will also interfere with the accuracy of this last parameter.

5. The sensitivity of proliferation assays is such that small errors in cell numbers will result in large differences in (^{3}H)-thymidine incorporation. When values obtained in triplicate cultures correspond poorly (for example, >5% differences in CPM values > 1000), technical problems such as cell clumping, dilution, and pipeting should be considered.

6. Excessively high values may be obtained from contaminated wells, as thymidine will be incorporated into replicating bacteria; therefore, it is a good practice to check the wells from microtiter plates under inverted microscope for contamination. Contamination may also interfere with proliferation of the activated lymphocytes. It is also useful to check the blast formation by microscopic examination of the cultures. Activating lymphocytes will tend to enlarge, and detection of blast will give a general indication of successful activation *(2)*.

7. The main problem that may occur with proliferative response assays is high levels of background (^{3}H)-thymidine incorporation in control cultures without antigen. This problem is frequently because of the FCS used to supplement the cultures which may be mitogenic for B cells. Different lots of FCS should be screened to select those that are nonstimulatory or only weekly stimulatory in the absence of any stimuli.

8. The culture period required for stimulation—after which the cells are to be labeled—varies for different laboratories, media, and types of responding and stimulator cells. Conditions eliciting weak responses such as most allergens will require a longer period of time (5–6 d) than those eliciting a higher frequency of responding T cells (3–4 d). Because laboratory conditions vary, it will be necessary to run a kinetic assay to determine the optimal time of T-cell proliferation. Addition of thymidine on days 2, 3, 4, 5, and 6 will provide a useful test. Further extension of culture periods will not yield any improvements, because of exhaustion of nutrients in the medium (yellow color indicating acidic condition).

References

1. Hudson, L. and Hay, F. C. (eds) (1989) *Practical Immunology.*Blackwell Scientific Publications, Oxford, UK.
2. Coligan, J. E., Kruisbeek, A. M., Margulies, D. H., Shevach, E. M., and Strober, W. (eds) (1996) *Current Protocols in Immunology.* Wiley, Hoboken, NJ.
3. Kahlert, H., Stüwe, H.-Th., Cromwell, O., and Fiebig, H. (1999) Reactivity of T cells with grass pollen allergen extract and allergoid. *Int. Arch. Allergy Immunol.* **120,** 146–157.
4. Yssel, H., De Vries, J. E., Koken, M., Blitterswijk, W. V., and Spits, H. (1984) Serum-free medium for generation and propagation of functional human cytotoxic and helper T cell clones. *J. Immunol. Methods* **72,** 219–227.
5. Rohde, T., Maclean, D. A., and Pedersen, B. K. (1996) Glutamine, lymphocyte proliferation and cytokine production. *Scand. J. Immunol.* **44,** 648–650.

6. Horig, H., Spagnoli, G. C., Filguerira, L., et al. (1993) Exogenous glutamine requirement is confined to late events of T cell activation. *J. Cell. Biochem.* **53,** 343–351.

7. Böyum, A. (1968) Isolation of mononuclear cells and granulocytes from human blood. Isolation of monuclear cells by one centrifugation, and of granulocytes by combining centrifugation and sedimentation at 1*g. Scand. J. Clin. Lab. Investig.* **97,** 77–89.

8. Raulf-Heimsoth, M., Chen, Z., Liebers, V., Allmers, H., and Baur, X. (1996) Lymphocyte response to extracts from different latex materials and to the purified latex allergen Hev b 1 (rubber elongation factor). *J. Allergy Clin. Immunol.* **98,** 640–651.

9. Werfel, T., Ahlers, G., Schmidt, P., Boeker, M., and Kapp, A. (1996) Detection of a κ-casein-specific lymphocyte response in milk-responsive atopic dermatitis. *Clin. Exp. Allergy* **26,** 1380–1386.

10. Karplus, T. E., Ulevitch, R. J., and Wilson, C. B. (1987) A new method for reduction of endotoxin conatmination from protein solutions. *J. Immunol. Methods* **105,** 211–220.

3

Production of T-Cell Lines

Helga Kahlert

Abstract

Allergen-specific T-cell lines established from allergic patients provide the opportunity of investigating T-cell functions at the poly- or oligoclonal level. T-cell lines are useful in determining the presence or absence of antigen-specific T-cell reactivity. However, to obtain detailed knowledge of the action of T cells with clearly defined features, for example epitope specificity or phenotype, T-cell clones are necessary.

The frequency of allergen-specific T cells in peripheral blood mononuclear cells (PBMC) tends to be low and so stimulation of PBMC with single allergens often results in low allergen-specific reactivity or requires high doses of the allergen. In contrast, the stimulation of PBMC with whole allergen extract results in stronger reactivity because a greater spectrum of T-cell specificities is addressed. Therefore, for the investigation of polyclonal reactivity toward single allergens it is useful to establish T-cell lines, which represent an allergen-specific enrichment of T cells from the respective individual. These T cells are poly- or oligoclonal and might possess different epitope specificities. The method described here is based on experiences with human T-cell lines and clones specific for several allergens from grass pollens and tree pollens.

Key Words: T cell; oligoclonality; T-cell line; clone; allergen.

1. Introduction

Growing antigen-specific human T cells in vitro offers the possibility of investigating the function and characteristics of T cells and determining the influence of substances which may modulate T-cell functions. Allergen-specific T-cell lines established from allergic patients are useful for investigating T-cell functions at the poly- or oligoclonal level and for determining the presence or absence of antigen-specific T-cell reactivity. However, to obtain detailed knowledge of the action of T cells with clearly defined features, for example epitope specificity or phenotype, T-cell clones are necessary (1). Growing T-cell lines is less time consuming than growing T-cell clones (1).

From: Methods in Molecular Medicine: Allergy Methods and Protocols
Edited by: M. G. Jones and P. Lympany © Humana Press Inc., Totowa, NJ

In general, T-cell response to allergens tends to be weak because of the low frequency of allergen-specific T cells in peripheral blood mononuclear cells (PBMC). Stimulation of PBMC with single major allergens often results in low allergen-specific reactivity or requires high doses of the allergen *(2–5)*. In contrast, the stimulation of PBMC with whole allergen extract results in stronger reactivity because a greater spectrum of T-cell specificities is addressed *(2,6)*. Therefore, for investigating polyclonal reactivity toward single allergens, it is useful to establish T-cell lines, which represent an allergen-specific enrichment of T cells from the respective individual. These T cells are poly- or oligoclonal and might possess different epitope specificities. It has been shown that single individuals can possess several T-cell specificities for one allergen *(7–11)*.

The method described here is based on experiences with human T-cell lines and clones specific for several allergens from grass pollens and tree pollens. The method starts as usual with the separation of PBMC from the blood of the patients. The PBMC are seeded in a 96-well culture plate and stimulated with the desired allergen. During the culture period of 14 ± 2 d the cells are fed at defined intervals with fresh medium and interleukin-2 (IL-2). After 14 ± 2 d a proliferation test is set up with the respective allergen, using irradiated autologous PBMC as accessory cells. The antigen-specific stimulation of T cells requires autologous antigen-presenting cells as antigen presentation is restricted by the MHC class II molecules of the respective individual. B lymphocytes, monocytes, and a very low proportion of dendritic cells constitute the antigen-presenting cell fraction in PBMC. Positive cultures are either combined to represent a T-cell line or expanded separately to represent different T-cell lines. This procedure differs from the more frequently described procedure in the literature *(3,7,12)*, where the initial stimulation with the antigen is performed in 24-well culture plates with a greater number of cells in the same well. The advantage of the method described here, which uses 96-well culture plates, is that T-cell lines with stronger reactivity for a certain major allergen could be obtained because wells including cells with no allergen-specific reactivity or unspecific reactivity can be excluded more efficiently right from the beginning. This is especially important when only a few patients with the respective allergy are available and when the frequency of T cells with specificity for a certain major allergen is low.

If T-cell clones are required then T-cell lines should be cloned immediately after selection. The expansion of T-cell lines involves sequential stimulation with allergen and autologous PBMC and unspecific stimulation with PHA and allogeneic PBMC.

2. Materials

2.1. General Equipment for Cell Culture

1. Laminar flow hood.
2. Cell incubator (37°C, 5% CO_2, humidified atmosphere).

3. Centrifuge with tube and microtiter plate carriers.
4. Microscope.
5. Single and 8-channel automatic pipets.
6. −80°C freezer and liquid nitrogen storage container for cryopreservation.

2.2. Separation of PBMC

1. Leucosep tubes, 50 mL (Greiner, Frickenhausen, Germany) (*see* **Note 1**).
2. Lymphocyte separation medium (density 1.077; PAA, Cölbe, Germany) (*see* **Note 2**).
3. Heparin as anticoagulant (Liquemin N 20.000; Hoffman-La Roche, Grenzach-Whylen, Germany), 1 mL containing in aqueous solution 20,000 I.E. Na-heparin (*see* **Note 3**).
4. 30–50 mL syringes and appropriate cannulas.
5. Medium for cell washing: RPMI 1640 (PAA) either with 10% fetal calf serum (FCS) (⇒ RPMI*) or without it (⇒ RPMI∅). Shelf life: 4 wk when stored at 4°C under sterile conditions.

2.3. Generation of Allergen-Specific T-Cell Lines

2.3.1. Patients

For the generation of allergen-specific T-cell lines, it is necessary to use PBMC from subjects with a positive clinical history of the respective allergy and high allergen-specific IgE level in blood (> 3.5 kU IgE/L). The availability of patients for subsequent blood donations must be confirmed before bleeding the patients to ensure a source of autologous PBMC (*see* **Notes 4** and **5**). The amount of blood taken from patients should in the first instance be a minimum of 100 mL; however, up to a maximum of 450 mL blood enables you to restimulate the T cells without having to subsequently bleed the patient for fresh cells.

2.3.2. Culture Medium

Grow the T-cell culture under serum-free conditions in Ultraculture medium (Cambrex, Verviers, Belgium) (*see* **Note 6**) supplemented with the following ingredients:

1. UltraGlutamine I (Cambrex) at a final concentration of 2 mM. Aliquot the stock solution of UltraGlutamine I (100×) to 5 mL and store at −20°C (*see* **Note 7**).
2. Antibiotic–antimycotic solution (Sigma, Taufkirchen, Germany) at a final concentration of 100 U/mL penicillin, 100 µg/mL streptomycin sulfate, and 0.25 µg/mL amphotericin B. Aliquot the 100-fold stock solution to 5 mL and store at −20°C.
3. Mercaptoethanol (Invitrogen, Karlsruhe, Germany) at a final concentration of 20 µM. Aliquot 50 mM stock solution to 250 µL and store at −20°C.
4. For preparation of the culture medium thaw an aliquot of each, UltraGlutamine I, antibiotic–antimycotic solution, and mercaptoethanol (200 µL), mix and add to 500 mL Ultraculture medium under sterile filtration through a 0.22-µm filter (Millex GV13; Millipore, Eschborn, Germany).
5. The prepared medium is stored at 4°C until use. The shelf life is 4 wk.

2.3.3. T-Cell Stimulation

1. Allergens are obtained from either purified natural extracts or recombinant technologies. Dilute allergen to a concentration of 100 µg/mL with Ultraculture medium without supplements and then filter through 0.22-µM filter (Millex GV4; Millipore) (The filter should be suitable for sterile filtration of aqueous solutions with very low protein-binding capacity and with small diameters.) Aliquot the allergen solution to 200 µL or any other desired volume and store at −20°C. Dilute the allergen extract to a final concentration of 1 mg/mL with Ultraculture medium and sterile filter in the same way as described above, aliquot, and store at −20°C (*see* **Note 8**).
2. Recombinant IL-2 may be obtained from different sources. The material used by the author (IL-2CC) was obtained from Strathmann Biotec (Hamburg, Germany). Reconstitute the 50,000 units/vial in Ultraculture medium without supplements to a concentration of 2500 U/mL, aliquot at 200–500 µL/vial or any other desired volume, and store at −20°C.
3. 96-well round-bottom culture plates (Greiner).

2.4. Testing of T-Cell Lines for Allergen Specificity

1. Centrifuge capable for centrifugation of 96-well culture plates, 96-well round-bottom culture plates (Greiner, Germany).
2. Cell harvester. The method described here uses a 96-channel harvester (PerkinElmer, Rodgau-Jügesheim, Germany).
3. Beta-Counter. The method described here uses a Microbeta scintillation counter (PerkinElmer).
4. Microplate heat sealer (PerkinElmer) (*see* **Note 9**).
5. [6-3H]-Thymidine, 37 MBq/mL (Amersham Biosciences, Freiburg, Germany).
6. Allergen (*see* **Section 2.3.3.** and **Note 8**).
7. Autologous PBMC from respective patients should be prepared for the presentation of allergen-derived peptides to T cells in the proliferation assays (*see* **Note 4**).
8. Harvest PBMC from the blood as described under **Section 3.1**. After counting of PBMC with a hematocytometer, freeze the cells in aliquots of 5×10^6 cells/mL freezing medium in 2-mL cryovials (Greiner), and store in liquid nitrogen (*see* **Section 3.5.**). Count cells following thawing to ensure that only viable cells are considered. Adjust cells to a maximum of 100×10^6 PBMC/10 mL RPMI* tissue culture tubes (Greiner) and irradiate with 30 Gy (*see* **Note 10**).

2.5. Expansion of T-Cell Lines

1. Reconstitute phytohemagglutinin (PHA) (Sigma) in Ultraculture medium without supplements to a final concentration of 240 µg/mL, aliquot, and store at −20°C.
2. For nonspecific stimulation with PHA, use a mixture of irradiated (30 Gy) allogeneic PBMC from at least five healthy individuals. Harvest and freeze the cells in the same way as described for autologous PBMC (*see* **Sections 2.4.** and **3.1.**).
3. 24-well culture plates (Nunc, Wiesbaden, Germany).

2.6. Cryopreservation of T-Cell Lines

1. Freezing medium: RPMI 1640 with 10% DMSO (Merck, Darmstadt, Germany) and 20% FCS. Mix all the components, aliquot (5–10 mL), and store at −20°C until use.
2. Cryovials (Greiner).

3. Methods

The whole procedure is summarized in **Fig. 1**.

3.1. Separation of PBMC

1. Draw blood from the patients by using heparin as anticoagulant. Prepare the 50-mL syringes with approximately 100 µL heparin (≈ 2000 I.E. heparin).
2. Centrifuge (1 min, 1000g) 15 mL of lymphocyte separation medium in Leucosep tubes. Following centrifugation, the lymphocyte separation medium is found under the filter disc of the Leucosep tubes.
3. Transfer 30 mL heparinized undiluted blood on the filter disc and centrifuge for 20 min at 800g.
4. Harvest the cells from the interface using a pasteur pipet.
5. Wash cells with RPMIØ (1 volume cell suspension:2 volumes of RPMIØ) and centrifuge for 10 min at 800g.
6. Wash cells twice with RPMI* (10 min, 200g) and count the cells with a hematocytometer (*see* **Notes 11** and **12**). 1 mL of blood yields approximately 1×10^6 PBMC.
7. Freeze remaining cells as a supply of autologous PBMC (*see* **Sections 2.4.** and **2.6.**).

3.2. Generation of Allergen-Specific T-Cell Lines

1. Incubate freshly isolated PBMC from allergic patients at a concentration of 1×10^5 per well in a 96-well round-bottom culture plate in a total volume of 100 µL Ultraculture medium with the desired concentration of the respective allergen (1–25 µg/mL) (*see* **Note 8**).
2. Incubate for 5–7 d. Allergen-stimulated cells develop to form clusters of proliferation and increase in number.
3. Add 100 µL of fresh culture medium with a final concentration of 5–10 units IL-2/mL (*see* **Note 13**).
4. After 3–4 d of culture, exchange half of the medium with fresh medium containing 5–10 U IL-2/mL and incubate for another 4 d.
5. Fourteen days (± 2 d) after setting up the culture, perform a proliferation assay as described under **Section 3.3.** and check for antigen specificity.

3.3. Testing of T-Cell Lines for Allergen Specificity

1. Sediment the cells of the 96-well culture plate by centrifugation at 200g for 5 min. Remove the supernatant and wash the cells with 100 µL RPMI*.
2. Repeat the washing step once with 100 µL RPMI* and then once with 100 µL Ultraculture medium.

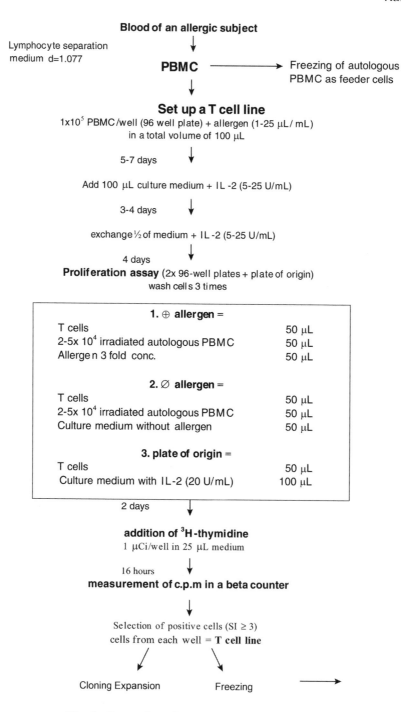

Fig. 1. Generation of allergen-specific T-cell lines.

3. Suspend the cells in 150 µL Ultraculture medium and divide the initial culture among three 96-well plates. Resuspend the cells in the well of the original plate and transfer 50 µL to corresponding wells of the two new culture plates using a multichannel pipet. These two plates represent the two test plates.

4. 50 µL of the cell suspension remains in the original plate for the continuation of the culture. Feed these cells with 100 µL Ultraculture medium containing IL-2 at a final concentration of 20 U/mL.

5. The proliferation test is performed with the two test plates. Add 5×10^4 irradiated autologous PBMC in a volume of 50 µL Ultraculture to each well of the two test plates.

6. Add the antigen in the optimal concentration in a volume of 50 µL to the wells of the antigen stimulation plate and 50 µL of culture medium without antigen to the control plate (*see* **Note 14**).

7. Incubate the plates for 48 h in the incubator with 5% CO_2, 37°C, and humidified atmosphere.

8. Add 1 µCi ^{3}H-thymidine (= 37 kBq) in 25 µL Ultraculture medium and incubate for another 16 h.

9. Harvest the cells onto a filter. The following steps of the method used by the author involves cell harvesting with a 96-channel cell harvester (PerkinElmer) on filter mats in 96-well plate format and the subsequent counting in a Microbeta scintillation counter (PerkinElmer).

10. Dry the filter mats (*see* **Note 15**) and apply a solid scintillator sheet on the filter, put it in a Microbeta sample bag (PerkinElmer), and allow the scintillator to melt into the filter mat using a microplate heat sealer (PerkinElmer).

11. Transfer the prepared filter into a 96-well filter mat cassette and then the cassette into the Microbeta counter for the measurement of the cpm (counts per minute).

12. Results are expressed as a stimulation index (SI), calculated as the quotient of the cpm of the allergen-stimulated wells and the cpm of the corresponding non-stimulated wells.

13. The cells from 10–16 wells with SI ≥ 3 should be combined to form a T-cell line. Several different T-cell lines can be collected from one 96-well plate depending on the stimulation indices for the individual.

14. Alternatively, if the amount of wells yielding appropriate SI is low or if a large panel of different T-cell lines is desired, the cells of individual wells may be expanded separately (*see* **Note 16**).

3.4. Expansion of Established T-Cell Lines

1. Transfer the T cells from the selected wells into a centrifugation tube and spin them down (10 min, 200*g*). Resuspend the cells in 500 µL Ultraculture medium and transfer them into a well of a 24-well culture plate.

2. Add 1×10^6–2×10^6 irradiated autologous PBMC. The ratio of T cells to PBMC should be approximately 2:5.

3. Add antigen in the desired concentration and start the expansion in a total volume of 1 mL.

4. After 3–4 d incubation, prepare a feeding mixture of 1×10^6–2×10^6 irradiated allogeneic PBMC, 2.5 µg PHA/mL, and 25 U IL-2/mL and add Ultraculture medium to make a total volume of 1 mL/well in a 24-well culture plate.
5. After 3–4 further days, exchange half of the medium with fresh Ultraculture medium containing 25 U IL-2/mL.
6. Continue the culture by exchanging half of the medium every third or fourth day with fresh medium and IL-2. When the medium becomes yellow and the cells are confluent, split the culture by dividing the cells between two wells with addition of fresh medium and IL-2.
7. Freeze as many cells as possible. This can be performed at any time-point of the culture, but a proliferation assay can only be set up 12–14 d after the last feeding with PBMC (*see* **Note 17**).
8. When the T cells are maintained in culture, antigenic stimulation with autologous PBMC is necessary every 28 d (*see* **Note 18**).

3.5. Cryopreservation of T-Cell Lines

1. Centrifuge the cells from the desired wells at 200*g* for 10 min. One to two fully grown wells of a 24-well plate are required for one cryovial.
2. Discard the supernatant, resuspend the cells in 1 mL cold (4°C) freezing medium, and transfer them to a cryovial.
3. Close the vial and transfer it immediately into a styropor box with approximately 2-cm-thick walls and place in a –80°C freezer or use temperature-controlled cell freezer when available.
4. Transfer the cryovials to liquid nitrogen after at least 1 d.

4. Notes

1. The advantage of Leucosep tubes is that the blood can be decanted directly onto the filter disc in the tube. This prevents the undesired mixing of the blood with the separation medium. Alternatively, the blood can be overlaid carefully over the separation medium in tubes without filter discs.
2. Any other lymphocyte separation medium with a density of 1.077 can be used as an alternative to the one used here.
3. When using heparin from other sources, it is wise to consider whether the heparin is free of preservatives, which may be harmful to the cells.
4. It is possible to establish Epstein-Barr virus (EBV)-transformed B-cell lines in order to have an unlimited supply of autologous MHC class II matched feeder cells for antigen presentation (for details *see* **ref. 13**). The use of EBV-transformed B cells leads to higher backgrounds in proliferation assays and needs antigen preincubation before irradiation. Their advantage, however, is that they are available in unlimited amounts.
5. The status of the patient is important for the outcome of the T-cell culture: Patients who are or were treated with allergen-specific immunotherapy will be increasingly unresponsive to the allergen because of tolerance induction (*3,14*). Furthermore, it is necessary to make sure that the patients have not used any symptomatic medication around the time-point of blood donation or in case of glucocorticoids approximately

6 wk before blood donation. When blood is drawn during an acute allergic phase (for example during the pollen season if grass pollen allergen-specific TCL are wanted) it has to be considered that the T cells might already be stimulated and that no difference between allergen and control stimulation might be observed in vitro.

6. It is also possible to use a medium supplemented with 5% human AB serum. The advantage of serum-free medium is that variations in background level because of components in AB serum are avoided. Because AB serum may vary from batch to batch serum-free medium offers the opportunity of more defined and stable culture conditions.

7. Glutamine may be used as an alternative. The advantage of using dipeptides such as UltraGlutamine I is that toxic degradation products of glutamine in medium are avoided.

8. The optimal concentration of the allergens for stimulation is generally in a range of 1–25 µg/mL (for grass or birch pollen major allergens) and has to be evaluated individually.

9. A microplate heat sealer is necessary when scintillation counting is performed with a Microbeta counter and when it is desirable to limit the amount of radioactive waste.

10. If irradiation facilities are not available, mitomycin C (Sigma) treatment of the PBMC can be used as an alternative *(12)*. In this case, PBMC should be adjusted to 5×10^6 cells/mL in sterile phosphate-buffered saline (PBS). Add 100 µL of a solution containing 0.5 mg/mL mitomycin C in PBS to 1 mL of the cell suspension and incubate for 20 min in the incubator at 37°C. Add RPMI* to a final volume of approximately 12 mL and centrifuge for 10 min at 200*g*. Repeat the washing procedure twice in order to remove any residual mitomycin C which might interfere with the T-cell proliferation. The solution should be prepared freshly each day prior to use. It should be considered that mitomycin C is very toxic and light sensitive.

11. Recommended dilution of freshly harvested PBMC is 1:20 in 3% acetic acid, to eliminate any remaining red blood cells, which makes counting easier.

12. In the last washing step, the same medium as needed for the T-cell stimulation should be used.

13. The low IL-2 concentration at this time-point in the culture setup is not capable of activating resting T cells and can only be utilized by T lymphocytes expressing large numbers of IL-2 receptors, which is typical for activated T cells. The activation under these conditions is induced mainly by the allergen.

14. The three components, T cells, autologous PBMC, and antigen, are added separately to the wells of the test plate. Therefore, the allergen solution has to be prepared threefold concentrated in order to achieve the final desired dilution in the plate. Always pipet in the following order: (1) T cells, (2) PBMC, (3) antigen.

15. It is important, for correct measurement, that the filters are completely dry. This can be achieved either with an electrical hair dryer or with a drying cabinet.

16. When expansion of single wells from the 96-well plate is desired, then first transfer the cells into wells of a 48-well plate and stimulate with 0.5×10^6–1×10^6 autologous or allogeneic PBMC/well and add allergen or PHA in the indicated concentration. Transfer to 24-well plate when cells are confluent and the medium is turning yellow.

17. It is recommended that detailed documentation about the culture status of a certain T-cell line is maintained. When freezing is performed 14 ± 2 d after the last stimulation with autologous/allogeneic PBMC, the cells could be used in a proliferation assay immediately after thawing.

18. Because the cells of a T-cell line are polyclonal, strong clones might overgrow weak clones and the feature of a T-cell line might change during the expansion process. Thus T-cell lines sometimes lose their specificity or at least their preliminary strong reactivity with the desired antigen during the expansion procedure. Other T-cell lines reveal progressively stronger antigen-specific proliferative responses with each expansion round.

References

1. Schramm, G., Kahlert, H., Suck, R., et al. (1999) 'Allergen engineering': variants of the timothy grass pollen allergen Phl p 5b with reduced IgE-binding capacity but conserved T cell reactivity. *J. Immunol.* **162**, 2406–2414.
2. Würtzen, P. A., van Neerven, R. J. J., Arnved, J., Ipsen, H., and Sparholt, S. H. (1998) Dissection of the grass allergen-specific immune response in patients with allergies and control subjects: T-cell proliferation in patients does not correlate with specific serum IgE and skin reactivity. *J. Allergy Clin. Immunol.* **101**, 241–249.
3. Ebner, C., Siemann, U., Bohle, B., et al. (1997) Immunological changes during specific immunotherapy of grass pollen allergy: reduced lymphoproliferative responses to allergen and shift from TH2 to TH1 in T-cell clones specific for Phl p 1, a major grass pollen allergen. *Clin. Exp. Allergy* **27**, 1007–1015.
4. Baskar, S., Parronchi, P., Mohapatra, S., Romagnani, S., and Ansari, A. A. (1992) Human T cell responses to purified pollen allergens of the grass, Lolium perenne. Analysis of relationship between structural homology and T cell recognition. *J. Immunol.* **148**, 2378–2383.
5. Sager, N., Feldmann, A., Schilling, G., Kreitsch, P., and Neumann, C. (1992) House dust-mite-specific T cell in the skin of subjects with atopic dermatitis: frequency and lymphokine profile in the allergen patch test. *J. Allergy Clin. Immunol.* **89**, 801–810.
6. Kahlert, H., Stüwe, H.–Th., Cromwell, O., and Fiebig, H. (1999) Reactivity of T cells with grass pollen allergen extract and allergoid. *Int. Arch. Allergy Immunol.* **120**, 146–157.
7. Spiegelberg, H. L., Beck, L., Stevenson, D. D., and Ishioka, G. Y. (1994) Recognition of T cell epitopes and lymphokine secretion by rye grass allergen Lolium perenne I-specific human T cell clones. *J. Immunol.* **152**, 4706–4711.
8. Ebner, C., Schenk, S., Szépfalusi, Z., et al. (1993) Multiple T cell specifities for Bet v 1, the major birch pollen allergen, within single individuals. Studies using specific T cell clones and overlapping peptides. *Eur. J. Immunol.* **23**, 1523–1527.
9. Van Neerven R. J. J., van t'Hof, W., Ringrose, J. H., et al. (1993) T cell epitopes of house dust mite major allergen Der p II. *J. Immunol.* **151**, 2326–2335.
10. Dormann, D., Montermann, E., Klimek, L., et al. (1997) Heterogeneity in the polyclonal T cell response to birch pollen allergens. *Int. Arch. Allergy Immunol.* **114**, 272–277.

11. Müller, W.-D., Karamfilov, T., Kahlert, H., et al. (1998) Mapping of T-cell epitopes of Phl p 5: evidence for crossreacting and non-crossreacting T-cell epitopes within Phl p 5 isoallergens. *Clin. Exp. Allergy* **28,** 1538–1548.

12. Müller, W.-D., Karamfilov, T., Fahlbusch, B., Vogelsang, H., and Jäger, L. (1994) Analysis of human T cell clones reactive with group V grass pollen allergens. *Int. Arch. Allergy Immunol.* **105,** 391–396.

13. O'Hehir, R. E., Askonas, B. A., and Lamb, J. R. (1993) Lymphocyte clones. In *Methods of Immunological Analysis* (Masseyeff, R. F., Albert, W. H., and Staines, N. A., eds), VCH Verlagsgesellschaft mbH, 120–138.

14. Baskar, S., Hamilton, R. G., Norman, P. S., and Ansari, A. A. (1997) Grass immunotherapy induces inhibition of allergen-specific human peripheral blood mononuclear cell proliferation. *Int. Arch. Allergy Immunol.* **112,** 184–190.

4

Production of Human T-Cell Clones

Adrienne Verhoef

Abstract

The study of monoclonal human T-cell populations has had a fundamental impact on our current knowledge of the function, specificity, and mechanisms of activation of these cells. The frequency of antigen-specific T cells in peripheral blood is low, necessitating several enrichment steps prior to the isolation of individual clones. Two different methods of limiting dilution cloning are described in this chapter, the choice of which depends on the availability of starting materials. After isolation, T-cell clones are expanded and then tested for specificity and cryopreserved, both of which are described.

Recently, time-saving variations to the above methods have emerged. However, they require the use of sophisticated equipment and reagents, making them less economical than the established techniques.

Key Words: T-cell clone; limiting dilution; antigen-presenting cells.

1. Introduction

The ability to study monoclonal human T-cell populations has had a fundamental impact on our current knowledge of the function, specificity, and mechanisms of activation of these cells. Several technological advances have facilitated the isolation and expansion of human T-cell clones. For example, the isolation and characterization of T-cell growth factor (interleukin-2 [IL-2]) represented a major step forward in generating T-cell clones in vitro (*1,2*). Furthermore, advances in determining the molecular structures of antigenic peptides, TCR, and MHC molecules have allowed the detailed analysis of the interactions among these molecules.

As the frequency of antigen-specific T cells in peripheral blood is low (for example, approximately 1:10,000 of peripheral T cells of a given individual recognizes house dust mite proteins *[3]*), several enrichment steps precede the isolation of individual clones. Unfractionated peripheral blood mononuclear cells

From: Methods in Molecular Medicine: Allergy Methods and Protocols
Edited by: M. G. Jones and P. Lympany © Humana Press Inc., Totowa, NJ

(PBMC) are incubated with the antigen of interest, allowing antigen-specific T cells to expand. This may be followed by several rounds of restimulation with the particular antigen and IL-2, resulting in an oligoclonal T-cell population (T-cell line). When satisfied that the T-cell line recognizes the antigen of interest, as measured in a proliferation assay, T-cell clones are isolated from the T-cell line by various methods. While 'limiting dilution cloning' was first described over 20 yr ago and has remained the method of choice, new technology has enabled more efficient cloning techniques to be developed. Two different methods of limiting dilution cloning are described in this chapter, the choice of which depends on the availability of starting materials. For both methods, a T-cell stimulatory or 'feeding mixture' is prepared consisting of irradiated, antigen-presenting cells (APC), antigen in a predetermined optimal concentration, IL-2, and a mitogen, depending on which method is used (*see* below). A set number of antigen-specific T cells are then added to the feeding mixture before plating out into wells of a tissue culture plate, aiming to dispense single T cells into individual wells.

Method A *(4)* is the preferred method when fresh, autologous (originating from the same donor as the T-cell line to be cloned) PBMC are readily available. This method has the added advantage of using significantly less in terms of reagents, as the cells are plated out into 'Terasaki' plates at 20 µL/well. Method B *(5)* is used when autologous PBMC are in short supply. As APC, autologous Epstein–Barr virus (EBV) transformed B cells (EBV-B cells; *see* **Section 2.2.**) are used together with allogeneic PBMC from two donors, to ensure that appropriate costimulation by different types of APC is provided.

After T-cell clones have been isolated they are transferred to larger tissue culture wells and expanded during several rounds of restimulation (*see* **Section 2.1.**). After sufficiently large numbers have been generated, T cells are tested for specificity in a T-cell proliferation assay and cryopreserved, both of which are described under **Section 3**.

Recently, variations to the above methods have emerged. For example, Turcanu et al. *(6)* describe a system of obtaining peanut-allergen-specific T-cell clones, based on labeling PBMC with the fluorescent dye, carboxyfluorescein diacetate (CFSE), prior to antigen stimulation. When T cells divide on antigen recognition, CFSE-labeled proteins are equally divided among daughter cells, thus resulting in a reduction of fluorescence. CFSE^{low} T cells (representing antigen-specific cells) are subsequently isolated by cell-sorting on a flow cytometer and cloned by limiting dilution cloning, thus avoiding multiple rounds of antigen-specific stimulation.

Additionally, with the advances of tetramer technology, antigen-specific T cells within unfractionated PBMC populations may be directly identified and isolated by labeling with antigen-specific tetramers *(7)*. However, although saving time, these new methods require the use of sophisticated equipment and reagents, making them less economical than the established techniques.

2. Materials

2.1. T-Cell Cloning, Expansion, and Maintenance (see Note 1)

1. Basic medium: RPMI-1640 supplemented with 2 mM L-glutamine (Invitrogen, Paisley, UK) (*see* **Note 2**).
2. AB medium: Basic medium with the addition of 5–10% screened, heat-inactivated human AB serum (Sigma, Poole, UK) (*see* **Notes 2** and **3**).
3. FCS medium: Basic medium with the addition of 10% heat-inactivated fetal calf serum (FCS; Invitrogen) (*see* **Notes 2** and **3**). Serum should be stored at −70°C.
4. Freezing mix: 85% FCS and 15% DMSO (Sigma).
5. Ficoll-Hypaque (Sigma).
6. Unfractionated PBMC, freshly obtained or stored in liquid nitrogen (*see* **Note 4**).
7. Recombinant IL-2 (R&D Systems, Abingdon; Peprotech, London).
8. Antigens (storage depends on manufacturer's instructions) (*see* **Note 5**).
9. Use of a γ-cell irradiator.
10. Phytohemagglutinin (PHA; Sigma).

2.2. EBV Transformation of B Cells

1. B95-8 EBV producing cell line (ECACC, Salisbury, UK).
2. Cyclosporin A (Sigma) or PHA (Sigma).

2.3. T-Cell Proliferation Assay for Testing T-Cell Antigen Specificity

1. ^{3}[H]-Thymidine (Amersham).
2. Cell harvester, β-plate counter.
3. Plastics: Terasaki plates, 96-well and 24-well plates, cryovials, tissue culture flasks (all Nunc, Fisher Scientific, Loughborough, UK).

3. Methods

3.1. EBV Transformation of B Cells (8)

3.1.1. Generating EBV Supernatant

1. Culture B95-8 cells according to the supplier's instructions. Harvest supernatant and filter through a 0.45-μm filter.
2. Store in 1 mL aliquots at −70°C until needed.

3.1.2. Transformation of Human B Cells with EBV Virus

1. Incubate 1×10^7 unfractionated fresh or frozen human PBMC with 1 mL of EBV supernatant in a 15-mL conical tube with loose cap, for 4 h in a 37°C, 5% CO_2 humidified incubator.
2. Add 8 mL of FCS medium to the tube, as well as 1 mL of cyclosporin A (1 μg/mL final concentration) to prevent T-cell proliferation. Mix well and dispense into five wells of a 24-well tissue culture plate at 2 mL/well.

3. Feed cultures weekly by removing 1 mL of supernatant from each well, without disturbing the cells, and replacing this with 1 mL of fresh FCS medium, and leave until foci of proliferating transformed B cells appear (usually after 2–4 wk).
4. Transfer growing cultures to a 75-cm^2 flask in 30 mL of FCS medium; when growth medium turns yellow, expand by transferring 15 mL of the growing culture to a new flask followed by addition of 15 mL of FCS medium and cryopreserve (*see* **Section 3.5.**).
5. For use as APC, the cells should be irradiated at 6000 rad.

3.2. T-Cell Cloning

Prior to cloning, T-cell lines are generated by incubating PBMC with the antigen of interest (1° line) followed by at least one round of restimulation with irradiated, autologous PBMC, antigen, and IL-2 to generate 2° and 3° lines, with the aim of increasing the precursor frequency of antigen-specific T cells. It is important to test the antigen-specific nature of the T-cell pool as soon as enough T cells have been generated (usually at the 3° stage), by using a range of antigen concentrations. This will also provide information on optimal antigen concentration to be used in the subsequent cloning procedure. Always include a negative control (APC + T cells) as it is not unusual for autoreactive T cells present in PBMC to be activated as a consequence of in vitro culture conditions. When antigen specificity has been determined (3° stage or beyond), the T-cell line is ready to be cloned. The T-cell line should be 'resting', i.e., 7 d after antigen-specific restimulation and 3–4 d after the last addition of IL-2.

3.2.1. Method A

Prepare feeding mixture in a total of 23 mL AB medium as follows:

1. Fresh, irradiated (3000 rad), autologous PBMC (0.5×10^6 per mL), antigen at predetermined optimal concentration, 10 ng/mL IL-2.
2. Prepare T cells as follows: recover T cells into suitable container and wash cells by filling up the tube with RPMI. Centrifuge ($160g$, 21°C, 10 min), remove medium, loosen the cell pellet, fill up the tube with RPMI, and centrifuge again.
3. Resuspend T cells in 5 mL AB medium at 1×10^6–2×10^6 per mL. Carefully layer the T-cell suspension onto an equal volume of Ficoll, in a 15-mL conical tube. Centrifuge ($280g$, 21°C, 10 min) and wash 2× with RPMI (as for step 2).
4. Recover the T cells from the interface of Ficoll gradient and wash 2× with RPMI (as for step 2).
5. Accurately count live T cells and add 3.6×10^5 cells to 1 mL AB medium (dilution 1). Make three subsequent serial dilutions of the T cells by adding 0.1 mL of dilution 1 to 0.9 mL of AB medium, resulting in a final dilution of 3.6×10^2 T cells in 1 mL. Add this to the feeder mixture, giving a final volume of 24 mL cloning mixture, containing 15 T cells/mL, resulting in a final concentration of 0.3 T cells/well.
6. Dispense mixture into 'Terasaki' plates at 20 µL/well and incubate for 7–10 d in a humidified 37°C, 5% CO_2 incubator.

7. Transfer contents of wells with expanding T-cell clones to 96-well flat bottom plates in the presence of autologous, irradiated PBMC (fresh or frozen; 1×10^5 cells/200 µL per well), antigen at optimal concentration and 10 ng/mL IL-2. Add 10 ng/mL IL-2 after 3–4 d; rapidly expanding clones (recognized by yellowing of AB medium) can be 'split' into two wells by transferring 100 µL of cell suspension into a new well and adding 100 µL of fresh AB medium to both wells.

8. Seven days after transfer to 96-well plates, the expanding T cells are transferred to 24-well plates, in the presence of a feeder mixture as described above, with 1×10^6 APC per well in a total volume of 2 mL/well.

3.2.2. Method B

1. Prepare feeding mixture as follows: irradiated allogeneic PBMC from two donors (1×10^6 total/mL), irradiated autologous EBV-B cells (1×10^5 per mL), antigen at optimal concentration, 1 µg/mL PHA in a total volume of 49 mL AB medium.

2. Prepare T-cell mixture as for method A with the following variations: add 1.67×10^5 T cells to AB medium in a final volume of 1 mL. Make three serial dilutions as for method A and add final dilution (167 T cells) to the feeding mixture, resulting in a final concentration of 3.33 T cells/mL of cloning mix.

3. Dispense cloning mixture into 96-well round bottom plates at 100 µL/well. Incubate in 5% CO_2 incubator at 37°C.

4. After 3–4 d, add 10 ng/mL IL-2, and make volume of wells up to 200 µL with AB medium.

5. Seven days after cloning, transfer expanding T cells to 24-well plates in the presence of a feeder mixture consisting of irradiated, allogeneic PBMC from two donors (1×10^6 per well), autologous irradiated EBV-B cells (1×10^5 per well), antigen at optimal concentration, PHA (1 µg/mL), and IL-2 (10 ng/mL), in a total volume of 2 mL/well.

3.3. T-Cell Expansion and Maintenance (see Note 6)

When T-cell clones have reached the 24-well stage, they can be maintained and expanded. T-cell clones should be maintained on a weekly feeding cycle, with irradiated autologous APC (1×10^6 per well for method A), antigen, and IL-2 (10 ng/mL), or with irradiated allogeneic APC (1×10^6 PBMC, 1×10^5 EBV-B), PHA, antigen, and IL-2 for method B, in a total volume of 2 mL/well of a 24-well plate; 3–4 d after each antigenic stimulation, 10 ng/mL IL-2 should be added to all wells, and rapidly expanding T-cell clones can be split at this stage. At the end of the 7-d feeding cycle when T cells are fully resting, they may be used for cryopreservation and functional assays.

3.4. T-Cell Proliferation Assay for Testing T-Cell Antigen Specificity

When sufficient numbers of T cells have been generated (at least 5×10^6), they should be tested for antigen specificity in a proliferation assay, with T cells incubated with APC in the absence of antigen as background control.

The T cells should be used at the end of the 7-d feeding cycle and be fully rested (*see* **Notes 7** and **8**).

1. Prepare and irradiate APC (autologous PBMC or EBV-B cells) and plate out in triplicate in a round bottom, 96-well plate at 2.5×10^4 per well.
2. Add antigen to appropriate wells at optimal concentration.
3. Add T cells at 2.5×10^4 cells/well.
4. Make volume of each well up to 200 µL with AB medium.
5. Incubate for 72 h with the addition of ^{3}[H]-thymidine (1 µCi /well) for the last 8–16 h.
6. Harvest and count plate.
7. Discard those T-cell clones that do not proliferate significantly as compared to background control.

3.5. Cryopreservation (see Note 9)

For long-term storage, cells are kept at −180°C, in the vapor phase of a liquid nitrogen freezer. To freeze cells:

1. Add cold freezing mix dropwise to an equal volume of cells suspended in complete medium (2×10^6–20×10^6 cells/mL, kept on ice).
2. Dispense 1 mL aliquots into cryovials and store at −70°C in a polystyrene container.
3. After 24 h, transfer the vials to a liquid nitrogen container, where they can remain viable for at least 10 yr.

4. Notes

1. As T-cell work requires long-term culture, contamination is an ever-present threat. Therefore, measures must be taken to prevent loss of valuable material. When there is uncertainty about the sterility of materials, they should be filter-sterilized (0.02-µM filter). Antibiotics (penicillin/streptomycin; 100 IU/mL) may be added to the tissue culture medium, but this does not prevent fungus or mycoplasma infection. The latter can also alter functional characteristics of T cells and thus lead to invalid experimental data. Routine mycoplasma testing, for which different kits are commercially available, is therefore recommended.
2. All media may be stored at 4°C for up to 2 wk.
3. Before embarking on T-cell cloning, some parameters should be established. Human serum should be tested for its ability to support T-cell growth (without causing nonspecific proliferation) at different concentrations, by measuring proliferation of PHA-stimulated PBMC in the presence of 2.5, 5, 7.5, and 10% serum containing RPMI, using serum from different batches as they can vary. This is not necessary for FCS, as this is not used for culturing human T cells.
   Alternatively, autologous plasma may be used to supplement media as a (low-cost) alternative to commercially available human serum. The preparation procedure is as follows: do not dilute donor blood before layering on Ficoll gradient, and after centrifugation, carefully transfer the top yellow layer (plasma) to a separate tube, taking care not to disturb the PBMC layer. Centrifuge plasma (1000*g*, 21°C, 15 min) and transfer plasma to new tube. Discard the pellet. Heat inactivate (55°C for 25–30 min)

and centrifuge again (1000g, 21°C, 15 min). Aliquot plasma and store at −20°C. Autologous plasma is generally used at a concentration ranging from 1 to 5%, but if important, optimal concentration should be assessed in a proliferation assay.

4. Initially, when generating antigen-specific lines, the following numbers of PBMC are needed: 1×10^7 for each T-cell line and an additional 1×10^6–5×10^6 PBMC for each round of restimulation. EBV transformation of B cells requires 1×10^7 PBMC; therefore, 50–100 mL of blood would provide sufficient starting material (as a rule of thumb: 1 mL of blood yields 1×10^6 PBMC on average). When cloning, an additional 50–100 mL of blood would ensure sufficient PBMC for fresh feeders and PBMC storage for subsequent stimulation of T-cell clones.

5. The optimal antigen dose should be determined by measuring the proliferation of PBMC incubated with increasing concentrations of the antigen. The dose which results in maximal proliferation should be used in subsequent procedures.

6. Once T-cell clones have been established by either method A or B, they may be restimulated for expansion and maintenance by method A or B depending on the continuous availability of materials. For example, if clones were generated using method A, but autologous PBMC are no longer available, method B can be used for further expansion. It is, however, not recommended to exclusively use method B for stimulation as this can lead to nonresponsiveness. Therefore, it is important to determine the MHC restriction of the T-cell clones so that PBMC from an HLA-matched donor may be used to replace autologous PBMC. Method A is the preferred method for several reasons: first, the T cells are stimulated in an antigen-specific way (in the absence of mitogenic stimulation as in method B), which results in a higher percentage of antigen-specific T-cell clones. Secondly, this method makes use of Terasaki plates which hold only 20 µL. Therefore, far less starting material is needed than in method B. The slight disadvantage of this method is the fact that the procedure only reaches the 96-well stage after 7–10 d, thus prolonging the procedure.

7. When identifying positive wells, it may be difficult to identify slow-growing clones and one may be tempted to select only fast-growing ones, thus introducing a bias. Therefore, it may be better to score clones 10 d after incubation.

8. T-cell cloning is not guaranteed to be successful first time around and may have to be repeated several times. When clones are obtained, low cloning efficiencies could result in very few clones, with even fewer antigen-specific ones. Another major problem is the inability to expand clones.

9. Early and continuous cryopreservation of T-cell clones is advisable because of the finite life span of T-cell clones in culture, with their potential to expand decreasing with time in culture.

References

1. Morgan, D. A., Ruscetti, F. W., and Gallo, R. (1976) Selective *in vitro* growth of T lymphocytes from normal human bone marrows. *Science* **193,** 1007–1008.
2. *Human T Cell Clones: A New Approach to Immune Regulation*, Eds: Feldmann, M.; Lamb, J. R.; Woody, J. N., Humana Press, New York, 1985.

3. Halvorsen, R., Bosnes, V., and Thorsby, E. (1986) T cell responses to a *Dermatophagoides farinae* allergen preparation in allergics and healthy controls. *Int. Archs. Allergy Appl. Immunol.* **80,** 62–69.
4. Lamb, J. R., Eckels, D. D., Lake, P., Johnson, A. H., Hartzman, R. J., and Woody, J. N. (1982) Antigen-specific human T lymphocyte clones: induction, antigen specificity and MHC restriction of influenza virus-immune clones. *J. Immunol.* **128,** 233–238.
5. van Schooten, W. C. A., Ottenhof, T. H. M., Klatser, P. R., Thole, J., de Vries, R. R. P., and Kolk, A. H. J. (1988) T cell epitopes on the 36K and 65K *Mycobacterium leprea* antigens defined by human T cell clones. *Eur. J. Immunol.* **18,** 849–854.
6. Turcanu, V., Maleki, S. J., and Lack, G. (2003). Characterization of lymphocyte responses to peanuts in normal children, peanut-allergic children, and allergic children who acquired tolerance to peanuts. *J. Clin. Investig.* **111,** 1065–1072.
7. Reijonen, H. and Kwok, W. W. (2003). Use of HLA class II tetramers in tracking antigen-specific T cells and mapping T-cell epitopes. *Methods* **29,** 282–288.
8. Miller, G. and Lipman, M. (1973) Release of infectious Epstein-Barr virus by transformed marmoset leucocytes. *Proc. Natl Acad. Sci. USA* **69,** 383–387.

5

Mapping of Human T-Cell Epitopes of Allergens

Thomas Zeiler and Tuomas Virtanen

Abstract

Allergens are characterized by their ability to be bound by gE. The Swiss-Prot protein database currently lists a partial or complete amino acid sequence of in excess of about 350 allergens. It is not clear how allergens participate in the process of allergic sensitization, the generation of specific T-helper type 2 (Th2) lymphocytes, which play a crucial role in stimulating B lymphocytes to produce allergen-specific IgE.

T-helper (Th) cells play a key role in the regulation of immune responses. The recognition of antigen by T cells is complex and it can trigger qualitatively differential signaling. Therefore, it is conceivable that epitopes or antigenic determinants recognized by Th cells may influence the quality of immune response. The aim of this chapter is to describe the way in which T-cell epitopes can be identified (mapped). This is particularly important because knowledge of the precise T-cell epitopes of allergens can give important information on the pathogenesis of allergy and can help to develop better preparations for the diagnostics and/or immunotherapy of allergy.

Key Words: Allergen; epitope; T-helper cell.

1. Introduction

Allergens are a special group of antigens characterized by their ability to be bound by IgE. Knowledge of the molecular biology of allergens has increased greatly during the past 10–15 yr. The Swiss-Prot protein database lists a partial or complete amino acid sequence of about 350 allergens at the moment (http://www.expasy.ch/cgi-bin/lists?allergen.txt; March 1, 2006). Despite the increased information, it is not clear how allergens participate in the process of allergic sensitization, the generation of specific T-helper type 2 (Th2) lymphocytes, which play a crucial role in stimulating B lymphocytes to produce allergen-specific IgE. Although several allergens are enzymes and this property appears

From: Methods in Molecular Medicine: Allergy Methods and Protocols
Edited by: M. G. Jones and P. Lympany © Humana Press Inc., Totowa, NJ

to be important for their allergenicity *(1)*, there is no evidence that any biological property in general would account for the allergenic capacity of proteins *(2,3)*.

The specific cells of the immune system that recognize antigens and allergens are B and T lymphocytes. Whereas B cells recognize three-dimensional molecular structures by their receptors *(4,5)*, T-helper (Th) cells (CD4[+]) recognize short linear fragments of allergens (approx. 10–20 amino acids) presented on the surface of antigen-presenting cells in association with the major histocompatibility complex (MHC) class II molecules *(6,7)*.

Th cells play a key role in the regulation of immune responses *(8)*. The recognition of antigen by T cells is not a simple on/off phenomenon and it can trigger qualitatively differential signaling *(9,10)*. Therefore, it is conceivable that the specific sites, epitopes, or antigenic determinants recognized by Th cells in allergens may influence the quality of immune response. In other words, the way how allergens are recognized by the cells of the immune system can be involved in favoring Th2 differentiation *(11–13)*. In this context, the interplay among the immune system, exogenous allergens, and endogenous proteins can be important *(11)*.

In addition to the fact that knowing the T-cell epitopes of allergens can give important information on the pathogenesis of allergy, it can help to develop better preparations for the diagnostics and/or immunotherapy of allergy. For the preparation to be used in immunotherapy, it is important that it contains all the important T-cell epitopes because the beneficial effects of immunotherapy are expected to be mediated via T cells *(14)*. This is especially true for modified preparations, such as T-cell epitope-containing peptides or their constructs *(15)*.

The conventional way of mapping T-cell epitopes is straightforward but requires basic knowledge of the methods of T-cell culture (*see* previous chapters). In brief, the optimal stimulation concentrations of peptides and allergens should be determined in advance. The mapping should be performed as soon as there are sufficient numbers of allergen-specific T cells, either clones or in lines, because the growth of T cells slows down after repeated stimulations. In some cases, the analysis can be done directly with peripheral blood mononuclear cells (PBMC) *(16,17)* but weak responses may preclude this approach *(18,19)*. T-cell epitopes are determined by stimulating the cells with peptides and measuring the responses by the incorporation of ^{3}H-thymidine in a proliferation test.

The mapping can be complemented by measuring the binding of allergen peptides to MHC class II molecules *(19)*. The analysis is valuable, for example, by identifying peptides which can bind to several MHC alleles.

A novel alternative for mapping T-cell epitopes is to use peptide/MHC class II tetramers *(20)*.

2. Materials

1. Allergens (*see* **Note 1**).
2. Peptides (*see* **Note 2**).
3. The allergen-specific T-cell lines and clones (*see* Chapters 3 and 4 and **Note 3**).

3. Methods

3.1. Measurement of Allergen-Specific Proliferation of T Cells

The responses of allergen-specific T-cell clones and lines on stimulation with peptides are usually measured by a standard proliferation assay as described in Chapter 2 (also *see* **Note 4**).

4. Notes

1. Natural or recombinant allergens are needed for creating allergen-specific T-cell lines and clones. It is advantageous that the preparation is pure; contaminants may be potent stimulants resulting in T-cell cultures of undesired specificities. For creating specific T-cell lines and clones, the optimal stimulation doses of allergens should be tested in advance with PBMC. It is often between 10 and 200 µg/mL.
2. Overlapping peptides can be obtained most conveniently from specialized commercial suppliers but they are quite expensive. A more economic way may be the in-house synthesis with the multipin technology (e.g., Mimotopes Pty Ltd). Another possibility is the use of allergen fragments. They can be produced by molecular biology methods or by the digestion of allergenic proteins with enzymes followed by a purification step with high-pressure liquid chromatography (HPLC). This approach yields fragments of various lengths which renders it difficult to localize the epitope accurately. One way to decrease the number of peptides needed can be the prediction of possible epitopes with computer programs like TEPITOPE *(21)* or through Internet (http://www.imtech.res.in/raghava/propred/, http://www.syfpeithi.de/) before the actual mapping experiments.

   Whereas the length of peptides presented in association with MHC II molecules varies from 10 to 20 amino acids *(6,7)* the length can influence the results of epitope mapping *(17)*. We have used 16mer peptides overlapping with 14 amino acids *(18,19)*. In this way, it is possible to detect the epitope-specific response with three to five peptides which increases the reliability of the results. With a shorter overlap, the response may be seen with only one or two peptides and if the response is weak, its detection can be difficult. The number of peptides needed for the mapping of T-cell epitopes can be calculated according to the formula $n = (l-o)/(p-o)$ in which n is the number of peptides needed (the nearest integer), l is the number of amino acids in the protein sequence, o is the number of amino acids in the overlap, and p is the number of amino acids in the peptide.

   The correct amino acid sequence of peptides to be used in mapping should be verified by mass spectrometry or by other methods. This is usually done by the manufacturer. If the preparation also appears pure by the analytical HPLC, it may be possible to use it directly for mapping. This is especially true for initial screening. However, because contaminants (e.g., peptide fragments) may affect the results, we have preferred to use peptides purified with HPLC.

Peptides may be poorly soluble in water because of their amino acid composition. In this case, the peptide may be first dissolved in a small volume of dimethyl sulfoxide (DMSO) and then diluted in the culture medium. The final concentration of DMSO on plates should be ≤0.1% (v/v).

Before use, the peptides can be sterilized by membrane filtration or by γ-irradiation. Storage is at −70°C.

3. Our experience suggests that the responses of PBMCs against allergens are often very weak. Therefore, we prefer to perform the mapping of T-cell epitopes with T-cell lines and clones.

   Epitope mapping with a T-cell line is likely to reveal a more comprehensive repertoire of epitopes than the mapping with T-cell clones only. In the mapping with clones, there is always the possibility that cloning and long-term T-cell culture result in the selection of a limited number of clones detecting few immunodominant epitopes. On the other hand, the responses of clones are usually clear-cut and allow a more detailed analysis of the T-cell response.

   It is easier to get well-responding T-cell lines from patients with clinically severe forms of allergy. Therefore, patients' reactivity to the allergen to be studied should be verified by skin prick tests and/or by measuring allergen-specific IgE.

4. A starting point for the optimal stimulation concentration for peptides can be deduced from the molar concentration of the allergen which produced the optimal results in tests with PBMCs (or T-cell lines or clones). For example, if the optimal concentration of an allergen with 160 amino acids is 100 µg/mL, the concentration for a 16mer peptide could be 10 µg/mL (the molar concentrations being roughly the same for the peptides and the allergen). Testing with lower and higher concentrations of peptides increases the reliability of the results.

   The results of a proliferation test (the counts per minute [cpm] obtained from scintillation counting) of a T-cell clone or line are usually expressed as a stimulation index (SI) according to the formula:

$$SI = \frac{(\text{mean cpm of wells with T cells, feeder cells, and allergen}) - (\text{mean cpm of wells with T cells only})}{(\text{mean cpm of wells with T cells and feeder cells}) - (\text{mean cpm of wells with T cells only})}$$

The SI with PBMCs is obtained simply by dividing the mean cpm of cells with allergen with the mean cpm of cells without allergen. Although no exact limit can be set for a positive response, SI ≥ 2 or 3 with PBMCs or T-cell lines and SI ≥ 5 with T-cell clones are often regarded as positive. Especially with PBMCs when the proliferative responses can be very weak, another possibility for determining positive responses is to assign a cutoff value calculated as the mean cpm value of several wells containing unstimulated cells plus three times the standard deviation. This allows the results of individual wells to be determined as positive or negative. Then the difference in the frequency of positive wells between stimulated and nonstimulated cultures (several replicates) is analyzed statistically *(17,22)*.

An alternative for measuring cellular responses in a proliferation assay is the measurement of cytokines from the cultures after stimulation.

References

1. Reed, C. E. and Kita, H. (2004) The role of protease activation of inflammation in allergic respiratory diseases. *J. Allergy Clin. Immunol.* **114,** 997–1008.
2. Virtanen, T. and Mäntyjarvi, R. A. (2005) Important mammalian respiratory allergens are lipocalins. In *Lipocalins* (Åkerström, B., Borregaard, N., Flower, D., and Salier, J.-P., eds), Landes Bioscience, Georgetown, *http://www.eurekah.com/abstract.php?chapid=2559&bookid=190&catid=15.*
3. Holt, P. G. and Thomas, W. R. (2005) Sensitization to airborne environmental allergens: unresolved issues. *Nat. Immunol.* **6,** 957–960.
4. Scheiner O. and Kraft, D. (1995) Basic and practical aspects of recombinant allergens. *Allergy* **50,** 384–391.
5. Dudler, T., Chen, W.-Q., Wang, S., Schneider, T., Annand, R. R., and Dempcy, R. O. (1992) High-level expression in *Escherichia coli* and rapid purification of enzymatically active honey bee venom phospholipase A_2. *Biochim. Biophys. Acta* **1165,** 201–210.
6. Schwartz, R. H. (1985) T-lymphocyte recognition of antigen in association with gene products of the major histocompatibility complex. *Annu. Rev. Immunol.* **3,** 237–261.
7. Germain, R. N. (1993) Antigen processing and presentation. In *Fundamental Immunology* (Paul, W. E., ed.), 3rd Ed., Raven, New York, pp. 629–676.
8. Abbas, A. K., Murphy, K. M., and Sher, A. (1996) Functional diversity of helper T lymphocytes. *Nature* **383,** 787–793.
9. Evavold, B. D. and Allen, P. M. (1991) Separation of IL-4 production from Th cell proliferation by an altered T cell receptor ligand. *Science* **252,** 1308–1310.
10. Sloan-Lancaster, J. and Allen, P. M. (1996) Altered peptide ligand-induced partial T cell activation: molecular mechanisms and role in T cell biology. *Annu. Rev. Immunol.* **14,** 1–27.
11. Virtanen, T., Zeiler, T., Rautiainen, J., and Mäntyjärvi, R. (1999) Allergy to lipocalins: a consequence of misguided T-cell recognition of self and nonself? *Immunol. Today* **20,** 398–400.
12. Kinnunen, T., Buhot, C., Närvänen, A., et al. (2003) The immunodominant epitope of lipocalin allergen Bos d 2 is suboptimal for human T cells. *Eur. J. Immunol.* **33,** 1717–1726.
13. Virtanen, T. and Mäntyjärvi, R. (2004) Mammalian allergens. In *Allergens and Allergen Immunotherapy* (Lockey, R. F., Bukantz, S. C., and Bousquet, J., eds), Marcel Dekker, Inc., New York, pp. 297–317.
14. Till, S. J., Francis, J. N., Nouri-Aria, K., and Durham, S. R. (2004) Mechanisms of immunotherapy. *J. Allergy Clin. Immunol.* **113,** 1025–1034.
15. Ali, F. R. and Larche, M. (2005) Peptide-based immunotherapy: a novel strategy for allergic disease. *Expert Rev Vaccines* **4,** 881–889.
16. Bungy, G. A., Rodda, S., Roitt, I., and Brostoff, J. (1994) Mapping of T cell epitopes of the major fraction of rye grass using peripheral blood mononuclear cells

from atopics and non-atopics. 2. Isoallergen clone 5A of Lolium perenne group I (Lol p I). *Eur. J. Immunol.* **24,** 2098–2103.

17. Reece, J. C., McGregor, D. L., Geysen, H. M., and Rodda, S. J. (1994) Scanning for T helper epitopes with human PBMC using pools of short synthetic peptides. *J. Immunol. Method.* **172,** 241–254.

18. Zeiler, T., Mäntyjärvi, R., Rautiainen, J., et al. (1999) T cell epitopes of a lipocalin allergen colocalize with the conserved regions of the molecule. *J. Immunol.* **162,** 1415–1422.

19. Immonen, A., Farci, S., Taivainen, A., et al. (2005) T cell epitope-containing peptides of the major dog allergen Can f 1 as candidates for allergen immunotherapy. *J. Immunol.* **105,** 3614–3620.

20. Novak, E. J., Liu, A. W., Gebe, J. A., et al. (2001) Tetramer-guided epitope mapping: rapid identification and characterization of immunodominant CD4+ T cell epitopes from complex antigens. *J. Immunol.* **166,** 6665–6670.

21. de Lalla, C., Sturniolo, T., Abbruzzese, L., et al. (1999) Cutting edge: identification of novel T cell epitopes in Lol p5a by computational prediction. *J. Immunol.* **163,** 1725–1729.

22. Taswell, C. (1984) Limiting dilution assays for the determination of immuno-competent cell frequencies. III. Validity tests for the single-hit Poisson model. *J. Immunol. Methods* **72,** 29–40.

6

Determining MHC Restriction of T-cell Responses

Mark Larché

Abstract

T-cell receptors (TcR) recognize short linear peptides (9–15 amino acid long), which have been processed by an 'antigen-presenting cell' and complexed to products of the major histocompatibility complex (MHC). Peptides of the appropriate shape and charge are able to bind within the groove of the MHC molecule and it is this complex which is recognized by the TcR. The MHC molecules are highly polymorphic, but each individual will only express one maternal and one paternal allele of HLA Class 1 molecule A, B, and C and HLA Class II DR, DP, and DQ. As a result of TcR specificity and MHC restriction, a clone of T cells will bear a specific receptor which has a very limited repertoire of targets (peptide–MHC complexes). When sufficient numbers of TcR are engaged on a T-cell surface, a cascade of signal transduction events is initiated which results in cellular activation.

When investigating the immune response, it may be advantageous to be able to identify which MHC molecules bind a particular peptide well and give rise to a vigorous T-cell response. Such information may be useful in generating effective vaccines. In this chapter, we provide examples of Epstein–Barr virus-transformed lymphoid cell lines and fibroblast cell lines to determine MHC restriction elements.

Key Words: MHC; T cells; peptides; MHC restriction.

1. Introduction
1.1. How Antigen-Specific Cells Recognize Antigen

The antigen-specific arm of the immune response is provided by T and B lymphocytes. Antigen recognition is affected by cell surface receptors whose specificity is generated by random rearrangement of multiple gene segments during development *(1)*. B lymphocytes express both soluble and membrane-bound antigen receptors. The soluble form is secreted and is otherwise known

From: *Methods in Molecular Medicine: Allergy Methods and Protocols*
Edited by: M. G. Jones and P. Lympany © Humana Press Inc., Totowa, NJ

as antibody or immunoglobulin (Ig). T-lymphocyte antigen receptors (T-cell receptor; TcR) are expressed in membrane-bound form only.

Although the receptors are closely related, the mechanics of T-cell and B-cell antigen recognition differ in a number of important ways. B-cell receptors recognize three-dimensional structure, which can include both linear and conformational protein sequences. The protein may be native (i.e., intact) or it may be partially degraded. However, as long as the area of the molecule that is recognized by the antigen receptor has retained conformational integrity, recognition can be achieved. Thus B-cell antigen receptors are able to bind to three-dimensional structures which have been generated by a linear series of amino acids in a protein or by the juxtaposition of two or more discontinuous sequences of amino acids in the tertiary structure of the protein.

T-cell antigen receptors recognize antigen in a very different and more selective manner. T cells are unable to recognize whole antigen molecules or, indeed, large fragments of protein. For recognition to occur, the TcR must engage short linear peptide sequences (epitopes) from the antigenic protein which are generally of the order of 9–15 amino acids in length. Furthermore, such peptides must be complexed to products of the major histocompatibility complex (MHC; so-called "tissue-typing" antigens; Ref. *[2]*). The MHC is a highly polymorphic locus located on chromosome 6 which encodes cell surface glycoproteins which are part of the Ig superfamily.

1.2. The Major Histocompatibility Complex and Its Products

In man, the products of MHC are referred to as human leukocyte antigens (HLA). The MHC locus contains three regions known as Class I, Class II, and Class III. The latter encodes components of the complement cascade and is irrelevant in this chapter. HLA Class I molecules are membrane-bound glycoproteins containing three Ig-like domains. Following protein synthesis and maturation within the cell, a fourth domain in the form of β2-microglobulin associates with the Class I glycoprotein. HLA Class II molecules are composed of a heterodimer of α and β chains, each containing two Ig-like domains, both of which are anchored in the membrane by a hydrophobic transmembrane domain.

A common feature of both Class I and Class II molecules is a membrane distal peptide-binding groove formed with a floor of β-pleated sheets and two α-helices. The structure is shown schematically in **Fig. 1**.

Peptides of the appropriate shape and charge are able to bind within the groove and it is this complex that is recognized by the TcR. Subtle differences exist between Class I and Class II molecules which are beyond the scope of this review. However, in general terms it can be said that MHC Class I molecules bind peptides generated in the intracellular microenvironment and loaded into the binding groove within the endoplasmic reticulum. Such peptides would

T cell

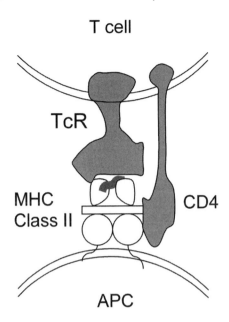

Fig. 1. The peptide binding groove of MHC molecules comprises a floor of β-pleated sheets and two α-helical walls in between which the peptide is bound. The TcR interacts with the peptide–MHC complex and the accessory molecule CD4, with framework regions of the MHC.

include those from self-molecules and also from intracellular pathogens such as viruses. In contrast, MHC Class II molecules generally bind peptides which have been generated by the proteolytic degradation of proteins which have been taken up from the extracellular environment into the lysosome pathway.

Ultimately, both forms of MHC molecules are displayed on the cell surface with bound peptide. When presented in this way on an appropriate cell type in sufficient numbers, MHC–peptide complexes can interact with specific TcR leading to T-cell activation. For effective activation to occur, additional cell surface structures such as accessory molecules must also be ligated. Two important accessory molecules for T-cell activation are CD4 and CD8. The former has affinity for framework regions of the MHC Class II molecule and the latter for MHC Class I molecules. For this reason, T cells expressing CD4 can recognize peptides bound to MHC Class II molecules and T cells expressing CD8 recognize peptides bound to MHC Class I molecules.

As a result of the extremely polymorphic nature of the MHC gene locus, there are several hundred HLA molecules of the Class I and Class II types. Each individual will only express a limited number of these molecules which are grouped together into families of similar genes. Thus, HLA Class I molecules are grouped into A, B, and C types and Class II into DR, DP, and DQ. In general terms, an individual will express one maternal allele of each of these groups and one paternal allele. There may also, however, be variable numbers of extra DR molecules expressed. The result of such polymorphism is that different individuals have different repertoires of HLA molecules. Because these molecules, by virtue of their different peptide-binding grooves, can bind different peptides from a variety of molecules there will be distinct differences in an individual's ability to recognize any given protein. Such diversity ensures that, at the species level, some individuals who are able to mount an adequate immune response to a specific pathogen or protein should always be present within the population.

1.3. MHC Restriction

Further complexity is generated by the fact that within an individual, TcR maturing in the thymus are only potentially useful to the host if they recognize combinations of peptide bound to "self"-MHC (rather than, for example, MHC molecules expressed by another individual). Thus, all other TcR specificities are deleted in the thymus in a process known as thymic education. The result, in a population expressing polymorphic MHC, is that T cells from one individual will generally not be capable of recognizing peptide presented by cells from another individual unless the two individuals share the relevant MHC molecule. For example, an individual expressing DR1 (an MHC Class II molecule) but not DR2 will not have T cells capable of recognizing peptides of antigen X when they are presented by DR2, but will have TcR capable of recognizing complexes of peptide from antigen X when they are bound to DR1. The combination of the limited ability of any given peptide to bind within a single peptide-binding groove and the ability of an individual's T cells to recognize peptides only when they are bound to self-MHC (or in some cases a complex that mimics self and peptide) is generally referred to as "MHC restriction". The definition of the MHC as the factor which restricted the ability of genetically disparate strains of mouse to mount immune responses to viruses earned Peter C. Doherty and Rolf Zinkernagal the Nobel Prize in 1996 for experiments performed 20 yr earlier *(3)*.

1.4. The Outcomes of T-Cell Activation

As a result of TcR specificity and MHC restriction, a clone of T cells will bear a specific receptor which has a very limited repertoire of targets (peptide–MHC complexes). When sufficient numbers of TcR are engaged on a T-cell surface, a cascade of signal transduction events is initiated which results in cellular activation *(4)*. The manifestations of T-cell activation are various but generally include cell division and elaboration of soluble factors such as cytokines. The latter, however, may vary in type and, as a consequence, if cytokine production is to be employed as a readout of T-cell activation, it is important to know which cytokines to look for. Cell surface markers may also change; CD69, for example, is often employed as a marker of cell activation. For practical purposes, however, cell division or proliferation is the most readily measurable outcome of T-cell activation and forms the basis of many functional assays.

1.5. Identification of MHC Restriction Elements

Individual MHC molecules are often referred to as "restricting elements" because they restrict the response of an individual to a given peptide. Peptides may be said to be recognized "in the context of" a particular restricting element, i.e., they bind to and are presented to the TcR by a particular MHC molecule.

When investigating the immune response to different pathogens or proteins it may be advantageous to be able to identify a restricting element that binds a particular peptide well and gives rise to a vigorous T-cell response. Such information may be particularly useful, for example, in generating effective vaccines.

Owing to the variety of MHC molecules expressed, determining MHC restriction can be a difficult process. A stepwise approach to narrow the possibilities can be considered. In order to determine whether peptides are recognized in the context of MHC Class I or Class II molecules it may be enough to simply determine the CD4/CD8 phenotype of the responding cells by flow cytometry, for example, or immunocytochemistry. This approach may be suitable for pools of cells which are relatively homogeneous such as T-cell clones or lines, but inappropriate for primary cultures of peripheral blood mononuclear cells. A further simple approach to narrowing down the possibilities is the addition of monoclonal antibodies directed against framework determinants of families of MHC molecules. For example, the addition of the appropriate concentration of antibodies (generally 1–10 µg/mL) directed against HLA-DR, DP, DQ into replicates of a T-cell culture should allow the identification of inhibition of the T-cell response by one of the three antibodies, HLA-DR, for example. This will indicate that the response is being restricted by HLA-DR. However, because an individual will possess more than one HLA-DR allele (two HLA-DR*B1 alleles and variable combinations of HLA-DR*B3, B4, and B5; B2 being nonfunctional), further experiments are required to determine the exact restricting element. At this stage, knowledge of the HLA genes expressed by the individual, in the form of a histocompatibility type (tissue type), is essential.

With the knowledge of which HLA genes are expressed by an individual, the investigator can then determine the potential molecules restricting a given response. What remains is to obtain cell lines expressing defined MHC molecules of each of these types and assay the ability of these cells to bind and present the peptide (or perhaps in some cases process and present whole antigen) in question to T cells of the appropriate specificity.

In order to provide the cleanest system, it is preferable to employ cell lines which have been engineered to express only one MHC molecule on their surface. Mouse fibroblast cell lines transfected with a variety of human MHC genes have been generated by a number of investigators and may be available directly from these researchers or through culture collections. Alternatively, Epstein–Barr virus (EBV)-transformed lymphoid cell lines (EBV-LCL) of defined HLA phenotype may be used in combination to define MHC restriction elements. EBV-LCL can be obtained from organizations such as the European Collection of Animal Cell Cultures (ECACC) or other culture collections. For further information see http://www.hgmp.mrc.ac.uk/GenomeWeb/culture-collections.html.

2. Materials

2.1. Isolation of Peripheral Blood Mononuclear Cells

1. Preservative-free heparin (Leo Laboratories, Bucks, UK).
2. Histopaque (Sigma, Poole, Dorset, UK).
3. Heparinized culture medium; RPMI-1640 L-glutamine free (*see* **Note 1**), HEPES buffered, supplemented with 2 mM L-glutamine, 100 U/mL penicillin, 100 µg/mL streptomycin (all Sigma), and 10 U/mL preservative-free heparin (Leo Laboratories).
4. Complete culture medium (*see* **Note 2**); RPMI-1640 L-glutamine free, bicarbonate buffered, supplemented with 2 mM L-glutamine, 100 U/mL penicillin, 100 µg/mL streptomycin, and 5% normal human AB serum (*see* **Note 3**) (all Sigma).
5. Serological sterile, plastic pipettes (10 and 25 mL; Greiner Laboratories Ltd, Stonehouse, Gloucester, UK).
6. 50-mL Cellstar polycarbonate tubes (Greiner).
7. Sterile, individually wrapped 3-mL pastettes (Greiner).
8. Trypan blue (0.4%) solution in saline (Sigma).

2.2. Transformation of B Cells with EBV

1. Complete culture medium; RPMI-1640 L-glutamine free, bicarbonate buffered, supplemented with 2 mM L-glutamine, 100 U/mL penicillin, 100 µg/mL streptomycin, and 10% FCS (all Sigma).
2. Marmoset cell line B95-8 (ECACC #85011419; *Proc. Natl Acad. Sci. USA* **70**, 190, 1973). This cell line secretes EBV into the culture supernatant.
3. Cyclosporin A (Sigma).
4. Sterile individually packed syringe filters 0.45 µM pore size (Sartorius AG, Gottingen, Germany).

2.3. Growth of Cell Lines

The materials for the growth of cell lines will vary slightly depending on the MHC expressing "presenting cells" employed. For example, murine fibroblasts transfected with human HLA molecules are generally adherent in culture and in order to propagate these cells it is necessary to remove them from the surface of the well or flask. This can be done with either EDTA or in more difficult cases with trypsin (or a mixture of the two). In contrast, EBV-transformed B cells and T-cell lines and clones grow in suspension.

1. Complete culture medium with FCS (*see* **Section 2.2.**).
2. Serological pipettes, polycarbonate tubes, pastettes, trypan blue (*see* **Section 2.2.**).
3. CO_2 incubator.
4. 24-well culture plates, 25 and 75-cm^2 tissue culture flasks (Nalgene Nunc International: through Life Technologies, Paisley, Scotland).
5. Di-sodium or tetra-sodium ethylene diamine tetra acetic acid (EDTA; BDH/Merck, Poole, UK) 0.02% solution in PBS (Life Technologies).
6. Trypsin solution for cell culture (Life Technologies).
7. Presenting cells must be prevented from proliferating and thus contributing to the readout of the assay. For transfected fibroblasts and other cells this can be achieved with the cytostatic agent mitomycin C which can be purchased from Sigma. However (*see* **Notes 4** and **5**), there are problems associated with the use of this agent in cell cultures and, when using EBV-LCL, it may be preferable to irradiate the cells prior to use. This can be achieved with a source of electromagnetic radiation such as a gamma source (commonly cesium or cobalt) or an X-ray tube. The latter are generally impractical to acquire merely for cell culture and the investigator would be advised to seek access to such a source either within their own institution or at another nearby. If a source of electromagnetic radiation is not available then mitomycin C may be used (*see* **Note 5**).

2.4. Proliferation Assays

1. Complete culture medium; RPMI-1640 L-glutamine free, bicarbonate buffered, supplemented with 2 mM L-glutamine, 100 U/mL penicillin, 100 µg/mL streptomycin, and 5% normal human AB serum (all Sigma).
2. Serological sterile, plastic pipettes (10 and 25 mL; Greiner Laboratories Ltd).
3. Repeater pipette (Eppendorf; through BDH, UK).
4. Repeater pipette tips (Ritips; Greiner).
5. 96-well flat-bottomed (*see* **Note 4**) culture plates (Nalgene Nunc International; through Life Technologies).
6. Antigen (protein/peptide) stock solution at a concentration of 1–10 mg/mL.
7. Tritiated [methyl-^{3}H]-thymidine, sterilized aqueous solution; 925 GBq/mmol (stock solution; Amersham International, Amersham, Bucks, UK). Diluted 1/20 in complete culture medium (working solution).
8. A 37°C cell culture incubator gassed with 5% CO_2 in air (for example, from manufacturers such as Gallenkamp and Leec).

9. Culture harvesting equipment (for example, Unifilter-96 harvester; Perkin Ellmer, Beaconsfield, Buckinghamshire, UK).
10. Liquid scintillation counter (for example, TopCount Microplate Scintillation Counter; Perkin Elmer).

3. Methods

3.1. Isolation of Peripheral Blood Mononuclear Cells

The method of choice for the isolation of peripheral blood mononuclear cell populations is density gradient centrifugation with products such as Histopaque (Sigma) and Ficoll-paque (Pharmacia). These solutions are largely carbohydrate-based and have a density of 1.077 g/L. This allows monocytes, lymphocytes, and basophils to remain at the blood/media interface whereas other blood cells pass through to form a pellet. A variable number of platelets may be retained at the interface along with the mononuclear cells and it is for this reason that heparinized medium is recommended for initial washing steps in order to avoid mononuclear cell clumping.

1. Whole peripheral blood is collected into either a heparinized syringe or into a tube containing heparin (final concentration of heparin should be 20 U/mL).
2. Using a wide-bore (i.e., 25-mL pipette), blood is slowly layered onto an equal quantity (*see* **Note 6**) of Histopaque (at room temperature) taking great care not to disturb the interface between the two liquids. Tilting the tube and passing blood slowly down the side of the tube is advisable.
3. Tubes are centrifuged at 700*g* (with the brake in the "off" position) for 20 min at room temperature.
4. Cells at the interface between the separation medium and plasma are collected using a 3-mL pastette. The interface cells form a thin white layer, which can be difficult to see. The pastette bulb should be emptied of air before passing into the solution in order not to disturb the integrity of the interface. Cells are collected into a tube together with a mixture of plasma and separation medium. Care should be taken (a) to ensure that all cells are collected and (b) that not too much of the separation medium is taken up. The latter, by virtue of its density, may make subsequent washing of the cells by centrifugation difficult.
5. Heparinized culture medium is added in at least equal volume to the cell suspension. Close the tube and invert several times to ensure adequate mixing. Centrifuge the suspension at 500*g* for 10 min with the brake "on".
6. Discard the supernatant, resuspend the cell pellet by briskly and firmly tapping the bottom of the tube. Refill the tube with heparinized medium and add plasma (*see* **Note 7**) to approximately 10% final concentration. Centrifuge the suspension at 300*g* for 10 min with the brake "on".
7. Resuspend the cell pellet as before. Bring the volume in the tube up to 10 mL with complete culture medium. Mix gently and remove 10 µL using a sterile pipette tip. Mix the 10 µL with 90 µL of Trypan Blue solution and load a Neubauer

(or similar) hemocytometer. Count cells and calculate both cell concentration in the solution and the total number of cells recovered.
8. If not used immediately, cell suspensions should be stored on ice prior to use in the proliferation assay.

3.2. Preparation of EBV Supernatants

1. Culture the marmoset cell line B95-8 in culture medium containing 10% FCS in 37°C CO_2 incubator. Use 25 or 75-cm^2 flasks as applicable to the volume required. Freeze stocks for future culture.
2. Collect culture supernatant when the medium is yellow using serological pipettes (i.e., the medium is spent). Centrifuge at 500*g* for 10 min at room temperature.
3. Filter the culture supernatant through a sterile 0.45-μM filter via a plastic syringe and freeze in 1 mL aliquots for future use. Store at −80°C.

3.3. Generation of EBV-Transformed B Cell/Lymphoid Lines (EBV-LCL)

1. Take 10 mL of PBMC (fresh or frozen) and wash twice with complete culture medium containing 10% FCS.
2. Resuspend the cell pellet and add 1 mL of EBV supernatant and mix thoroughly.
3. Place in a 37°C incubator for 1 h or more with frequent shaking. Ensure adequate gas exchange by having the tube lid slightly loose.
4. Add 9 mL of culture medium with 10% FCS and add cyclosporin A to a final concentration of 10 μg/mL.
5. Culture for 3 d prior to transfer to a 24-well plate (1–2 mL/well).
6. Feed each well by removing 50% of the medium and replacing it with the same volume of fresh culture medium with 10% FCS every 3–4 d.
7. When cells are confluent, transfer to a tissue culture flask. Split cells regularly and freeze stocks at the earliest opportunity (see other chapters).

3.4. Preparation of Presenting Cells

3.4.1. Fibroblast Cell Lines Transfected with Human MHC Genes

The generation of fibroblast cell lines (FCL; and transfection protocols) is beyond the scope of this chapter. The cell lines can be acquired from individual investigators or through cell line repositories as described earlier. The genes of interest, in this case HLA genes, are transfected in a plasmid expression vector which also contains a gene sequence conferring resistance to a chemical compound such as an antibiotic. Common examples would be resistance to Hygromycin or G418. In order to maintain high levels of expression of the gene of interest it is necessary to grow these cell lines constantly in the drug to which the presence of the plasmid vector confers resistance. In the absence of the drug, cells lose copies of the plasmid and the expression of the transfected gene wanes to levels which are below the threshold required for the assay to be performed.

FCL are generally adherent and should be grown in culture flasks and propagated with either EDTA and/or trypsin. These compounds work in different ways. EDTA chelates Mg^{2+} and Ca^{2+} ions, which are essential for cell adherence (an active process), whereas trypsin is a proteolytic enzyme, which cleaves the adhesion molecules that facilitate attachment to the extracellular matrix. Care must be taken with the concentration of trypsin used and the length of exposure because other molecules (notably the very MHC molecules on which the assay relies) may also be removed. In order to be sure that the conditions applied are appropriate for each individual cell line, regular checks on levels of expression of HLA molecules should be made by flow cytometry.

For removal of adherent cells with EDTA solution, all culture medium should be removed, and sufficient EDTA solution to cover the floor of the flask should be added. The flask should then be incubated at 37°C in the incubator. Subsequently, the cells may be recovered by pipeting the solution in the flask up and over the cells in a washing manner. This action will remove the cells from the surface of the flask, a process which can often be observed with the naked eye as the translucent appearance of the cell monolayer is replaced by clear plastic. Cells which adhere with greater tenacity may be removed by adding trypsin to the EDTA solution or by using trypsin alone. Serum contains potent inhibitors of trypsin and so all culture medium should be removed from the flask and the monolayer of cells rinsed with serum-free culture medium prior to the addition of the trypsin solution. Enough trypsin should be added to merely wet the surface of the cells and any excess material should be removed. Cells should be incubated at 37°C as previously described. Cells should be washed off the surface of the flask with complete culture medium which, by virtue of its serum content, will stop the proteolytic reaction.

Inhibition of proliferation of FCL is achieved with the cytostatic agent mitomycin C. The procedure is as follows:

1. Having removed adherent cells with either EDTA or trypsin, cells should be washed by centrifugation at 500*g* for 10 min in serum-free medium at room temperature. This procedure should be repeated once more.
2. Resuspend cells in a plastic 15-mL test tube (maximum 10^7 cells/mL) in 900 μL of serum-free medium.
3. Add 100 μL of mitomycin C (final concentration 50 μg/mL).
4. Incubate at 37°C for 45 min with gentle shaking every 15 min.
5. Wash at least three times in complete medium containing AB serum.
6. Keep cells on ice prior to use in proliferation assay. Cells should be used within the hour where possible.

3.4.2. EBV-Transformed Lymphoid Cell Lines

These cells express high levels of MHC molecules and do not require drugs to maintain these levels because they have not been transfected with the genes encoding HLA molecules. The cells grow very rapidly in suspension and, thus, do not require EDTA or trypsin for passage. In order to prevent proliferation of these transformed cells during the proliferation assay it is necessary to irradiate immediately prior to use. In the absence of a radioactive source, mitomycin C may be used as above but this compound has toxicity problems, which are described in **Section 4**. However, because these cells are transformed and grow vigorously in culture, they often require a high dose of radiation in order to prevent high background proliferation levels within the assay. This varies from line to line and should be determined empirically by irradiating samples of the cells for varying times and monitoring proliferation by the addition of tritiated thymidine to the culture for 24 h or so. The length of exposure required to achieve the required dose will vary depending on the source employed. Again this should be determined empirically. As a rough guide, PBMC require approximately 3000 rad to prevent proliferation. EBV-LCL may require twice this dose or more. In some cases the dose required is so high that the cells disintegrate very shortly after exposure and in such cases mitomycin C may be the preferred option.

Cells should be prepared in complete culture medium and placed in a suitable tube for the radiation source (usually a 15 or 30-mL plastic tube). The tube is exposed under the appropriate conditions and close attention is paid to the safety requirement associated with the use of the source. Cells should then be washed twice in complete culture medium and stored on ice prior to use in the proliferation assay. Again cells should be used within 1 h where possible.

3.4.3. Antigen Loading

In order to function as antigen-presenting cells, FCL or EBV-LCL must be exposed to antigen or antigenic peptide prior to the proliferation assay. FCL lack any substantial ability to take up and process whole antigen proteins and thus should be used exclusively with short peptide sequences (up to 25 amino acids, for example). These may be synthesized or made to order by a variety of commercial sources. EBV-LCL are capable of pinocytosing proteins in solution and processing these proteins to generate functional MHC–peptide complexes.

In both cases (FCL and EBV-LCL), sufficient time must be allowed for either the peptide to bind to the MHC molecules on the surface of the cell (FCL) or for the antigen to be taken up, processed, and presented on the cell surface. For most purposes this can be an overnight incubation although substantially shorter periods of time can be employed with the lower limit for efficient presentation being in the order of 2 h.

Following incubation with antigen/peptide, cells should be washed at least twice. This is important, particularly in the case of cells incubated with peptides, because excess free peptide can interact with T cells in the subsequent proliferation assay and in some cases induce a state of hyporesponsiveness in those cells. Following cell washing, procedures to prevent proliferation (mitomycin C or irradiation) can be undertaken.

3.5. Proliferation Assays

Proliferation assays should be meticulously planned prior to execution. Component solutions should be prepared at concentrations which take into account subsequent dilution by the addition of other reagents. For example, in the dose determination experiment described below, the assay includes two component solutions which are added to wells in equal volume (100 µL). As a result, the final concentration of each solution is halved. For this reason, particularly with more complex experiments, it is important to consider the number of solutions being included in the assay and their ultimate concentration therein. For an experiment with two solutions (such as cell suspension and antigen solution), each must be added to the well at twice the required final concentration. Similarly, if three or four components are required, quadruple strength solutions will be required. In my own experience, a three-component assay is best treated as four, with the fourth solution being culture medium. Such an approach will allow stock solutions to be prepared and stored at convenient concentrations. It is rare that an experiment will have more than four component parts but in such a case, solutions of higher concentration can be prepared in a similar fashion.

In addition to preparation of solutions, the layout of the experiment should be decided, recorded in the investigator's notebook, and finally, drawn onto the lid of the 96-well plate to be used for the assay. The number of wells employed for each culture condition should be decided bearing the earlier considerations in mind.

1. Adjust cell suspension to 2×10^6 mL and dispense 100 µL into the selected wells of the plate. The procedure can be carried out rapidly and with relative accuracy using a repeater pipet as listed in **Section 2**.
2. Incubate the plate for 48–72 h in the first instance or, for a time-course study, prepare several identical plates and incubate for differing periods such as 1, 2, 3, 4 d.
3. Between 8 and 16 h before the end of the prescribed culture period, add approximately 37 kBq (1 µCi) of tritiated thymidine per well (*see* **Note 8**).
4. Harvest the contents of each well onto a suitable surface following the manufacturer's instructions.
5. Count the incorporated radioactive label using a scintillation counter according to the manufacturer's instructions.
6. Determine the mean and standard deviation (or standard error) for each antigen concentration and plot these values on the *y*-axis against antigen concentration on the *x*-axis. An example of a typical dose–response curve is shown below.

Determination of the optimal cell concentration for use in the assay should also be carried out. We have found that high cell concentrations in an assay may favor cytokine production at the expense of the proliferative response. Plates should be prepared such that antigen-presenting cell numbers remain constant between plates whereas responder cell concentration varies from plate to plate. A suitable range of responder cell concentrations (per mL) would be 0.5×10^5, 1×10^5, 2×10^5, and finally 5×10^5.

3.5.1. Assay Example: Determination of the MHC Restriction of a Proliferative Response to a Peptide Using FCL

In this hypothetical example, it has been determined in cultures of PBMC, with a variety of peptides, that a particular peptide is able to elicit a proliferative response in certain individuals. After tissue typing of the subjects who are able to mount a proliferative response, it is observed that a number of these individuals share expression of the HLA-DRB1*0101 molecule and thus FCL expressing this molecule are chosen in order to assay the ability of this molecule to present the peptide to T cells. FCL are incubated overnight with 100 µg/mL of the peptide. Cells are then harvested, washed three times in serum-free medium, and incubated with mitomycin C as described earlier. After extensive washing, cells are resuspended in complete medium containing AB serum at a concentration of 10^6 per mL; 100 µL of cell suspension is added to the wells of a 96-well culture plate. To these wells are added 100 µL of responder T cells (from stock solutions between 10^5 cells/mL and 10^6 cells/mL). The responder cell population will usually be a T-cell clone or T-cell line, which is specific for the peptide or the whole protein from which the peptide is derived. Furthermore, the responder population will be derived from one of the individuals that, in this example, responded to the peptide and expressed the DRB1*0101 molecule. In any event, the responder population should be enriched in some way for cells of the appropriate specificity. Such T-cell populations will be generated prior to the MHC restriction experiments by methods described in other chapters of this book. Cells will be cultured for 48–72 h prior to the addition (for the final 8–16 h of the culture) of 37 kBq of tritiated methyl thymidine. Finally cultures are harvested onto glass fiber filters and incorporated label measure by liquid scintillation spectroscopy (for example, using the Perkin Elmer TopCount system). If the peptide-specific proliferative responses of the individuals tested are restricted by DRB1*0101, a proliferative response will be generated in the assay. Inclusion of the appropriate controls is of great importance. For example, an irrelevant peptide should be included with some of the FCL wells to assess the background interaction of the T cells and the FCL. Additionally, if possible, an established T-cell population with known restriction to a peptide in the context of DRB1*0101 should be used with the appropriate peptide in order to generate a positive control response to demonstrate that the FCL population are capable of presenting a peptide to T cells. This sort of control may not be easily available but the

Table 1
MHC Restriction Assay Plate Plan

	Wells 1–6	Wells 7–12
A	FCL with medium alone	FCL with test peptide
B	FCL with test peptide + T-cells	FCL with irrelevant peptide + T-cells
C	FCL with positive control peptide	FCL with positive control peptide + positive control T-cell line/clone*
D		
E		
F		
G		
H		

*An example of such a positive control T-cell clone and peptide in the context of DRB1*0101 would be a T-cell clone specific for the influenza haemagglutinin peptide HA 307–319 (*5*).

investigator should bear such controls in mind. A negative proliferative response in the assay in the absence of a positive control does not necessarily mean that the peptide response is not restricted by the MHC molecule in question (**Table 1**).

3.5.2. Example Assay: Determination of MHC Restriction Using EBV-LCL

As they are diploid human cells, EBV-LCL express the full complement of MHC molecules. Thus, both maternal and paternal alleles will be expressed for three Class I molecules and three (or more as described earlier) Class II molecules. This may mean that, for example, at the DR locus, a cell line expresses DR1 from one allele and DR3 from the other. Clearly this makes determination of precise restriction very difficult because even if an antibody to DR blocks the response to the peptide or protein in question, it is not possible to say whether the response was restricted by DR1 or DR3. These issues become further complicated when one considers the presence (albeit generally at lower cell surface density) of other DR molecules such as DRB3, B4, and B5. However, homozygous cell lines are available, for example, from the ECACC whose MHC expression has been defined and demonstrated to be homozygous at certain alleles. Thus, for example, a cell line which is homozygous for DRB1*0101 may be used to determine restriction specificity with greater accuracy although the potential confounding influence of other DR molecules such as DRB3 may require that the assay is performed with several different cell lines and a process of elimination employed to define the presenting molecule.

EBV-LCL are prepared as described earlier. Following incubation with antigen/peptide and irradiation they are plated into the wells of a 96-well plate at a concentration of 10^6 cells/mL (100 μL/well) in complete culture medium with AB serum. Responder cells are prepared as for FCL although in the case of

EBV-LCL a more crude source of T cells may be assayed (for example, T cells enriched from PBMC using nylon wool or T-cell enrichment columns; R&D Systems, Abingdon, UK). Following culture for 48–72 h, cultures are labeled and harvested as for FCL cultures. The requirement for adequate positive controls is as important here as with FCL although in the case of EBV-LCL, positive controls may be easier to obtain because these cells can process whole antigen and the same requirement for specific T-cell lines or clones does not hold for EBV-LCL as enriched PBMC T cells can be employed.

4. Notes

1. L-Glutamine is labile in solution. Sigma Chemical Company have conducted a study addressing the stability of glutamine solutions at various temperatures. Even at 4°C, after approx. 3 wk, only 60% remains. This figure falls to only 10% after storage for the same period at 35°C. See the Sigma catalog for more details.

2. Some investigators use mercaptoethanol (2-ME) at $5{\times}10^{-5}$ M to enhance proliferative responses in vitro *(6)*.

3. For experiments in which proliferative responses of human cells are being measured it is preferable to use human AB serum rather than FBS because background counts tend to be lower in AB serum. However, when cells are being grown in bulk culture prior to assay the use of FBS rather than AB serum provides a less expensive alternative. Furthermore, different batches of serum (AB and FBS) may vary considerably in their properties in cell culture. Some give high backgrounds in proliferation assays and occasionally may be cytotoxic. For these reasons, new batches of serum should be screened prior to purchase.

4. A variety of shapes are available for the 96-well format. The most common are flat-bottomed, U-bottomed, and V-bottomed. For proliferation assays, flat and U are the most useful, V-bottomed being used in cytotoxicity assays predominantly. The issue of which plate to use centers on cell density. T-cell activation requires the interaction of T cell with antigen-presenting cell and thus cells must be cultured in close proximity to one another. If a small number of cells are being used in each well, a U-bottomed plate will "concentrate" the cells in a relatively small area allowing interaction. Too many cells, however, may lead to overcrowding and subsequent restriction of gas and nutrient exchange for the cells at the bottom of the well. In higher cell density situations, therefore, it is advisable to use the flat-bottomed variety. A comparison of both within the same system can yield useful information when establishing an assay.

5. Mitomycin C has been known to leak out of cells during the culture period and inhibit the proliferation of responding cells. This is why it is important to wash the cells several times after incubation with the drug.

6. Manufacturers of density gradient separation media such as Histopaque and Ficoll-paque generally suggest that prior to layering, blood should be diluted 1:1 with culture medium and subsequently layered over equal volumes of separation medium. Whereas this does give the best yields, it is also expensive and in many cases (particularly where cell yield is not vitally important), it is not economically viable.

In our laboratory, PBMC are separated from whole blood without dilution. Separation is usually carried out in 50-mL tubes in which 20–25 mL of blood is layered onto 15 mL of separation medium. This is effectively 140% less media than is recommended per unit whole blood and provides a considerable saving.

7. When washing cells in heparinized medium, save some of the autologous plasma from the cell separation which may be added back to the cell suspension at approximately 10% to act as a protein source for the cells during washing. This means that relatively expensive AB serum or FCS is not required.

8. Alternative methods for determination of cell proliferation are available. Most recently, cell division-tracking dyes such as carboxyfluoroscein succinimidyl ester (CFSE; Invitrogen-Molecular Probes) have been applied to measure cellular proliferation. However, such technology requires access to flow cytometry facilities for analysis. Incorporation of the thymidine analogue 5-bromodeoxyuridine has been employed *(7)* and may be particularly useful when restrictions prevent the use of radioactive isotopes or where sophisticated liquid scintillation spectroscopy equipment is not available. More recently, vital techniques have been employed to quantify live cells following a period of stimulation in culture (for example, CytoLite, Packard Bioscience B.V., Groningen, Netherlands). It should be stressed, however, that this approach is not suitable for use on heterogeneous populations such as PBMC. The technique is effective with more homogenous cell sources such as T-cell clones or lines.

References

1. Tonegawa, S., Steinberg, C., Dube, S., and Bernardini, A.. (1974) Evidence for somatic generation of antibody diversity. *Proc. Natl Acad. Sci. USA* **71**, 4027–4031.
2. Bjorkman, P. J., Saper, M. A., Samraoui, B., Bennett, W. S., Strominger, J. L., and Wiley, D. C. (1987) The foreign antigen binding site and T cell recognition regions of class I histocompatibility antigens. *Nature* **329**, 512–518.
3. Zinkernagel, R. M. and Doherty, P. C. (1974) Restriction of in vitro T cell-mediated cytotoxicity in lymphocytic choriomeningitis within a syngeneic or semiallogeneic system. *Nature* **248**, 701–702.
4. Boniface, J. J., Rabinowitz, J. D., Wulfing, C., Hampl, J., Reich, Z., and Altman, J. D. (1998) Initiation of signal transduction through the T cell receptor requires the peptide multivalent engagement of MHC ligands. *Immunity* **4**, 459–466.
5. Lamb, J. R., Skidmore, B. J., Green, N., Chiller, J. M., and Feldmann, M. (1983) Induction of tolerance in influenza virus-immune T lymphocyte clones with synthetic peptides of influenza hemagglutinin. *J. Exp. Med.* **157**, 1434–1447.
6. Iwata, S., Hori, T., Sato, N., Ueda-Taniguchi, Y., Yamabe, T., and Nakamura, H. (1994) Thiol-mediated redox regulation of lymphocytes proliferation. *J. Immunol.* **152**, 5633–5642.
7. Pera, F., Mattias, P., and Detzer, K. (1977) Methods for determining the proliferation kinetics of cells by means of 5-bromodeoxyuridine. *Cell Tissue Kinet.* **10**, 255–264.

7

Short-Term Culture of CD8 Cells and Intracellular Cytokine Staining

Beejal Vyas and Alistair Noble

Abstract

CD8 T cells play an important role in the regulation of allergic disease. Human and murine CD8 T cells have been shown to be capable of differentiating into distinct subsets defined by cytokine profiles analogous to the Th1 and Th2 subsets and termed T cytotoxic 1 (Tc1, IFN-γ producing) and 2 (Tc2, IL-4 producing).

Effector cell phenotype can be analyzed in vitro on a single cell basis using intracellular cytokine staining and flow cytometry or analysis of other phenotypic markers. Human PBMC usually contain only very low percentages of effector cells which produce relatively high levels of cytokines required for this kind of analysis. It is therefore necessary to activate the T cells to induce rapid accumulation of cytoplasmic cytokines before analysis. This makes it difficult to analyze the antigen specificity of responding T cells but will indicate the type 1/type 2 bias of the population, reflecting previous exposures to antigen. In this chapter, we provide protocols for the generation of polarized populations of CD8 T effector cells using polyclonal stimulation and for their subsequent analysis by intracellular cytokine staining.

Key Words: Effector cells; intracellular cytokine staining; Tc1; Tc2; CD8 T cells.

1. Introduction

In general, the techniques and conditions required for both short-term CD8 T-cell culture and generation of CD8 T-cell clones are the same as those used for CD4 T cells, because both subsets are able to undergo rapid clonal expansion on engagement of the TcR in the presence of IL-2 or IL-4. However, there are some special considerations when using CD8 T cells. First, CD8 cells generally produce very low levels of IL-2 or IL-4 upon activation and so their continued growth is more dependent on provision of exogenous cytokine. Secondly, CD8 T cells produce cytotoxic mediators and are more susceptible

From: *Methods in Molecular Medicine: Allergy Methods and Protocols*
Edited by: M. G. Jones and P. Lympany © Humana Press Inc., Totowa, NJ

to activation-induced cell death than their CD4 counterparts and may therefore undergo high levels of apoptotic death after prolonged culture and/or restimulation. CD8 T cells recognize MHC class I-associated peptide antigens, so generation of antigen-specific CD8 cells is inefficient when using crude antigen preparations added to the culture. Use of specific peptides or transfection of antigen-presenting cells with the antigen or gene encoding it may be beneficial. An alternative strategy is the use of dendritic cells instead of PBMC as antigen-presenting cells in the culture, as they efficiently cross-present soluble antigens in the MHC class I pathway. Lastly, although CD8 cells respond well to mitogens such as PHA, anti-CD3 antibodies, or superantigens, their requirements for costimulatory signals may be different. It is thought that CD8 cells are less dependent on costimulation through CD28 and more so through LFA-1 (*[1]*; B.V., unpublished) or cytokine receptors (*2*). This is an important consideration when culturing purified CD8 cells in the absence of antigen-presenting cells. In these circumstances, a combination of anti-CD3 and anti-LFA-1 antibodies may prove the most effective primary stimulus, whereas IL-7 and IL-15 are most effective at preventing CD8 cell apoptosis.

1.1. CD8 T-Cell Subsets

Functional heterogeneity within the CD8 subset of T cells has long been recognized, and they have often been classified as cytotoxic or suppressor (immunoregulatory) T cells. However, in contrast to CD4 T cells, these functions have not been clearly associated with distinct cytokine profiles. More recently, CD8 T cells have been shown to be capable of differentiating into distinct subsets defined by cytokine profiles analogous to the Th1 and Th2 subsets and termed T cytotoxic 1 (Tc1) and 2 (Tc2) (*3–5*). Tc1 and Tc2 cells have been demonstrated in both rodents and humans and are defined according to IFN-γ (Tc1) and IL-4 (Tc2) production. Tc1 cells secrete very high levels of IFN-γ in comparison to Th1 cells and low levels of IL-2. Tc2 cells produce IL-4, IL-5, IL-6, IL-10, and IL-13, often at similar or greater levels than Th2 cells. Such a clear-cut analogy between the cytokine profiles of CD4 and CD8 subsets has been challenged by studies which demonstrated patterns of cytokine production in CD8 populations that did not fit the Th1/Th2 paradigm (*6–8*).

As their name suggests, Tc1 and Tc2 effector cells are capable of cytotoxicity at similar levels, although it has been shown that murine Tc1 cells use both Fas and perforin pathways for killing target cells, whereas Tc2s are restricted to perforin killing (*9*). "Suppressor" functions of CD8 T cells have been associated with IFN-γ, IL-4, IL-10, and TGF-β in various models and therefore cannot be ascribed to a single CD8 subset (*6,7,10,11*). This is not surprising because these regulatory CD8 cells can control immune reactivity associated with both Th1 inflammatory reactions and Th2-associated antibody-mediated immunopathology and are therefore likely to require different effector mechanisms. Further research is required to dissect the functional roles of Tc1 and Tc2 cells in different disease states.

The conditions under which Tc1 and Tc2 cells are generated during an immune response are also analogous to those for CD4 T cells. IL-12 and IL-4 are the major differentiation factors for Th1 and Th2 cells, although IFN-γ can replace IL-12 in human T-cell differentiation *(12)*. Murine Tc1 and Tc2 cells were initially generated using IL-12 + anti-IL-4 and IL-4 + anti-IL-12, respectively, as for CD4 cells. It has since been shown that murine Tc1 development is not dependent on IL-12 *(13)*; whether this is true in humans is unclear.

An important distinction between CD4 and CD8 T-cell differentiation lies in the distinct bias of CD8 cells toward the Tc1 pathway *(5)*. In CD4 cells, most TcR-dependent stimuli induce a mixture of Th1 and Th2 effectors initially, unless stringent polarizing conditions are employed. In the case of CD8 cells, most stimuli induce rapid development of Tc1 cells with few, if any, Tc2s. Induction of human Tc2 cells usually requires appropriate TcR-dependent signals, IL-4, and the presence of IL-12-neutralizing antibody and varies greatly between donors. This difficulty in generating Tc2 cells accounts for their relatively recent discovery and for their apparent rarity in vivo. It is also possible that current cloning procedures favor the generation of Tc1 clones.

1.2. CD8 Subsets and Allergic Disease

Although CD4 Th2 cells directed against environmental antigens are the major inducers of the allergic phenotype, it has long been recognized that CD8 T cells play an important role in the regulation of allergic disease. During antigen processing of allergens, certain peptide epitopes can be presented via MHC class I molecules to CD8 T cells *(14,15)*. These cells have the effect of suppressing the subsequent IgE response to the allergen, probably via skewing of the CD4 T-cell response toward a Th1 phenotype; such regulatory CD8 cells typically have a Tc1 cytokine profile *(16)*. The role of Tc2 cells in allergy is far less clear, but there is evidence for the presence of such cells in the asthmatic lung *(17)*, where they may be involved in disease pathogenesis *(18,19)*. Further studies of Tc1/Tc2 development are likely to reveal divergent roles for CD8 T cells in the immunoregulatory and inflammatory pathways of allergic disease.

1.3. Use of Intracellular Cytokine Staining to Characterize CD8 T Cells

Preferential outgrowth of different CD8 subsets during long-term culture procedures can be avoided by using short-term cultures to generate effector cells. The phenotype of such effector cells can be analyzed on a single cell basis using intracellular cytokine staining and flow cytometry or analysis of other phenotypic markers. Such analysis is likely to more closely reflect the patterns of cytokine production from effector cells generated in vivo. Human PBMC usually contain only very low percentages of effector cells which produce relatively high levels of cytokines required for this kind of analysis, because such cells are short-lived and rapidly recruited into tissues. It is therefore necessary to activate the T cells for several days in culture with antigen or mitogen to generate fresh effector cells in vitro, then restimulate them in the presence of a protein transport inhibitor to induce rapid accumulation of cytoplasmic cytokines before fixation and flow cytometric analysis. This approach makes it difficult to analyze the antigen specificity of responding T cells but will indicate the type 1/type 2 bias of the population, reflecting previous exposures to antigen. The technique cannot be conducted in vivo and hence requires cells to be removed from their immunological milieu. Moreover, this application is limited only to those tissues from which viable T cells can be isolated. Unlike previous methods which detected cytokine secretion into supernatants, this approach has the following advantages: (i) percentages of cytokine-secreting cells as well as levels of production per cell can be assessed simultaneously; (ii) coexpression of multiple cytokines can be detected, allowing analysis of subsets such as Th0/Tc0; (iii) reutilization of secreted cytokines from the medium is prevented; and (iv) only one monoclonal anti-cytokine antibody is required.

A recent development arising from intracellular cytokine staining techniques has been the cytokine secretion assay. This allows the purification of rare antigen-specific cells from PBMC, based on their cytokine secretion in response to antigen, and is particularly suitable for CD8 T cells because of their propensity for high-level IFN-γ production. This technique is described elsewhere *(20)*. In this chapter, we provide protocols for the generation of polarized populations of CD8 T effector cells using polyclonal stimulation and for their subsequent analysis by intracellular cytokine staining. The intracellular staining protocol is equally useful for the analysis of CD4 effector cells or T-cell clones.

2. Materials

1. Hanks balanced salt solution (HBSS), phosphate-buffered saline (PBS), RPMI-1640 medium, fetal calf serum (Invitrogen, Paisley, UK).
2. Whole blood buffy coat (N. Thames blood transfusion service, London, UK) or heparinized venous blood.
3. Lymphoprep (Robbins Scientific, W. Midlands, UK).
4. CD8 Dynabeads™, Detach-a-bead™ solution (Dynal Ltd, Wirral, UK).
5. Complete medium: RPMI-1640 + 10% human AB serum (Serotec, Oxford, UK) + 1% nonessential amino acids (Sigma, Poole, UK) + 1% sodium pyruvate (Sigma) + 50 µg/mL gentamycin (Sigma).
6. Anti-CD3 UCHT1, anti-IFN-γ-FITC (clone 25723.11), anti-IL-4-PE (clone 3010.211), anti-IL-2-PE (clone 5344.111) (BD Biosciences, Oxford, UK).
7. Anti-CD28 (Eurogenetics, Hampton, UK).

8. Recombinant human cytokines: IL-2, IL-4 (Serotec); IL-12 (R&D Systems, Cambridge, UK).
9. Anti-IL-4 (BD Biosciences), anti-IL-12 (R&D Systems).
10. 4% formaldehyde fixative: 30% stock solution (Sigma) diluted to 4% in 1.5× strength PBS (using 10× PBS), stored room temperature <6 wk.
11. 1% (w/v) paraformaldehyde solution: dissolved in PBS at 60°C + one drop concentrated NaOH.
12. PMA, ionomycin, brefeldin A (Sigma): dilute freshly from 10,000× concentrated stock solutions in absolute ethanol, stored at −20°C.
13. Permeabilizing buffer: PBS + 1% bovine serum albumin (BSA; Sigma) + 0.5% saponin (Sigma). If stored for any length of time, 0.1% sodium azide preservative should be added.

3. Methods

3.1. Generation of Tc1/Tc2-Polarized Populations of Human CD8 T Cells from Peripheral Blood

3.1.1. Protocol for Purification of CD8 T Cells from Peripheral Blood or Buffy Coats

1. Dilute whole buffy coat 1:4 with HBSS or if using peripheral blood dilute 1:2 with HBSS.
2. Isolate PBMC by Lymphoprep density gradient centrifugation at 800g for 20 min at 18°C. Wash cells with cold HBSS at 600g for 10 min at 4°C.
3. Determine viable cells by trypan blue exclusion, then wash twice with HBSS at 200g for 10 min at 4°C and resuspend at 1×10^7 per mL in PBS containing 2% fetal calf serum.
4. Calculate the volume of Dynabeads required using a 3:1 bead to target ratio, assuming CD8 target cells make up 25% of PBMC. Prior to use, wash Dynabeads™ as follows: transfer the desired amount of Dynabeads™ to an Eppendorf tube, place on a magnetic particle concentrator (MPC; Dynal Ltd) for 1 min, and aspirate the fluid. Resuspend the beads in 1 mL of washing buffer (PBS containing 2% FCS), reapply to the MPC for 30 s, and discard the wash buffer. This washing procedure should be repeated twice, each time ensuring that the tube remains firmly on the MPC.
5. Transfer the washed beads to the PBMC suspension and mix by rotation for 1 h at 4°C.
6. Collect the attached cells using the MPC and decant off the unbound cells. Resuspend the beads in wash buffer and return to the MPC for a further 1 min. Discard the wash and repeat the whole washing procedure a further four times. It is important to ensure that all air bubbles are carefully removed following each wash using a sterile pastette as these may contain contaminating cells.
7. In order to elute the bound CD8 T cells, resuspend pelleted cells/beads in wash buffer and add Detach-a-bead™ antibody (1/30) for 60 min at room temperature with mild agitation.

8. Place the tube on the MPC for 2 min and collect the released cells. Wash the attached cells with 1 mL of complete medium and reapply to the magnet for a further 30 s. Transfer the medium into a clean sterile tube and repeat this procedure twice. Pool the washes together.
9. To remove any residual Detach-a-bead™ solution, centrifuge the isolated T cells at 200g for 10 min and resuspend at 1×10^6 cells/mL in complete medium. Take 10^5–10^6 of these cells and stain for CD3, CD8, CD4, CD14, or CD19 using fluorochrome-labeled antibodies. Acquire samples by flow cytometry to determine the precise purity of the isolated populations.

3.1.2. Protocol for Generating Polarized Populations of Tc1 or Tc2 Effector Cells in Short-Term Cultures for Cytokine Analysis, Further Characterization, or Cloning

1. Coat a sterile 24-well tissue culture plate with purified anti-CD3 at a concentration of 5 μg/mL in PBS and anti-CD28 at a concentration of 2 μg/mL in PBS (0.25 mL/well) either overnight at 4°C or for 3 h at 37°C (*see* **Note 1**).
2. Wash the plate three times with PBS to remove any excess unbound antibody.
3. Plate out the cells at a density of 1×10^6 cells/mL (1 mL/well) and culture for 4 d. To generate Tc1 cells add recombinant IL-2 at a concentration of 20 U/mL, recombinant IL-12 at 200 U/mL, and anti-IL-4 (5 μg/mL). To generate Tc2 cells, add recombinant IL-2 (20 U/mL), recombinant IL-4 (100 U/mL), and anti-IL-12 (5 μg/mL) (*see* **Notes 2–4**).
4. Culture the cells in a humidified incubator at 37°C, 5% CO_2 for approximately 6 d.

3.2. Stimulation of CD8 Effector Cells and Intracellular Cytokine Analysis

The method for analyzing cytokine production by single cells was originally described by Jung et al. *(21)* who demonstrated the feasibility of using intracytoplasmic staining and flow cytometry to determine the frequency of cytokine-producing cells in a heterogeneous population (*see* **Note 5**). The basic protocol consists of in vitro stimulation of T cells in the presence of a protein transport inhibitor. This is followed by cell fixation, permeabilization, and then intracytoplasmic staining of accumulated cytokines.

3.2.1. Restimulation of Effector Cells to Induce High-Level Cytokine Production

1. Generate effector CD8 T cells under the appropriate conditions as previously described. Each sample should contain approximately 2×10^5–1×10^6 viable cells.
2. Gently resuspend the cells, transfer to 5-mL tubes, wash three times, and resuspend in 1 mL complete medium.
3. Restimulate cells by addition of either PMA (10 ng/mL) and ionomycin (400 ng/mL) to the medium or by coating the 24-well plates with anti-CD3 (5 μg/mL) and

anti-CD28 (2 µg/mL) as described previously (*see* **Note 6**). Include an unrestimulated control sample containing effector cells cultured in only the medium.
4. Culture the cells overnight. Add brefeldin A protein transport inhibitor to a final concentration of 5 µg/mL and culture for a further 6 h. Following incubation, transfer cells to 5-mL Falcon tubes and wash three times with PBS/0.5% BSA.

3.2.2. Staining of Restimulated Cells with Anti-cytokine Monoclonal Antibodies

1. Having stained for any necessary cell surface markers, proceed to fixing the cells. Pellet the cells by centrifugation and resuspend in 1 mL of 4% formaldehyde solution, vortex each tube immediately, and leave to stand at room temperature for 20 min in the dark.
2. Wash once in 2 mL PBS/0.5% BSA and centrifuge at $200g$ for 10 min at 4°C.
3. Permeabilize the cells by adding 2 mL of PBS containing 0.5% saponin and 1% BSA for 10 min at room temperature in the dark. Vortex periodically and centrifuge at $200g$ for 10 min at 4°C. The effects of saponin are reversible; therefore ensure its presence during each antibody incubation and washing step to maintain membrane permeability. Wash the cells once more in permeabilizing buffer, centrifuge at $200g$ for 10 min at 4°C, and resuspend pelleted cells (50–100 µL per tube).
4. Add 0.1–0.5 µg per tube of each fluorochrome-labeled anti-cytokine antibody: e.g., anti-IFN-γ-FITC + anti-IL-4-PE (*see* **Note 7**). Add the same quantity of isotype control antibodies to the control samples. It is advisable to titer each reagent for use. Leave cells to incubate for 30 min at room temperature in the dark.
5. Wash cells with 2 mL of PBS/0.5% saponin/1% BSA and centrifuge at $200g$ for 10 min at 4°C.
6. Resuspend cells in 1 mL PBS/0.1% BSA for direct flow cytometric analysis. If cells are not to be acquired immediately, resuspend in 1% paraformaldehyde in PBS and store at 4°C for up to 1 wk.
7. Acquire samples on a flow cytometer such as a FACScalibur (BD Biosciences) and analyze using the appropriate software.

3.3. Flow Cytometric Analysis and Expected Results

1. CD8 T-cell yields and purities: 50 mL of blood typically yields approximately 10^7 CD8 T cells. These should be >98% CD8+, >98% CD3+, <1% CD4+, 1% CD19+.
2. Cytokine staining results: typical staining profiles obtained from polarized CD8 populations are shown in **Fig. 1**. A gate should be set on the forward scatter vs side scatter plot to include only viable, nonapoptotic cells in the cytokine profile. Apoptotic cells often appear during culture and restimulation because of activation-induced cell death; they can be distinguished by their greater side scatter and reduced forward scatter compared to viable effectors (*see* **Note 8**). IFN-γ and IL-4 are used as the definitive Tc1 and Tc2 cytokines, respectively, but other cytokines can be analyzed simultaneously. Proportions of cytokine-positive cells are usually in the range of 10–50%, but vary greatly between donors. It should be noted that there is a large stochastic element to the acquisition of cytokine production in

Tc1   **Tc2**

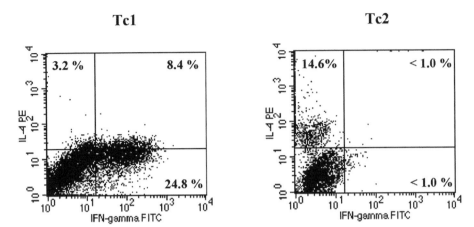

Fig. 1. Typical cytokine profiles of polarized Tc1 (left) and Tc2 (right) populations. Peripheral blood CD8 T cells from a single donor were polarized into Tc1 and Tc2 effectors as described and restimulated after 4 d with PMA + ionomycin in the presence of brefeldin A. Cells were stained with anti-IFN-γ-FITC and anti-IL-4-PE and analyzed on a FACScalibur™ flow cytometer using Cellquest software. Quadrant markers were set according to isotype control antibody-stained samples and unrestimulated controls, which had <1% positive staining.

effector T cells (*1,22,23*) and therefore 100% positive staining for any cytokine is rarely observed except in long-term T-cell clones. It is extremely important to perform sufficient negative controls, such as effector cells which are not restimulated but are stained with anti-cytokine antibodies, and restimulated cells stained with isotype-matched control antibodies. Single color controls are also advisable to ensure correct compensation settings (*see* **Note 9**).

4. Notes

1. The choice of primary stimulus for inducing CD8 T-cell growth can obviously be altered to address specific questions. Use of certain mitogens such as PHA and superantigens requires the presence of accessory cells in the culture in addition to CD8 cells. A convenient source of accessory cells is the CD8-depleted PBMC fraction which should be irradiated at 4000 rad before addition to culture.
2. Generation of Tc2 effectors is sometimes problematic and varies greatly between donors. We have observed that addition of steroids to the cultures, or use of PMA + ionomycin as a primary stimulus, can greatly enhance development of Tc2 cells. Extending the initial culture period (7–10 d) may also favor Tc2 generation, because this subset is less prone to activation-induced cell death.
3. Generation of allergen-specific CD8 cells is highly problematic resulting from low precursor frequencies and donor-to-donor variation. In this case, the concentration of purified CD8 cells should be increased and the culture supplemented with

autologous, irradiated PBMC as a source of antigen-presenting cells. Introduction of the protein allergens into the cytoplasm of antigen-presenting cells using transfection reagents or electroporation before addition of T cells will enhance MHC class I presentation and thus amplify the proliferative response. Longer culture periods will be required to allow sufficient expansion of antigen-specific cells.

4. If accessory cells are present in the primary culture, it may be necessary to stain effector cells for CD8 and/or CD3 in addition to intracellular cytokines. Because all components of the TCR complex are rapidly downregulated after effector cell activation, the cells should be labeled with fluorochrome-labeled CD8 or CD3 antibody at the end of the *primary* culture, then washed, and restimulated. The fluorochrome will then remain detectable after receptor downregulation.

5. A disadvantage of this technique is that it is only semiquantitative in terms of the titers of cytokines produced per cell, because fluorescence intensities of individual cells are detected. Another limitation is that not all cells may produce a given cytokine synchronously and therefore the timing between stimulation and fixation is important. It would therefore be beneficial to determine the kinetics of synthesis and secretion of a given cytokine. It should also be remembered that although the presence of a cytokine may be detected within cells this does not necessarily mean that it will be secreted.

6. The secondary restimulation of effector cells prior to intracellular staining can be performed using immobilized anti-CD3 and anti-CD28 antibodies. However, the choice of secondary stimulus can affect the cytokine staining profile.

7. If suitable fluorochrome-labeled antibodies are unavailable for a cytokine of interest, biotin-labeled antibodies can be substituted. The cells should then be washed in permeabilizing buffer and stained with fluorochrome-labeled streptavidin before analysis. However, not all monoclonal antibodies are effective for intracellular staining because certain epitopes are destroyed by fixation.

8. Populations of cells grouped along the x–y axis of FL1 vs FL2 plots after compensation are indicative of nonspecific binding by dead or apoptotic cells, rather than genuine cytokine-positive cells. They should be eliminated by adjusting the gate in the forward scatter vs side scatter window.

9. The choice of fluorochromes depends on the setup of the flow cytometer to be used. For a single 488-nm laser FACScalibur™, use FITC or Alexa Fluor™ 488 (FL1 channel), PE (FL2 channel), and PerCP or PE-Cy7 (FL3). For a dual laser FACScalibur™ with an additional 635-nm laser, APC or Alexa Fluor™ 647 (FL4 channel) can be added to give simultaneous detection of four cytokines or markers.

References

1. Kelso, A. and Groves, P. (1997) A single peripheral CD8[+] T cell can give rise to progeny expressing type 1 and/or type 2 cytokine genes and can retain its multipotentiality through many cell divisions. *Proc. Natl Acad. Sci. USA* **94**, 8070–8075.
2. Sepulveda, H., Cerwenka, A., Morgan, T., and Dutton, R. W. (1999) CD28, IL-2-independent costimulatory pathways for CD8 T lymphocyte activation. *J. Immunol.* **163**, 1133–1142.

3. Croft, M., Carter, L., Swain, S. L., and Dutton, R. W. (1994) Generation of polarized antigen-specific CD8 effector populations, reciprocal action of interleukin IL-4 and IL-12 in promoting type 2 versus type 1 cytokine profiles. *J. Exp. Med.* **180,** 1715–1728.

4. Sad, S., Marcotte, R., and Mosmann, T. R. (1995) Cytokine-induced differentiation of precursor mouse CD8+ T cells into cytotoxic CD8+ T cells secreting Th1 or Th2 cytokines. *Immunity* **2,** 271–279.

5. Vukmanovic-Stejic, M., Vyas, B., Gorak-Stolinska, P., Noble, A., and Kemeny, D. M. (2000) Human Tc1 and Tc2/Tc0 CD8 T-cell clones display distinct cell surface and functional phenotypes. *Blood* **95,** 231–240.

6. Salgame, P., Convit, J., and Bloom, B. R. (1991) Immunological suppression by human CD8+ T cells is receptor dependent and HLA-DQ restricted. *Proc. Natl Acad. Sci. USA* **88,** 2598–2602.

7. Inoue, T., Asano, Y., Matsuoka, S., Furutani-Seiki, M., Aizawa, S., and Nishimura, H. (1993) Distinction of mouse CD8+ suppressor effector T cell clones from cytotoxic T cell clones by cytokine production and CD45 isoforms. *J. Immunol.* **150,** 2121–2128.

8. Noble, A., Macary, P. A., and Kemeny, D. M. (1995) IFN-γ and IL-4 regulate the growth and differentiation of CD8+ T cells into subpopulations with distinct cytokine profiles. *J. Immunol.* **155,** 2928–2937.

9. Carter, L. L. and Dutton, R. W. (1995) Relative perforin- and Fas-mediated lysis in T1 and T2 CD8 effector populations. *J. Immunol.* **155,** 1028–1031.

10. Noble, A., Zhao, Z., and Cantor, H. (1998) Suppression of immune responses by CD8 cells, 2. Qa-1 on activated B cells stimulates CD8 cell suppression of T helper 2 responses. *J. Immunol.* **160,** 566–571.

11. Chen, Y., Inobe, J., and Weiner, H. L. (1995) Induction of oral tolerance to myelin basic protein in CD8-depleted mice, both CD4+ and CD8+ cells mediate active suppression. *J. Immunol.* **155,** 910–916.

12. Farrar, J. D., Smith, J. D., Murphy, T. L., and Murphy, K. M. (2000) Recruitment of Stat4 to the human interferon-alpha/beta receptor requires activated Stat2. *J. Biol. Chem.* **275,** 2693–2697.

13. Carter, L. L. and Murphy, L. M. (1999) Lineage-specific requirement for signal transducer and activator of transcription Stat4 in interferon-γ production from CD4+ versus CD8+ T cells. *J. Exp. Med.* **189,** 1355–1360.

14. Rock, K. L., Gamble, S., and Rothstein, L. (1990) Presentation of exogenous antigen with class I major histocompatibility complex molecules. *Science* **249,** 918–921.

15. McMenamin, C. and Holt, P. G. (1993) The natural immune response to inhaled soluble protein antigens involves major histocompatibility complex (MHC) class I-restricted CD8+ T cell-mediated but MHC class II-restricted CD4+ T cell-dependent immune deviation resulting in selective suppression of immunoglobulin E production. *J. Exp. Med.* **178,** 889–899.

16. MacAry, P. A., Holmes, B. J., and Kemeny, D. M. (1998) Ovalbumin-specific, MHC class I-restricted, alpha beta-positive, Tc1 and Tc0 CD8+ T cell clones mediate the in vivo inhibition of rat IgE. *J. Immunol.* **160,** 580–588.

17. Ying, S., Humbert, M., Barkans, J., Corrigan, C. J., Pfister, R., and Menz, G. (1997) Expression of IL-4 and IL-5 mRNA and protein product by CD4+ and CD8+ T cells, eosinophils, and mast cells in bronchial biopsies obtained from atopic and nonatopic (intrinsic) asthmatics. *J. Immunol.* **158,** 3539–3544.

18. Stanciu, L. A., Shute, J., Promwong, C., Holgate, S. T., and Djukanovic, R. (1997) Increased levels of IL-4 in CD8$^+$ T cells in atopic asthma. *J. Allergy Clin. Immunol.* **100,** 373–378.

19. Sawicka, E., Noble, A., Walker, C., and Kemeny, D. M. (2004) Tc2 cells respond to soluble antigen in the respiratory tract and induce lung eosinophilia and bronchial hyperresponsiveness. *Eur. J. Immunol.* **34,** 2599–2608.

20. Brosterhus, H., Brings, S., Leyendeckers, H., Manz, R. A., Miltenyi, S., and Radbruch, A. (1999) Enrichment and detection of live antigen-specific CD4$^+$ and CD8$^+$ T cells based on cytokine secretion. *Eur. J. Immunol.* **29,** 4053–4059.

21. Jung, T., Schauer, U., Heusser, C., Neumann, C., and Rieger, C. (1993) Detection of intracellular cytokines by flow cytometry. *J. Immunol. Methods* **159,** 197–207.

22. Bucy, R. P., Karr, L., Huang, G. Q., Li, J., Carter, D., and Honjo, K. (1995) Single cell analysis of cytokine gene coexpression during CD4$^+$ T-cell phenotype development. *Proc. Natl Acad. Sci. USA* **92,** 7565–7569.

23. Kelso, A., Groves, P., Troutt, A. B., and Francis, K. (1995) Evidence for the stochastic acquisition of cytokine profile by CD4$^+$ T cells activated in a T helper type 2-like response in vivo. *Eur. J. Immunol.* **25,** 1168–1175.

8

Isolation, Flow Cytometric Analysis, and Suppression Assay of CD4+CD25+ T-Regulatory Cells

Hayley Jeal

Abstract

Allergy and asthma are characterized by airway hyperresponsiveness and chronic mucosal inflammation mediated by CD4+ Th2 lymphocytes and their cytokines. It is unclear why allergic individuals make a Th2-type T-cell response whereas other (nonallergic) individuals do not. Recently, attention has focused on regulatory mechanisms, such as T-regulatory cells, preventing IgE responses to allergens in nonatopic individuals. Regulatory CD4+CD25+ T cells have been described in both mice and humans. The suppressive phenotype of these cells has been associated with the expression of the forkhead transcription factor, Foxp3. It has been suggested that allergic disease may arise from an inappropriate balance between allergen activation of regulatory CD4+CD25+ T cells and effector Th2 cells or from the impairment in the suppressive activity of these so-called T-regulatory cells.

The isolation of these T-regulatory cells is described in order to further our understanding of the role of these cells in allergic disease and asthma and allow us to design novel therapies.

Key Words: T-regulatory cells; tolerance; T-cell proliferation.

1. Introduction

Allergy and asthma are characterized by airway hyperresponsiveness and chronic mucosal inflammation mediated by CD4+ Th2 lymphocytes and their cytokines. It is unclear why allergic individuals make a Th2-type T-cell response whereas other (nonallergic) individuals do not. For many years, an imbalance between Th2 and Th1 cytokines has been considered to be the basis for allergic disease; however, more recently, attention has focused on regulatory mechanisms, such as T-regulatory cells, preventing IgE responses to allergens in nonatopic individuals.

From: *Methods in Molecular Medicine: Allergy Methods and Protocols*
Edited by: M. G. Jones and P. Lympany © Humana Press Inc., Totowa, NJ

Regulatory CD4+CD25+ T cells were first characterized in mice, and the transfer of these cells has been shown to reduce the pathology of experimentally induced diseases such as thyroiditis, gastritis, and colitis (1) whereas their depletion results in the development of systemic autoimmune disease (2). A similar population of cells has since been described in human beings (3–5). The suppressive phenotype of these cells has been associated with the expression of the forkhead transcription factor, Foxp3. The CD4+CD25+ T-regulatory cell population constitutes approximately 10% of the CD4+ T-cell population.

It has been suggested that allergic disease may arise from an inappropriate balance between allergen activation of regulatory CD4+CD25+ T cells and effector Th2 cells or from the impairment in the suppressive activity of these so-called T-regulatory cells (6). In a murine model of asthma, a diminished presence of CD25+ T-regulatory cells resulted in increased airway hyper-reactivity (7). Other studies have failed to find differences in the number or functionality of these cells between atopic and nonatopic individuals. An upregulation of CD4+CD25+ T-regulatory cells has been observed in individuals following specific allergen immunotherapy (8–10).

Understanding the exact role of these cells in allergic disease and asthma will allow us to design novel therapies that are capable of targeting the direct T-regulatory cell pathway and thus leading to useful prevention and treatment of allergic disease.

2. Materials

2.1. Isolation of Peripheral Blood Mononuclear Cells

1. Dulbecco's phosphate-buffered saline (Sigma, Poole, Dorset, UK).
2. Ficoll Paque (GE Healthcare Ltd, Bucks, UK).
3. Culture medium (RPMI-1640-L-glutamine) (Sigma).
4. Sterile, individually wrapped 3-mL pastettes (VWR international, Leicestershire, UK).
5. Serological sterile, plastic pipets: 10 and 25 mL (Sarstedt, Leicester, UK).
6. 50-mL sterile centrifuge plastic tubes (Starlab Ltd, Milton Keynes, UK).
7. Trypan blue (0.4% in saline) (Sigma).
8. Nebauer hemocytometer (e.g., from Jencons, Leighton Buzzard, UK).
9. Microscope (Jencons).

2.2. Isolation of CD4+CD25+ Regulatory T Cells Using Magnetic Cell Sorting – MACS®

1. CD4+CD25+ regulatory T-cell isolation kit (Miltenyi Biotec, Surrey, UK, MACS® 130-091-301) which contains:
   1 mL CD4+ T-cell biotin-antibody cocktail, human
   2 mL Anti-Biotin MicroBeads
   1 mL CD25 MicroBeads

2. Separation buffer (degassed): 100 mL Dulbecco's PBS (Sigma) containing 0.5% BSA and 2 mM EDTA (note: EDTA can be replaced by other supplements such as anti-coagulant citrate dextrose formula-A (ACD-A) or citrate phosphate dextrose (CPD). BSA can be replaced by other proteins such as gelatine, HSA, or fetal calf serum).
3. MACS magnets (MidiMACS™ and MiniMACS™ separation unit) and MACS columns (LD and MS).
4. Ice box.

2.3. Extracellular Flow Cytometry Staining

1. Flow cytometry tubes (BD Biosciences).
2. PBS-BSA-azide: 100 mL Dulbecco's PBS (Sigma) containing 0.1% BSA and 0.09% sodium azide.
3. Labeled antibodies and isotype controls to CD4 and CD25 (Dako UK Ltd, Cambridgeshire, UK).
4. Flow cytometer (Becton Dickinson, Cowley, Oxford, UK).

2.4. Proliferation Assay

1. Complete culture medium; RPMI supplemented with 2 mM L-glutamine, 100 U/mL penicillin, and 100 µg/mL streptomycin (all Life Technologies, Paisley, UK) and 5% vol/vol human AB serum (Sigma).
2. Sterile repeater pipet (Jencons).
3. 96-well flat bottomed culture plates (Nunc, Fisher Scientific, Loughborough, UK).
4. Antigen solution.
5. Phytohemagglutinin (PHA) positive control (Life Technologies, Gibco, Paisley, UK).
6. Tritiated [methyl-3H]-thymidine (Amersham Pharmacia Biotech, Little Chalfont, UK), diluted 1:20 in RPMI culture medium.
7. 37°C humidified 5% CO_2 cell culture incubator (e.g., from manufacturers such as RS Biotech Laboratory Equipment Ltd, Scotland, UK).
8. Cell culture harvester (e.g., Unifilter-96, Canberra Packard, Pangbourne, Berks, UK).
9. Liquid scintillation counter (e.g., TopCount Microplate Scintillation Counter, Canberra Packard).
10. Laminar flow hood (e.g., Jencons).
11. CO_2 incubator (e.g., Jencons).

2.5. Cytokine Analysis

1. Th1/Th2 human CBA kit (BD Bioscience, Pharmingen, Oxford, UK).
2. 5-mL flow cytometry tubes (BD Biosciences, Oxford, UK).
3. Flow cytometer (e.g., BD Biosciences).

3. Methods
3.1. Isolation of PBMCs

The isolation of peripheral blood mononuclear cells (PBMCs) is an important preanalytical step for many downstream laboratory procedures such as in vitro culture assays or flow cytometry. Typically, the isolation of PBMCs is carried out using density gradient centrifugation, which takes advantage of the different sizes of the cell types and their differential migration through solutions, such as Ficoll, following centrifugation. Different layers form as a result and erythrocytes and granulocytes sediment at the bottom of the tube whereas lymphocytes, mono-cytes, and platelets are not dense enough to penetrate into the separation solution and thus form a concentrated band at the interface between the original blood sample and the Ficoll. This enables these cells to be easily recovered in a small volume. It is important for this step to be carried out efficiently so that good yields of PBMCs are obtained.

1. Peripheral whole blood (150 mL) is collected in either heparinized vacutainers or syringes coated with heparin (0.5 mL – 500 units).
2. Blood is diluted 1:2 with Dulbecco's PBS.
3. 20 mL of Ficoll Paque (at room temperature) is poured into 50-mL tubes (Falcon).
4. Using a 25-mL pipet, the tube is tilted and blood (25 mL) is carefully trickled down the side and layered onto the Ficoll Paque.
5. Tubes are centrifuged at room temperature at $300g$ for 20 min (with the brake off).
6. Using a 3-mL pastette, cells at the interface, which form a thin white layer, are collected and placed into a fresh tube. Ensure that all cells are collected without taking up too much separation medium.
7. PBS is added to wash the cells, which are then centrifuged at 4°C at $300g$ for 10 min (with the brake off).
8. The supernatant is discarded by careful pipeting and the cells are resuspended by firmly tapping the base of the tube.
9. Add 40 mL of RPMI medium to the cells, mix well, and then remove 20 µL, and add to 20 µL of Trypan Blue. Store the cells on ice while counting cells.
10. Load the cells/Trypan Blue mix into a Nebauer hemocytometer, then count the cells, and calculate the number of cells per milliliter and the total cells in solution (*see* **Note 1**).
11. Once the cell count is completed, remove 2×10^6 cells for the proliferation assay (e.g., 2 divided by cells per milliliter to give volume for removal), 1×10^6 for staining and 9×10^6 for irradiation. Cells should be made up with complete medium and then stored on ice until needed. Autologous mononuclear cells should be made up to 2×10^6 cells/mL before being irradiated. These cells are used as antigen-presenting cells.

3.2. CD4+ Cell Separation Using MACS® – Negative Selection

The isolation of CD4+CD25+ cells is performed in a two-step procedure using a MACS® CD4+CD25+ Treg isolation kit. First, a depletion step takes place whereby non-CD4+ cells are labeled using a cocktail of biotin-conjugated antibodies and then subsequently with Anti-Biotin MicroBeads (*see* **Fig. 1**). The cells are depleted by separation over a MACS® column and the flow-through

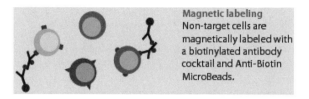

Magnetic labeling
Non-target cells are magnetically labeled with a biotinylated antibody cocktail and Anti-Biotin MicroBeads.

Fig. 1. Magnetic labeling of non-CD4+ cells.

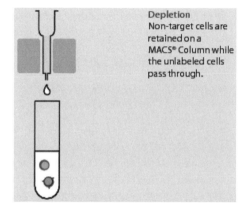

Depletion
Non-target cells are retained on a MACS® Column while the unlabeled cells pass through.

Fig. 2. Depletion of non-CD4+ cells.

fraction contains the enriched CD4+ cells (*see* **Fig. 2**). It is important during the next couple of steps to work quickly, keep the cells cold, and use precooled solutions. This will prevent cell loss, the capping of antibodies on the cell surface, and nonspecific labeling.

Volumes for magnetic labeling are for up to 10^7 cells; scale up accordingly for higher cell numbers, and for lower cell volumes use the same volumes as stated.

1. After the removal of PBMCs for the proliferation assay, staining, and irradiation, the cells are washed by adding RPMI and then centrifuged at 300*g* for 10 min at 4°C.
2. The supernatant is removed completely by careful pipeting and the cells are resuspended by firmly tapping the base of the tube.
3. 90 µL of separation buffer is added per 10^7 cells. (It is necessary to ensure the cell suspension is well mixed to prevent the clumping of cells, which may clog the column.)
4. Add 10 µL of CD4+ T-cell biotin-antibody cocktail per 10^7 cells and incubate for 10 min at 4–8°C.
5. 20 µL of Anti-Biotin Microbeads are added per 10^7 cells. The cells are mixed well and incubated for an additional 15 min at 4–8°C (*see* **Note 2**).

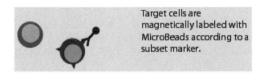

Fig. 3. Magnetic labelling of CD4+CD25+ regulatory T-cells.

6. The cells are washed by adding 1–2 mL of separation buffer and centrifuged at 300g for 10 min at 4°C. Remove the supernatant carefully using a 3-mL pastette.
7. Resuspend up to 10^8 cells in 500 µL of buffer (for larger volumes, scale up accordingly).
8. Proceed to magnetic separation (*see* **Section 3.2.1.**).

3.2.1. Depletion of Non-CD4+ Cells with a MACS® LD Column

1. An LD column is placed into a MidiMACS Separator, 2 mL of separation buffer is run through the column, and the effluent is discarded.
2. The cell suspension is added to the column and the unlabeled cells which pass through the column are collected (these are the CD4-rich, negatively selected cells).
3. The column is washed with 2 × 1 mL of separation buffer and the buffer is added successively as soon as the column reservoir is empty.
4. The CD4+ flow-through fraction is made up to 14 mL with separation buffer and a cell count is carried out.
5. 2 × 10^6 cells are removed for the cell proliferation assay and 0.5×10^6 cells are removed for staining on a flow cytometer and kept on ice until needed.
6. Proceed to the positive selection of CD4+CD25+ cells.

3.2.2. CD25 Cell Separation Using MACS® – Positive Selection

In the second step of this T-cell separation, CD4+CD25+ T cells are directly labeled with magnetic beads specific for the CD25 low-affinity IL-2 receptor (*see* **Fig. 3**). They are isolated by positive selection from the pre-enriched CD4+ T cells (*see* **Fig. 4**).

Volumes given are for an initial cell number of 10^7. For larger initial cell numbers, scale up accordingly.

1. The CD4+ cells are centrifuged at 300g for 10 min at 4°C (with the brake off).
2. The supernatant is removed and discarded using a 3-mL pastette.
3. The cell pellet is resuspended in 90 µL (per 10^7 cells) of separation buffer.
4. Add 10 µL (per 10^7 cells) of CD25 MicroBeads to the cells, mix well, and incubate for 15 min at 4–8°C (*see* **Note 2**).
5. The cells are washed with 10–20 times labeling volume of separation buffer and centrifuged at 300g for 10 min at 4°C (with the brake off). The supernatant is discarded as before.

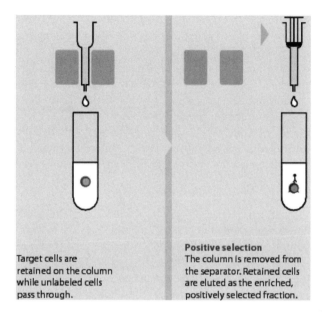

Target cells are retained on the column while unlabeled cells pass through.

Positive selection The column is removed from the separator. Retained cells are eluted as the enriched, positively selected fraction.

Fig. 4. Magnetic separation: Positive selection of CD4+CD25+ regulatory T cells.

6. Resuspend up to 10^8 cells in 500 µL of separation buffer.
7. Proceed to the positive magnetic selection stage (*see* **Section 3.2.3.**).

3.2.3. Positive Selection of CD25+ Cells Using a MACS® MS Column

1. Place the MS column in a MiniMACS Separator.
2. The column is rinsed with 500 µL of separation buffer and the effluent is discarded.
3. Just before the buffer has finished running through the column reservoir, add the cell suspension.
4. Collect the unlabeled cells, which flow through the column (these are the CD25– cells).
5. Wash the column with 3×500 µL of separation buffer. Perform the washing step by adding the next wash just as the column reservoir is empty.
6. After completing the last washing step, remove the tube labeled CD25– and add 10 mL of separation buffer and centrifuge for 10 min at 300*g* at 4°C (with the brake off).
7. Meanwhile, the column is removed from the magnet and placed over a tube labeled CD25+ cells.
8. Pipet 1 mL of buffer onto the column and plunge the buffer through the column (thereby removing the CD25+ cells) by firmly applying the plunger supplied with the column.
9. A cell count of the CD25+ cells is carried out. 2×10^6 cells/mL are needed for the cell proliferation assay and 0.2×10^6 cells/mL for staining. If a large volume of

cells are recovered at the positive selection stage a second column run can be carried out where the eluted cells from the first column can be run down a second MS column. This will increase the purity of the CD4+CD25+ cells.

10. The second MS column is prepared in the same way by rinsing with 500 μL of buffer and the eluted CD25+ cells are run down the column and a further 3×500 μL washes are performed. The flow-through fraction is discarded and the CD25+ cells are flushed through in the same way as before.

11. A cell count is carried out and 0.2×10^6 cells are removed for staining. The CD25+ cells are centrifuged at $300g$ for 10 min at 4°C and resuspended in the appropriate volume of complete medium to give 2×10^6 cells/mL.

3.2.4. Increasing the Purity of the CD25– Cells

1. Following centrifugation the supernatant is discarded using a pastette and the CD25– cells are resuspended in 500 μL of buffer.

2. An LD column is placed in a MidiMACS Separator and rinsed with 2×1 mL of separation buffer.

3. The CD25– cells are run down the column and 2×1 mL washes are performed.

4. The flow-through fraction is collected (this contains the pre-enriched CD25– cells).

5. Make the volume of cells up to 14 mL with separation buffer and carry out a cell count.

6. Remove 0.5×10^6 cells/mL for staining, then centrifuge the cells at $300g$ for 10 min at 4°C (with the brake off), and resuspend the CD25– cell pellet in the appropriate volume of complete medium to give 2×10^6 cells/mL.

7. Proceed to the cell proliferation assay (*see* **Section 3.3.**).

3.3. Proliferation Assay

Several factors should be considered before T-cell proliferation assays are carried out. First, it is necessary to determine the optimal antigen concentration and length of incubation by carrying out a number of experiments using a variety of antigen concentrations and time intervals. The antigen dose and incubation time that gives the highest proliferation can be considered optimal conditions for proliferation.

Positive and negative controls should be incorporated into the assay. PHA, a mitogen, is a good positive control as it induces blastogenesis in vitro. Cells incubated with the medium alone serve as a good negative control.

In order to compare the suppressive activity of CD4+CD25+ T cells on allergen-stimulated T-cell proliferation and cytokine production in vitro it is necessary to set up a coculture assay whereby both regulatory T cells and effector T cells (CD4+CD25– cells) are incubated together in vitro with the allergen of choice. Suppression of proliferation can be determined by comparing proliferation in the coculture system to that of the effector cells alone.

Table 1
Plate Layout for Suppression Assay

	1	2	3	4	5	6	7	8	9	10	11	12
A	PBMCs 2×10^6 cells/mL						Medium only			Rat antigen		
B	CD4+ cells only 2×10^6 cells/mL						Medium only			Rat antigen		
C	CD25- cells only 2×10^6 cells/mL						Medium only			Rat antigen		
D	CD25+ cells only 2×10^6 cells/mL						Medium only			Rat antigen		
E	CD25- cells 2×10^6 cells/mL CD25+ cells 1×10^6 cells/mL						Medium only			Rat antigen		
F	CD25- cells only 3×10^6 cells/mL						Medium only			Rat antigen		
G	Irradiated cells only 2×10^6 cells/mL						Medium only			Rat antigen		
H	PBMCs PHA			CD4+ PHA			CD25- PHA					

Planning the layout of the experiment is an important stage; *see* **Table 1** for an example plate set up to examine the effect of regulatory T cells on proliferation to rat allergen.

Proliferation assay:

1. The previously identified optimal concentration of antigen is added to the appropriate wells.
2. 20 µL of PHA (diluted 1:100 with RPMI medium) is added to the appropriate wells.
3. All cells are incubated with medium and antigen in triplicate.
4. 100 µL of each cell type is added to the appropriate wells (*see* **Note 3**). 100 µL of complete medium is added to the wells containing the PBMCs.
5. 100 µL of autologous irradiated mononuclear cells are added to wells containing all other cells.
6. For the coculture, 100 µL of CD25+ cells at 1×10^6 cells/mL and 100 µL of CD25– cells at 2×10^6 cells/mL are added to the same wells and then 100 µl of irradiated mononuclear cells (total volume in well = 300 µL).
7. For the CD25– cells at 3×10^6 cells/mL, add 150 µL of cells, 100 µL of irradiated cells, and 50 µL of complete medium (total volume in well = 300 µL).
8. For the irradiated cells only, add 100 µL of irradiated cells and 100 µL of complete medium.
9. Incubate the plate for the number of days shown to be optimal for proliferation, e.g., 7 d at 37°C in an incubator with 5% CO_2.
10. On the last day of culture, e.g., day 7, remove 50 µL of supernatant from each well and store at –80°C until cytokine analysis can be carried out.
11. Add 5 mCi of tritiated thymidine to each well at the end of 7 d and incubate for approximately 16 h.
12. Harvest the contents of the wells according to the manufacturer's instructions.

13. Count the incorporation of radioactivity using a scintillation counter according to the manufacturer's instructions.
14. Determine the mean counts per min (c.p.m.) in allergen-stimulated wells and medium controls wells.
15. Subtract the counts for the control wells from the allergen-stimulated wells.
16. Suppression of proliferation by CD4+CD25+ cells can be calculated as a difference in c.p.m. from mixed CD4+CD25+/CD4+CD25– cultures as a percentage of c.p.m. obtained with CD4+CD25– T cells alone, e.g.,

$$\frac{(CD4 + CD25 - c.p.m.) - (mixed\,CD4+25 - /CD4+25+c.p.m.)}{CD4+CD25-c.p.m.} \times 100$$

3.4. Extracellular Staining Using a Flow Cytometer

Cytometry refers to the measurement of the chemical and physical properties of cells. Flow cytometry is the method by which such measurements are made as the cells pass in a fluid stream through a measuring point surrounded by an array of detectors. In this way, the purity of the various cell types isolated using the MACS® regulatory t-cell isolation kit can be determined. It is necessary to include isotype controls in flow cytometry whereby nonreactive monoclonal antibodies of the same isotype and those conjugated with the same fluorochrome can measure the amount of conjugate binding that is unrelated to the target antigen of the human cells.

1. Label eleven 5-mL flow cytometry tubes as follows:

PBMCs 1 = unstained
        2 = CD4 FITC
        3 = CD25 RPE
        4 = CD4 FITC/CD25 RPE
        5 = IgG$_1$ FITC/IgG$_1$ RPE

CD4+ cells 1 = CD4 FITC/CD25 RPE
           2 = IgG$_1$ FITC/IgG$_1$ RPE

CD4+CD25– cells 1 = CD4 FITC/CD25 RPE
                2 = IgG$_1$ FITC/IgG$_1$ RPE

CD4+CD25+ cells 1 = CD4 FITC/CD25 RPE
                2 = IgG$_1$ FITC/IgG$_1$ RPE

2. 0.2×10^6 of each cell type is placed into the appropriate tubes and 2 mL of buffer is added.
3. The tubes are centrifuged at 4°C for 5 min at 400g.
4. Pour off the supernatant and resuspend cells by flicking the bottom of the tube.
5. Add the relevant diluted primary antibody (e.g., FITC-conjugated CD4 antibody/RPE-conjugated CD25 antibody) to the appropriate tubes in 20–50 µL of buffer according to the manufacturer's instructions.

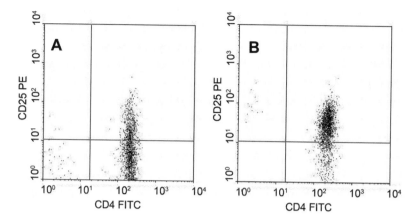

Fig. 5. Example of extracellular staining of (**A**) pre-enriched CD4+ T-cells after depletion of non-CD4+ cells and (**B**) isolated CD4+CD25+ regulatory T-cells.

6. Incubate on ice for 15–30 min in the dark.
7. The supernatant is discarded and the cells resuspended by flicking the bottom of the tube.
8. Add 2 mL of buffer to each tube and centrifuge at 4°C for 5 min at 400g.
9. Pour off the supernatant and resuspend cells by flicking the tube.
10. Add 200–400 µL to each tube and analyze on a flow cytometer to determine cell purity (*see* **Fig. 5**).

4. Notes

1. Cell calculations: The number of cells counted in the 25 squares of the hemocytometer should be multiplied by 2 (as they are diluted 1:2 with Trypan Blue), then by 10^4 (for the volume of the graticule); this will give cells per milliliter. A further multiplication (for the total volume of sample) is required to ascertain the total cell count in solution:

   e.g., 300 cells counted $\times$ 2 $\times$ 10^4 = 600 $\times$ 10^4 = 6 $\times$ 10^6 cells/mL $\times$ 40 = 24,000 $\times$ 10^4 = 2.4 $\times$ 10^8 in total.

2. Working on ice may require increased incubation times. Higher temperatures and/or longer incubation times lead to nonspecific cell labeling.
3. CD25– cells are incubated alone at a concentration of 3 $\times$ 10^6 cells/mL to control for amplified cell density of the CD25+/CD25– cultures.

References

1. Read, S., Malmstrom, V., and Powrie, F. (2000) Cytotoxic T lymphocyte-associated antigen 4 plays an essential role in the function of CD25(+)CD4(+) regulatory cells that control intestinal inflammation. *J. Exp. Med.* **192**, 295–302.

2. Sakaguchi, S., Fukuma, K., Kuribayashi, K., and Masuda, T. (1985) Organ-specific autoimmune diseases induced in mice by elimination of T cell subset. I. Evidence for the active participation of T cells in natural self-tolerance; deficit of a T cell subset as a possible cause of autoimmune disease. *J. Exp. Med.* **161,** 72–87.
3. Baecher-Allan, C., Brown, J. A., Freeman, G. J., and Hafler, D. A. (2001) CD4+CD25 high regulatory cells in human peripheral blood. *J. Immunol.* **167,** 1245–1253.
4. Dieckmann, D., Plottner, H., Berchtold, S., Berger, T., and Schuler, G. (2001) Ex vivo isolation and characterisation of CD(+)CD25(+) T cells with regulatory properties from human blood. *J. Exp. Med.* **193,** 1303–1310.
5. Stephens, L. A., Mottet, C., Mason, D., and Powrie, F. (2001) Human CD4(+) CD25(+) thymocytes and peripheral T cells have immune suppressive activity in vitro. *Eur. J. Immunol.* **31,** 1247–1254.
6. Ling, E. M., Smith, T., Nguyen, X. D., et al. (2004) Relation of CD4+CD25+ regulatory T-cell suppression of allergen-driven T-cell activation of atopic status and expression of allergic disease. *Lancet* **363,** 608–615.
7. Doganci, A., Eigenbrod, T., Krug, N., et al. (2005) The IL-6R alpha chain controls lung CD4+CD25+ Treg development and function during allergic airway inflammation in vivo. *J. Clin. Invest.* **115,** 313–325.
8. Akdis, C. A., Blesden, T., Akdis, M., Wuthrich, B., and Blaser, K. (2003) Role of interleukin 10 in specific immunotherapy. *J. Clin. Invest.* **102,** 98–106.
9. Francis, J. N., Till, S. J., and Durham, S. R. (2003) Induction of IL-10+CD4+ CD25+ T cells by grass pollen immunotherapy. *J. Allergy Clin. Immunol.* **111,** 1255–1264.
10. Varney V. A., Hamid, Q. A., Gaga, M., et al. (1993) Influence of grass pollen immunotherapy on cellular infiltration and cytokine mRNA expression during allergen-induced late-phase cutaneous responses. *J. Clin. Invest.* **92,** 644–651.

9

Monocyte-Derived Dendritic Cells as Antigen-Presenting Cells in T-Cell Proliferation and Cytokine Production

Sun-sang J. Sung

Abstract

Dendritic cells (DC) are widely considered to be the major antigen-presenting cell (APC) type in immune responses. These cells are obtained from adherent cells or are purified CD14[+] monocytes from peripheral blood mononuclear cells (PBMC) by in vitro stimulation with granulocyte, macrophage-colony-stimulating factor (GM-CSF) plus interleukin (IL)-4. They express high levels of MHC class II and costimulatory molecules, internalize Ag rapidly via Fc receptors and mannose receptors, and, by macropinocytosis, produce large amounts of IL-12 on CD40 ligation, and are potent in presenting soluble Ag and in stimulating allogeneic mixed-leukocyte reactions.

To study primary T-cell responses and cytokine production in allergy patients, we have developed an in vitro system by using highly purified T cells as responder cells and monocyte-derived DC (MDC) as the APC. MDC provide a convenient and potent APC source for T-cell response studies.

Key Words: Antigen-presenting cells; dendritic cells; T-cell proliferation; cytokines.

1. Introduction

Dendritic cells (DC) are widely considered to be the major antigen (Ag)-presenting cell (APC) type in immune responses *(1)*. In human, the best studied DC type is the monocyte-derived DC (MDC) *(2,3)*. These cells are obtained from adherent cells or are purified CD14[+] monocytes from peripheral blood mononuclear cells (PBMC) by in vitro stimulation with granulocyte, macrophage-colony-stimulating factor (GM-CSF) plus interleukin (IL)-4. They express high levels of MHC class II and costimulatory molecules, internalize Ag rapidly via Fc receptors and mannose receptors, and, by macropinocytosis *(4)*, produce large amounts of IL-12 on CD40 ligation *(5)*, and are potent in presenting soluble Ag and in stimulating allogeneic mixed-leukocyte reactions *(2,3)*. MDC

From: *Methods in Molecular Medicine: Allergy Methods and Protocols*
Edited by: M. G. Jones and P. Lympany © Humana Press Inc., Totowa, NJ

are considered immature DC *(1–3)*. They can be induced to develop into mature DC with elevated MHC class II expression, decreased Ag uptake, and increased Ag presentation potency by stimulation with inflammatory cytokines such as TNF and IL-1, bacterial products such as endotoxin, and T-cell ligands such as CD40 ligand *(2,3,5,6)*. MDC have been useful in studying the mechanism of Ag presentation *(1,2)* and in clinical trials in the treatment of viral infections and cancer *(3,7,8)*.

In the past, human Ag-specific T-cell response studies have been severely limited by the lack of suitable potent autologous APC. The great majority of T-cell response studies utilize total PBMC and rely on macrophages and B cells in the cultures to function as the APC. However, this cell mixture can detect only strong to moderate T-cell proliferative responses. Furthermore, T-cell cytokine production is influenced by the different cell types present in the cultures, making the results difficult to interpret. MDC have provided a convenient, readily available, and potent APC source for T-cell response studies. To study primary T-cell responses in allergy patients, we have developed an in vitro system by using highly purified T cells as responder cells and MDC as the APC *(9)*. This method has been successfully applied to studies on T-cell proliferation and cytokine production in response to allergens and allergen peptides and should be generally applicable to in vitro studies on T-cell and APC functions.

2. Materials

2.1. PBMC Isolation

1. Anticoagulant acid citrate dextrose (ACD-A) solution: 22 g/L trisodium citrate·2H_2O, 8 g/L citric acid·H_2O, 24.5 g/L dextrose. Sterilize by filtration (0.20-µm filter; Nalgene, Rochester, NY) and store at 4°C (*see* **Note 2**).
2. Ficoll-paque, density 1.077 g/L (Amersham Pharmacia, Piscataway, NJ). Store at 4°C.
3. Ca^{2+}–Mg^{2+} solution: 0.25 M $CaCl_2$, 0.078 M $MgCl_2$, sterilize by filtration.
4. Phosphate-buffered saline (PBS): 1 part endotoxin-free 10× PBS without Ca^{2+} and Mg^{2+} and 9 parts endotoxin-free H_2O (Irvine Scientific, Santa Ana, CA).

2.2. Isolation of CD14+ Monocytes and MDC Derivation

1. Anti-CD14 monoclonal antibody (mAb) 63D3 (ATCC, Bethesda, MD).
2. Goat-anti-mouse IgG magnetic microbeads (Miltenyi, Auburn, CA).
3. Miltenyi LS column and VarioMACS magnetic cell separation assembly.
4. Wash buffer for cell separation columns (PBS/BSA/EDTA): 0.5% bovine serum albumin (BSA), 5 mM EDTA in PBS. Store at 4°C. When ready to use, filter solution through a 0.2-µm 115-mL filter unit (Nalgene). Leave solution in vacuum in the filter unit for 15 min at room temperature to deaerate solution and store buffer on ice.
5. Human recombinant GM-CSF (Peprotech, Rocky Hill, NJ); 1×10^7 units/mg protein. Dissolve in RPMI 1640 with 10% fetal bovine serum at 10 µg/mL to 1 mg/mL

of GM-CSF. Aliquot into sterile freezing or Eppendorf tubes and store at −70°C (*see* **Note 3**).

6. Human recombinant IL-4 (Peprotech): 2×10^7 units/mg protein. Dilute and aliquot as in GM-CSF.

7. Complete medium: RPMI 1640 (Invitrogen, Carlsbad, CA), 2 mM L-glutamine, 100 U/mL penicillin, 100 μg/mL streptomycin, and 10% heat-inactivated (56°C, 30 min), defibrinated autologous plasma (from stock 70% plasma; *see* **Section 3.1., step 4**).

2.3. T-Cell Purification for Ag-Specific Responses

1. Monoclonal antibodies against human CD19 (Pharmingen, San Diego, CA), CD56 (B159.5.2, Dr G. Trinchieri, Wistar Institute, Philadelphia, PA), CD13 *(9)*, and CD83 (Coulter Immunotech, Miami, FL).

2. Goat-anti-mouse IgG magnetic microbeads (Miltenyi), LS columns, VarioMACS magnetic sorting assembly, and PBS/BSA/EDTA column washing solution as described in **Section 2.2., step 4**.

2.4. MDC Antigen Presentation in T-Cell Proliferation

Ags: recombinant Der p 2 *(9)* at 2 mg/mL; tetanus toxoid at 1.4 mg/mL and diphtheria toxoid at 0.5 mg/mL (Massachusetts Department of Health, Jamaica Plains, MA), dialysed against PBS and sterile filtered; and phytohemagglutinin (PHA, Wellcome Diagnostics, Dartford, England) at 9 mg/mL.

2.5. T-Cell Ag-Specific Cytokine Production

1. Recombinant IL-2 (Hoffmann LaRoche, Nutley, NJ): Dissolve IL-2 in RPMI 1640 with 10% fetal calf serum (FCS) at 10,000 U/mL. Aliquot in 2500 U/vial and store at −70°C.

2. Ag as described in **Section 2.4**.

3. Der p 2 20 mer overlapping set: A set of thirteen 20 mer Der p 2 peptides (University of Virginia Biomolecular Research Facility) with 10 amino acid overlap between adjoining peptides is dissolved in H_2O at 1 mM and stored at −20°C.

2.6. Assay of Th1 and Th2 Cytokines in Supernatants of Stimulated T Cells by ELISA

1. Immulon 4 plates, 96 well (Dynatech, Chantilly, VA).

2. Paired anti-human (hu) IFN-γ (Endogen, Woburn, MA), anti-huIL-4 (Pharmingen), and anti-huIL-5 (Pharmingen) capture and biotinylated detecting mAb. Store in aliquots at −20°C.

3. Standard recombinant huIFN-γ, huIL-4, and huIL-5 (all from Endogen): Dissolve as 0.2 μg/mL in RPMI 1640 containing 10% FCS and store in 25-μL aliquots at −70°C. Larger aliquots (e.g., 0.5 mL) can be used as stock aliquots and later realiquoted.

4. Streptavidin-horseradish peroxidase (HRP; Pharmingen).

5. Coating buffer: 0.1 M sodium bicarbonate solution, pH 8.2.

6. Plate-blocking solution: 5% BSA in PBS and 0.05% Tween 20 (Fisher Scientific, Pittsburgh, PA). Prepare fresh and stir solution for 1–2 h to allow BSA to dissolve before use.
7. PBS/Tween plate-washing solution: 0.05% Tween 20 in PBS.
8. HRP substrate: 0.4 mg/mL *O*-phenylenediamine (Sigma Chemical Co., St Louis, MO) in citrate–phosphate buffer, pH 5.0 (24.3 mL of 0.1 M citric acid and 25.7 mL of 0.2 M dibasic sodium phosphate per 100 mL buffer), and 80 μL H_2O_2 per 100 mL substrate solution. Prepare fresh for each measurement.
9. Stop solution: 3 N HCl.

3. Methods

The described procedure requires two donations of 200 mL of blood each with donations 7 d apart. Monocytes are purified from the PBMC of each donation for MDC generation. T-responder cells are purified from the second donation. A complete experiment spans 13 and 17 d for T-cell proliferation and cytokine production, respectively.

3.1. PBMC Isolation (see Note 4)

1. Draw 7.5 mL ACD-A into each of four 60-mL syringes with a 18-G needle.
2. Using a 19-G butterfly needle (Abbott Laboratories, N. Chicago, IL), draw 50 mL of blood in each syringe from the arm by venipuncture. Mix contents after each syringe is filled.
3. Put the blood into 50-mL conical centrifuge tubes. Spin blood at 450*g* for 15 min at 4°C. Pipet out plasma and pool in 50-mL conical tubes. Avoid disturbing the white buffy coat cells on top of the packed red cells. Note the volumes of plasma and total blood.
4. To the plasma, add Ca^{2+}–Mg^{2+} solution (in mL) calculated by the empirical formula: 8.4 × plasma volume/total plasma plus red blood cell volume. Incubate plasma at 37°C. If no clotting occurs after 1 h, add increments of 0.2 mL of Ca^{2+}–Mg^{2+} solution and continue the incubation. Defibrinated plasma is pipeted out, aliquoted, and stored at −20°C. Use this plasma as 70% autologous plasma (*see* **Note 5**).
5. Pool the packed cells in a 500-mL sterile bottle. Add cold PBS to 420 mL.
6. Pipet 12 mL of Ficoll-paque into each of twelve 50-mL conical polypropylene tubes (Falcon 2070, B–D). Gently overlay the Ficoll-paque with 35 mL of diluted packed cells.
7. Centrifuge at 1400*g* at 15°C for 20 min.
8. Pipet out interface cells (PBMC) with a cotton-plugged pasteur pipet into 50-mL conical tubes. Dilute cells at least twofold with cold PBS. Spin cells down at 200*g* at 4°C for 10 min.
9. Suction off supernatant. Pool all PBMC into one 50-mL conical tube with 50 mL cold PBS and spin cells down again.
10. Resuspend cells in 5 mL cold PBS. Count a 20× diluted aliquot of cells with a hemocytometer.

3.2. Isolation of CD14⁺ Monocytes and MDC Derivation (see Note 6)

1. Transfer the washed PBMC to an 8-mL round bottom tube (Falcon 2027). Rinse the original 50-mL tube with 2 mL cold PBS and pool all the cells. Spin cells down at $200g$ at 4°C for 10 min.
2. Resuspend cells in 4 mL cold complete medium (*see* **Section 2.2.**). Add 80 µg purified anti-CD14 mAb 63D3. Rotate in the cold for 30 min (*see* **Note 7**).
3. Centrifuge cells down at $200g$ for 10 min at 4°C. Wash off free mAb in cell suspension twice with cold PBS.
4. To the cell pellet add 50 µL heat-inactivated autologous plasma (*see* **Note 8**), 50 µL PBS/BSA/EDTA, and 80 µL goat-anti-mouse IgG magnetic microbead. Incubate in the refrigerator for 15 min.
5. To purify CD14⁺ monocytes, set up a VarioMACS assembly in a laminar flow hood with a LS column mounted in the column holder. The column is equilibrated with 5 mL cold PBS/BSA/EDTA followed by 0.5 mL of ice-cold autologous heat-inactivated plasma to block nonspecific binding (*see* **Note 8**). In this and subsequent steps, maintain sterility of cells by ensuring all reagents and supplies are sterile, and work aseptically.
6. To the magnetic bead-treated cells, add 1 mL cold PBS/BSA/EDTA and load the cells to the LS column with a cotton-plugged pasteur pipet. Wash tubes by the addition of 0.5 mL PBS/BSA/EDTA solution. Wait until all the cells have drained into the column. Load the wash solution (PBS/BSA/EDTA). Collect the flow-through cells in an 8-mL tube. Repeat washing with 2-mL aliquots of PBS/BSA/EDTA solution until 6 mL of flow-through wash solution are collected.
7. Remove the column containing the magnetically selected CD14⁺ cells from the VarioMACS unit. Connect the bottom outlet of the column to a 10-mL syringe with a sterile three-way stopcock. Flush cells out by pushing through 6 mL of PBS/BSA/EDTA in 2-mL aliquots with the syringe, and collect the column washes at the column top with a pasteur pipet (*see* **Note 9**). Pool cells.
8. Count cells and culture CD14⁺ monocytes in complete medium supplemented with 50 ng/mL GM-CSF and 50 ng/mL IL-4 at 1×10^6 cells/mL, 4 mL/well in 6-well plates (Falcon 3046).
9. At the end of 4 d refeed cells by taking out 2 mL of medium and adding 2 mL of fresh medium containing GM-CSF and IL-4 (*see* **Note 10**).

3.3. T-Cell Purification for Ag-Specific Responses

In this section, Ag-specific response measurements using T cells purified from PBMC from the second donation by negative selection and MDC from the first donation are described.

1. Seven days after the first blood donation, collect another 200 mL blood from the same donor. Process cells and plasma as in the first collection (*see* **Section 3.1.**).
2. After fractionating the cells through the separation column into CD14⁺ monocytes and CD14⁻ PBMC (*see* **Section 3.2.**), the CD14⁺ cells are incubated in complete

medium (*see* **Section 2.2.7.**) containing GM-CSF and IL-4 for MDC generation for use in T-cell cytokine production studies (*see* **Section 3.5.**).

3. T cells are purified from the CD14$^-$ cell fraction by negative selection. Resuspend the cells in 1 mL complete medium. Add anti-CD19, anti-CD56, anti-CD13, and anti-CD83 mAb to a final concentration of 20 µg/mL each. Rotate the cells in the cold room for 30 min.

4. Wash cells twice with PBS/BSA/EDTA and spin cells down at 200g for 10 min at 4°C. Resuspend cell pellet in 50 µL autologous heat-inactivated plasma, 50 µL PBS/BSA/EDTA, and 80 µL goat-anti-mouse IgG magnetic microbeads. Incubate in the refrigerator for 15 min.

5. Load cells in a LS column and select magnetic microbead-bound cells with a VarioMACS sorting assembly. Collect the flow-through T cells and wash columns as in **Section 3.2.**, **step 6**. Count the T cells with a hemocytometer.

3.4. MDC Ag Presentation in T-Cell Proliferation

1. Detach MDC by washing medium over cells with a cotton-plugged pasteur pipet. Wash cells twice with cold PBS and centrifuge washed cells down at 200g, 4°C for 10 min. Resuspend in complete medium (**Section 2.2.7.**) at 1×10^6 cells/mL (*see* **Note 11**).

2. Resuspend purified T cells at 2×10^6 cells/mL in complete medium. To 96-well plates (Falcon 3072) add 100 µL of T cells into quadruplicate wells.

3. Add graded number of MDC at T:DC ratios of 1000:1, 300:1, 100:1, 30:1, 10:1 in a final volume of 50 µL complete medium. Add allergen to 10 µg/mL in 50 µL medium. The final culture volume per well is 200 µL.

4. For allergen dose–response studies, use a T:DC ratio of 10:1 and add graded amounts of allergen from 0.1 to 10 µg/mL. For the measurement of T-cell responses to overlapping Der p 2 peptides, 4 µL of 1 mM peptides was added to give a final concentration of 20 µM peptide.

5. Include negative and positive controls. Negative control wells contain no Ag. Positive control wells contain 3 µg/mL tetanus toxoid or 20 µg/mL PHA.

6. Incubate the plates at 37°C, 5% CO_2 for a total of 5 d. At the end of the incubation period, add 50 µL [^{3}H]-thymidine (20 µCi/mL, 6.7 Ci/mmol; PerkinElmer, Boston, MA) and pulse cells for 8 h.

7. Harvest cells by a multiwell cell harvester and count [^{3}H]-thymidine incorporation in a scintillation counter.

3.5. T-Cell Ag-Specific Cytokine Production

1. Resuspend purified T cells at 4×10^6 per mL. To 16-mm wells in 24-well plates (Falcon 3047), add 250 µL T cells.

2. Add 100 µL of 0.5×10^6 per mL 7-d MDC (**Section 3.4.1.**).

3. To each of the wells add 100-µL graded amounts of allergens (0.3–10 µg/mL final concentration) or 100 µL of 0.1 mM peptide in duplicate and add complete medium (**Section 2.2.7.**; 50 µL) to make the final volume of 500 µL. Incubate cells for 7 d to activate memory T cells to become effectors.

4. At the end of 7 d, add 1.5 mL of RPMI 1640 to each well to wash. Centrifuge the 24-well plates in microtiter plate carriers at $150g$ at 4°C for 5 min. Pipet out 1.6 mL supernatant carefully with a 1-mL pipeter (pipetman).

5. Repeat washing and pipet out 1.6 mL supernatant again. Add 100 µL of 0.5×10^6 per mL fresh DC, 100 µL of fresh Ag, and 10 µL of rIL-2 (2500 U/mL) to induce cytokine production by effector T cells. Incubate cells for 48 h for IL-4 and 72 h for IL-5 and IFN-γ production measurements.

3.6. Assay of Th1 and Th2 Cytokines in Supernatants of Stimulated T Cells by ELISA

1. Coat Immulon 4 plates with 50 µL of 2 µg/mL anti-huIFN-γ, anti-huIL-4, or anti-huIL-5 capture mAb in 0.1 M sodium bicarbonate solution, pH 8.2 at 4°C overnight.
2. Wash plate three times with PBS/Tween.
3. Add 250 µL of 5% BSA in PBS/Tween to block plates for 2 h at room temperature.
4. Spin debris in cell supernatants down in a microfuge at $12,000g$ for 15 min.
5. Dilute supernatants with complete medium at 3×, 10×, 30×, and 100× for IFN-γ and IL-5 measurements. Use undiluted supernatants for IL-4 measurements.
6. Prepare standard curves for cytokines by making 200 µL for each dilution of 3, 1, 0.3, 0.1, and 0.03 ng/mL of standard cytokine in complete medium.
7. Wash plates three times with PBS/Tween. Add 50 µL supernatants or cytokine standard in duplicates for each dilution. Cover plates with plastic wrap. Incubate at room temperature for 2 h.
8. Discard supernatants and wash plates three times with PBS/Tween.
9. Add 50 µL of 0.2 µg/mL biotinylated detecting anti-huIFN-γ, anti-huIL-4, or anti-huIL-5 mAb. Cover plates with plastic wrap. Incubate at room temperature for 2 h.
10. Wash plates three times with PBS/Tween. Add 1:5,000 diluted streptavidin-HRP for 1 h.
11. Wash plates three times and add 100 µL of substrate solution and incubate for 15 min at room temperature (*see* **Note 12**).
12. Add 50 µL 3 N HCl to stop the reaction. Measure absorbance at 492 nm.

4. Notes

1. T-cell proliferative responses to the presentation of tetanus toxoid or diphtheria toxoid by MDC derived from adherent cells (*10*) or low-density Percoll fractionated monocytes (*11*) are shown in **Fig. 1.** MDC from adherent cells and Percoll-purified monocytes comprised only 70 and 85% of the total cell population, respectively. The small contaminating lymphocytes could not be purified from the MDC easily by magnetic depletion. Ag presentation of these MDC is compared with that by E⁻ cells obtained by the depletion of CD2⁺ T cells by E-rosetting of PBMC with neuraminidase-treated sheep erythrocytes followed by centrifugation over a Ficoll-paque cushion as described in **Section 3.1** (**Fig. 1.**) and can be compared with that by MDC from CD14⁺ monocytes as shown in **Ref.** (*9*). T-cell IFN-γ or IL-5 production in response to MDC presentation of either protein Ag (Der p 2) or Ag peptides is shown in **Fig. 2.**

A TT   **B** DT

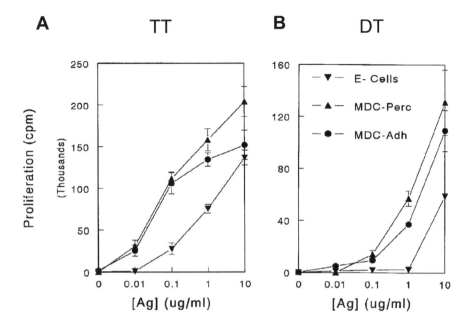

Fig. 1. T-cell proliferation in response to graded doses of Ag presented by MDC. T-cell proliferation was performed as described in **Section 3**. MDC were cultured from Percoll-purified low-density monocytes *(11)* (MDC-Perc) or from the adherent cells in PBMC *(10)* (MDC-Adh). The Ag presentation of MDC was also compared with that by sheep erythrocyte negative non-T cells (E⁻ cells) added at 6×10^4 cells/well. The Ags used were tetanus toxoid in **(A)** and diphtheria toxoid in **(B)**.

2. Human blood monocytes are exquisitely sensitive to endotoxin stimulation. Solutions are prepared from endotoxin-free water and stored in endotoxin-free containers. Glass bottles and heat-resistant caps are baked overnight at 180°C before use.

3. Avoid repeated freezing and thawing of cytokines and always dilute cytokines in serum-containing solutions to avoid cytokine denaturation.

4. The method described is designed for the collection of two blood donations of 200 mL each over a period of 8 d. Volunteers participating in this protocol donate blood for a maximum of eight experiments per year, with 400 mL blood donated per experiment. The method can be scaled down for less blood collected, in which case yellow cap (ACD-A) 8-mL vacutainer tubes (B–D, San Jose, CA) can be used.

5. Autologous plasma is used for lower background proliferation and cytokine production. The Ca^{2+}–Mg^{2+} solution used to defibrinate the plasma should be kept at minimal amounts. Excessive amount of Ca^{2+} in plasma will lead to the precipitation of $Ca_3(PO_4)_2$ on culture.

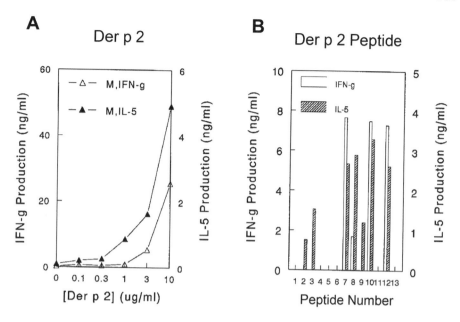

Fig. 2. IFN-γ and IL-5 production by T cells stimulated with house dust mite allergen Der p 2 or Der p 2 peptides. Purified T cells were stimulated with Der p 2 (**A**) or Der p 2 overlapping 20 mer peptides (**B**) as described in **Section 3**. MDC from CD14⁺ monocytes were used as the APC. The results are representative of four experiments from the same individual.

6. The key to the isolation of pure CD14⁺ monocytes is to block nonspecific binding on columns with plasma, keep the column washing solution cold and deaerated, and incubate the mAb-coated cells with goat-anti-mouse IgG magnetic microbead at refrigerator temperatures with minimal bead volumes of 20%.
7. Hybridoma supernatants at 1:2 dilution can be used instead of purified mAb.
8. It is important to heat-inactivate the plasma or serum used with magnetic microbead-coated cells. Otherwise the beads which are made of dextran will activate complement by the alternative pathway, resulting in cell killing. For heat inactivation, heat serum or plasma at 56°C in a water bath for 30 min.
9. It is more efficient to collect positively selected cells by pushing wash solutions from the bottom of the separation column and pipetting cells out from the top than to allow the cells to drip out from the bottom by gravity, especially when the columns are partially clogged.
10. More frequent feeding with cytokines may increase MDC yield.
11. Strongly adherent cells can be detached by incubation in PBS/BSA/EDTA on ice for 30 min followed by pipeting with a pasteur pipet.
12. The color development time can be varied so as to obtain the optimal absorbance readings.

References

1. Banchereau, J., Briere, F., and Caux, C., et al. (2000) Immunobiology of dendritic cells. *Annu. Rev. Immunol.* **18,** 767–811.
2. Rossi, M. and Young, J. W. (2005) Human dendritic cells: potent antigen-presenting cells at the crossroads of innate and adaptive immunity. *J. Immunol.* **175,** 1373–1381.
3. O'Neill, D. W., Adams, S., and Bhardwaj, N. (2004) Manipulating dendritic cell biology for the active immunotherapy of cancer. *Blood* **104,** 2235–2246.
4. Sallusto, F., Cella, M., Danieli, C., and Lanzavecchia, A. (1995) Dendritic cells use macropinocytosis and the mannose receptor to concentrate macromolecules in the major histocompatibility complex class II compartment: downregulation by cytokines and bacterial products. *J. Exp. Med.* **182,** 389–400.
5. Cella, M., Scheidegger, D., Palmer-Lehmann, K., Lane, P., Lanzavecchia, A., and Alber, G. (1996) Ligation of CD40 on dendritic cells triggers production of high levels of interleukin-12 and enhances T cell stimulatory capacity: T-T help via APC activation. *J. Exp. Med.* **184,** 747–752.
6. Cella, M., Engering, A., Pinet, V., Pieters, J., and Lanzavecchia, A. (1997) Inflammatory stimuli induce accumulation of MHC class II complexes on dendritic cells. *Nature* **388,** 782–787.
7. Dhodapkar, M. V., Krasovsky, J., Steinman, R. M., and Bhardwaj, N. (2000) Mature dendritic cells boost functionally superior CD8(+) T-cell in humans without foreign helper epitopes. *J. Clin. Invest.* **105,** R9–R14.
8. Thurner, B., Haendle, I., Roder, C., et al. (1999) Vaccination with mage-3A1 peptide-pulsed mature, monocyte-derived dendritic cells expands specific cytotoxic T cells and induces regression of some metastases in advanced stage IV melanoma. *J. Exp. Med.* **190,** 1669–1678.
9. Sung, S. J., Taketomi, E. A., Smith, A. M., Platts-Mills, T. A., and Fu, S. M. (1999) Efficient presentation of house dust mite allergen Der p 2 by monocyte-derived dendritic cells and the role of beta 2 integrins. *Scand. J. Immunol.* **49,** 96–105.
10. Sung, S. S., Nelson, R. S., and Silverstein, S. C. (1985) Mouse peritoneal macrophages plated on mannan- and horseradish peroxidase-coated substrates lose the ability to phagocytose by their Fc receptors. *J. Immunol.* **134,** 3712–3717.
11. Wright, S. and Silverstein, S. (1982) Tumor-promoting phorbol esters stimulate C3b and C3b′ receptor-mediated phagocytosis in cultured human monocytes. *J. Exp. Med.* **156,** 1149–1164.

10

Ultrasensitive ELISA for Measurement of Human Cytokine Responses in Primary Culture

William P. Stefura, J. Darren Campbell, Renée Douville,
Monique J. Stinson, F. Estelle Simons, Allan B. Becker,
and Kent T. HayGlass

Abstract

ELISAs offer excellent specificity and, once fully optimized, sensitivity that rivals that of bioassays. The major variables that need to be experimentally determined when developing an ELISA are the optimal number of fresh cells required per well, the optimal antigen concentrations for stimulation, period of culture, and the anticipated intensity of the response. In this chapter, we review the major factors to be considered in the development and application of ultrasensitive ELISAs to the analysis of human immune responses. We specify the conditions we have found to be optimal for quantifying a number of cytokines of demonstrated relevance to human immune regulation and discuss the major pitfalls inherent in this approach.

Key Words: Cytokine; ELISA; primary culture; antigen-specific; human.

1. Introduction

Over the last 15 yr, there has been a shift from reliance on assessment of human serum Ig levels as indicators of immune status to analysis of human cytokine production and mechanisms of immune regulation. The major approaches taken include (i) derivation of human T-cell lines and clones, (ii) polyclonal stimulation of freshly derived lymphocytes directly ex vivo, (iii) short-term antigen-stimulated primary culture, and (iv) analysis of mRNA synthesis by RT-PCR and/or in situ hybridization. Each of these approaches is considered in detail elsewhere in this volume.

Experimental approaches available for quantitation of human cytokine protein levels have evolved from reliance on bioassays (which have superb sensitivity but are inherently more variable from assay to assay and have the potential for

From: *Methods in Molecular Medicine: Allergy Methods and Protocols*
Edited by: M. G. Jones and P. Lympany © Humana Press Inc., Totowa, NJ

specificity problems) to ELISA. ELISAs offer excellent specificity and, once fully optimized, sensitivity that rivals that of bioassays. In this contribution, we review the major factors to be considered in the development and application of ultrasensitive ELISAs to the analysis of human immune responses. We specify the conditions we have found to be optimal for quantifying a number of cytokines of demonstrated relevance to human immune regulation and discuss the major pitfalls inherent in this approach.

Whereas detailed methodology for Ag-specific stimulation is dealt with in detail elsewhere in this volume, the need for optimization of culture conditions prior to embarking on analysis must be reiterated. The major variables that need to be experimentally determined are the optimal number of fresh cells required per well, the optimal antigen concentrations for stimulation, period of culture, and the anticipated intensity of the response. Culturing an arbitrary number of cells for a single time period and then harvesting and analyzing one large lot of supernatant is convenient, but provides misleading results. Our experience has been that preliminary experiments carried out with peripheral blood mononuclear cells (PBMC) of five to seven donors usually provides a sufficiently complete picture to establish the experimental conditions required for the remainder of the study. Given that the supply of blood, hence PBMC, is invariably less than the number of experimental conditions that one wishes to investigate, a balance needs to be struck between using as few cells and little antigen as necessary while having sufficient of each to generate readily quantified, reproducible responses. In practice, we find that 2.5–5.0×10^5 PBMC/well, using a 96-well plate, is sufficient for antigens that range from "weak" (food allergens, single recombinant allergens such as Der p 1) to recall antigens that yield very strong responses (streptokinase, Candida).

The optimal antigen concentration needs to be determined empirically for each individual antigen, usually by testing it over a range of five half log dilutions. Fortunately, the range that stimulates strong responses is typically broad (at least one order of magnitude) and individuals do not differ dramatically in the Ag concentration that is required to yield maximal stimulation. Hence, in characterizing the cytokine response to streptokinase, one does not find that some individuals yield maximal responses at 10 pg/mL, whereas others respond best at 1000 or 50,000 pg/mL. The practical consequence of this is that once the optimal Ag concentration is determined, it can be used for all individuals in the subsequent study.

The third major variable that needs to be determined prior to undertaking a major study is the kinetics of the response. It is well established that different cytokines peak in their production at different times. Hence, in response to Ag-driven stimulation, IL-2 and IL-4 levels are generally maximal at 24–48 h whereas IFNγ and IL-13 do not reach maximal levels until day 5–day 7.

Harvesting all supernatants at, for instance, 48 h would suggest a strong IL-4 and undetectable IL-13 response whereas harvesting all supernatants at day 5 would indicate the opposite. We have found minimal differences between different individuals in the kinetics of their responses. The practical consequence is that one can establish one set of cultures to be harvested at 24 h for subsequent analysis of certain cytokines, an identical set for harvest at 48 h, and a third set for harvest at 5 d. Cytokine concentrations are then determined by the methods described below only in the relevant supernatants.

Spontaneous production of cytokine in antigen-unstimulated cultures needs to be considered. For some cytokines (i.e., IL-2, IL-4) culture in medium alone for periods of up to 10 d, well past the peak antigen-driven response, virtually never yields detectable levels. Other cytokines (notably IL-10, IL-13) are routinely detectable in control cultures at low but significant levels by days 4–6 of culture. Whereas the intensity of the antigen-stimulated cytokine production is much larger than that seen in the negative control, such cytokine production needs to be dealt with. One approach is to subtract the values obtained in control wells from antigen-stimulated wells. An alternative is to report both values independently (i.e., mean IL-13 production of 141 pg/mL in unstimulated wells vs 875 pg/mL following antigen stimulation).

Finally, we do not find significant differences in analyses of samples kept at −20 or −80°C for periods of up to 3 mo. The major concern is sublimation, which would of course dramatically alter cytokine concentrations in the remaining supernatant. This is dealt with by ensuring that the plate used to store the culture supernatants does not have large numbers of empty wells (using sterile distilled water to fill extra wells), tightly wrapping the plates with plastic wrap before storage, and prompt analysis of the cultures following completion of the experiment.

1.1. Sample Handling for Ultrasensitive ELISA

The availability of ultrasensitive ELISAs is a double-edged sword. Its sensitivity allows widespread use of physiologically relevant ligands (antigens, peptides, etc.) in the analysis of antigen-specific responses rather than pharmacologic reagents (PMA/calcium ionophore, anti-CD3, PHA) that yield intense cytokine production by virtually all T cells rather than only those specific for the nominal antigen. Given that the frequency of T cells specific for any single (nonallogeneic) antigen represents only a tiny fraction (usually <<1%) of total T cells, antigen-specific stimulation is clearly a preferable method to characterize such responses. At the same time, any ultrasensitive technique is highly sensitive to experimental error. Because measuring small volumes by micropipetor is such a routine procedure, it is not always carried out with precision.

To reinforce the need for accuracy and to provide a quantifiable indicator of that individual's variability for the supervisor, we routinely have all trainees quantify the variability in their technique when first entering the laboratory.

1.2. Strategies for Enhancing Sensitivity

A few strategies are useful to further enhance sensitivity. The assays described are configured using the minimum concentrations of the reagents required in order to minimize cost. Use of higher concentrations of capture and development reagents often increases sensitivity by one or twofold. Similarly, there is a linear relationship between how long an ELISA is allowed to develop and the sensitivity of that assay. For cytokines such as IL-5 or IL-13, produced at relatively high concentrations (typically 10-1000 pg/ml levels) following stimulation with strong recall antigens, the ELISA can sometimes be read at 1 h. For cytokines produced at levels where sensitivity is a major issue, such as IL-4, the assay is allowed to develop for up to 9 h. In all cases, the greater the difference between the absorbance of the maximum concentration of the recombinant standard and the background (all reagents except the cytokine), the better the precision of the assay.

Use of chemiluminescent detection systems rather than absorbance in ELISA results in additional 10 to 30-fold increases in sensitivity. The caveat is that an additional plate reader capable of quantitating chemiluminescence is required and the detection reagents for such assays are approximately 10-fold more expensive.

2. Materials

2.1. Buffers (see Note 1)

1. Coating buffer: 1.59 g Na_2CO_3, 2.93 g $NaHCO_3$ made up to 1 L with double distilled water. Add NaN_3 to 0.02% and adjust pH to 9.6.
2. Blocking buffer: PBS containing 0.17% BSA, 0.02% NaN_3. Adjust pH to 7.4.
3. Wash buffer: PBS containing 0.05% Tween-20. Adjust pH to 7.4.
4. Dilution buffer: PBS containing 0.085% BSA, 0.05% Tween-20, 0.02% NaN_3. Adjust pH to 7.4.
5. Substrate buffer: 122 mg $MgCl_2 \cdot 6H_2O$, 117 mL diethanolamine.

$MgCl_2$ should be dissolved in 800 mL double distilled water prior to addition of diethanolamine.

Diethanolamine may require warming at 37°C to liquefy. Adjust final pH to 9.8 and volume to 1 L. Keep this buffer in a dark bottle at 4°C as it is light sensitive. We utilize one *p*-nitrophenyl phosphate (PNPP) tablet (Sigma #S0942-200TAB) per 5 mL buffer.

The antibodies listed below are available from multiple sources including BD Pharmingen (http://www.bdbiosciences.com), Biolegend (http://www.biolegend.com), eBioscience (http://www.ebioscience.com), R&D Systems (http://www.rndsystems.com), and Serotec (http://www.serotec.co.uk). Prices vary considerably for the same products. In several instances, the clones producing the Abs are available from the ATCC (http://www.atcc.org) providing a more cost-effective approach for labs which will make use of particular assays at high frequency. Here, we have listed combinations of clones, and conditions, that we find provide highly sensitive assays.

2.2. Measurement of Human IFNγ Levels

1. Capture antibody: mouse anti-human IFNγ monoclonal (clone MD-1).
2. Standard: human recombinant gamma interferon catalog number Gxg01-902-535. Available from NCI at 80,000 IU/ampoule.
3. Detection antibody: biotinylated mouse anti-human IFNγ monoclonal (clone 4S.B3).

2.3. Measurement of Human IL-2 Levels

1. Capture antibody: rat anti-human IL-2 monoclonal (clone MQ1-17H12).
2. Standard: interleukin-2, human, Jurkat derived 86/504 at 100 IU/ampoule available from NCI or NIBSC or recombinant IL-2 human, ISRO 851 at 1000 IU/ampoule available from NCI.
3. Detection antibody: biotinylated mouse anti-human IL-2 monoclonal (clone B33-2).

2.4. Measurement of Human IL-4 Levels

1. Capture antibody: mouse anti-human IL-4 monoclonal (clone 8D4-8).
2. Standard: recombinant IL-4 WHO standard 88/656 available from NCI or NIBSC at 1000 U/ampoule.
3. Detection antibody: biotinylated rat anti-human IL-4 monoclonal (clone MP4-25D2).

2.5. Measurement of Human IL-5 Levels

1. Capture antibody: rat anti-mouse/human IL-5 monoclonal (clone JES1-39D10).
2. Standard: human recombinant IL-5 or recombinant IL-5 WHO standard 90/586 from NCI or NIBSC at 5000 U/ampoule.
3. Detection antibody: biotinylated rat anti-human IL-5 monoclonal (clone JES1-5A10).

2.6. Measurement of Human IL-6 Levels

1. Capture antibody: mouse anti-human IL-6 monoclonal (clone MQ2-13A5).
2. Standard: human recombinant IL-6 (i.e., Peprotech #200-06).
3. Detection antibody: biotinylated mouse anti-human IL-6 monoclonal (clone MQ2-39C3).

2.7. Measurement of Human IL-10 Levels

1. Capture antibody: rat anti-human IL-10 monoclonal clone JES3-19F1 (HB 10487, from American Type Culture Collection or purchased from commercial source.

2. Standard: interleukin-10 WHO Reference Reagent 93/722 available from NIBSC at 5000 U/ampoule or human recombinant IL-10 from commercial source.
3. Detection antibody: clone JES-12G8 (HB 11676 from the American Type Culture Collection) or purchased.

2.8. Measurement of Human IL-11 Levels

1. Capture antibody: mouse anti-human IL-11 monoclonal (clone 22616.1).
2. Standard: human recombinant IL-11.
3. Detection antibody: biotinylated mouse anti-human IL-11 polyclonal (i.e., R&D Systems #BAF218).

2.9. Measurement of Human IL-13 Levels

1. Capture antibody: rat anti-human IL-13 monoclonal (clone JES10-5A2).
2. Standard: human recombinant IL-13 (Peprotech 200-13) or recombinant human IL-13 DNA WHO Reference Reagent 94/622 available from NIBSC at 1000 U/ampoule.
3. Detection antibody: biotinylated mouse anti-human IL-13 monoclonal (clone B69-2).

2.10. Measurement of Human TGFβ Levels

1. Capture antibody: rat anti-mouse/human/pig TGFβ1 monoclonal (clone A75-2.1).
2. Standard: recombinant human TGFβ1 (Peprotech 100-21R) or transforming growth factor β-1, human, rDNA standard 89/514 at 3000 U/ampoule from NCI or NIBSC.
3. Detection antibody: biotinylated rat anti-mouse/human/pig TGFβ1 monoclonal (clone A75-3.1).

2.11. Measurement of Human TNFα Levels

1. Capture antibody: mouse anti-human TNFα monoclonal (i.e., Biolegend clone MAb-1).
2. Standard: human recombinant TNFα (Peprotech #300-01A).
3. Detection antibody: biotinylated mouse anti-human TNFα monoclonal (clone MAb11).

3. Methods

3.1. Assessment of Intra-assay Variability Because of Pipeting Error

Pipeting errors are cumulative, compounding the reduction in assay sensitivity by increasing variability in the assay. For this reason, the coefficient of variation (CV) of pipeting should be ≤3% at each step. To assess this, ELISA solution from previous assays is used as a source of chromogen. For PNPP, a substrate for alkaline phosphatase, this yields a bright yellow solution. It is used to generate readings in the microplate plate reader, allowing one to determine how precisely and reproducibly one measures volumes.

For a diagram of suggested plate design and sample data, *see* **Table 1**.

Table 1
Determination of Coefficient of Variation: Sample Data

Row	Absorbance (405–690 nm)						
	1	2	3	4	5	6	7
A	0.899	0.919	1.779	1.764	3.887	3.866	3.869
B	0.934	0.887	1.766	1.779	3.28	3.251	3.276
C	0.912		1.757		1.66	1.682	1.697
D	0.927		1.762		0.869	0.871	0.861
E	0.907		1.771		0.437	0.429	0.43
F	0.893		1.77		0.229	0.225	0.223
G	0.905		1.747		0.121	0.122	0.115
H	0.919		1.802		0.067	0.067	0.061
Mean absorbance	0.912	0.903	1.769	1.772			
CV (%)	1.5	2.5	0.9	0.6			

1. Using P200 or similar equipment, pipet eight 50-μL and eight 100-μL volumes of expired ELISA solution into 96-well ELISA plates, using columns 1 and 3, respectively (running up and down plate).
2. In column 2, pipet two 50-μL volumes of expired ELISA solution in the top two wells.
3. In column 4, pipet two 100-μL volumes of expired ELISA solution in the top two wells.
4. In columns 5–7, add 50 μL of dilution buffer to all 24 wells (three columns of eight wells each), then pipet 50 μL of expired ELISA solution into the top three wells. Carry out twofold dilutions of this solution down the plate. Discard the 50-μL extra from the last well.
5. Using microplate reader, determine the absorbance values at 405 nm (or more commonly 405–690 nm background) for each data set.
6. Using plate reader software (or by transferring data to SPSS, Excel, or similar software), determine the "CV" – the variability in dispensing and titrating samples – as a check on pipeting technique. Because errors are cumulative and ELISA is a multistep process, errors in dispensing samples and reagents need to be below 3% for maximal sensitivity.

3.2. Ultrasensitive ELISA

Having established that operator technique will add minimal variability to the assay, the optimized assay conditions below will provide excellent sensitivity (*see* **Note 2**). The specific capture and development reagents, standards, and their suggested concentrations are described below (*see* **Note 3**):

1. ELISA plate should be coated with 50 μL capture antibody in a high pH coating buffer at a predetermined optimal concentration, generally between 50 ng/mL and 2 μg/mL (*see* **Note 4**). For maximum sensitivity, this incubation is carried out overnight at 40°C in tightly wrapped foil.
2. Plates with a sealing lid should be kept in a plastic box lined with wet paper towels to minimize evaporation, hence variability in edge wells (*see* **Note 5**).
3. Blocking, using 75 μL/well, should be carried out at 37°C for 1–3 h in a moist box (*see* **Note 6**). We find no difference in background between these times. This time period is used to prepare samples for the next step. Wash four times manually or using a plate washer. Afterwards, bang plate dry three times on paper towels to avoid random dilution of the next series of reagents added to the plate.
4. A standard curve of cytokine standard in dilution buffer is generated on each assay plate (*see* **Notes 7** and **8**). The titration range is determined by the anticipated intensity of your experimental values.
5. Each experimental sample should be titrated in dilution buffer from an empirically determined optimal starting dilution (typically between 1:2 and 1:10) for a series of four twofold 50-μL dilutions running down the plate (i.e., 1:2, 1:4, 1:8, 1:16) (*see* **Notes 9** and **10**). This allows ~20 sample titrations per plate. The initial dilutions should not sit in the starting well for more than 2 or 3 min before carrying out this titration, usually with a multichannel pipetor, or the resulting curves will not be linear. A sample of dilution buffer alone is generally included in wells A2, A3, and A4.
6. Sample incubation can be 3 h at 37°C or overnight at 40°C. Maximal sensitivity is obtained following overnight incubation. Wash 4× as previously. Bang dry on paper towels.
7. Biotinylated development antibody in dilution buffer is added at a predetermined optimal concentration, generally between 50 ng/mL and 2 μg/mL, using 50 μL/well (*see* **Note 11**). Incubation can be 3 h at 37°C or overnight at 40°C. Maximal sensitivity is obtained following overnight incubation. Wash 4×, banging dry 3× on paper towels afterwards.
8. Streptavidin–enzyme conjugate is added at a predetermined optimal concentration to maximize signal while minimizing background. In our experience, streptavidin–alkaline phosphatase used at 1:1000 to 1:5000 with 50 μL/well is useful. This incubation (45 min at 37°C) is followed by washing (4×), banging dry (3×), and addition of 50 μL/well PNPP in substrate buffer at room temperature.
9. Progress of the assay is monitored visually, with readings (405–690 nm) taken at periods between 45 min and 6 h of assay development, depending on the sensitivity required.
10. A standard curve is prepared using the data obtained by serial dilution of the standard, with the cytokine concentration on the x axis (log) and the absorbance on the y axis (linear) to generate a sigmoidal curve.

When carrying out sample data analysis, the mean of at least two points (generally three or four points) *falling on the linear component of the standard curve* of that plate is required. These values should not differ from one another by more than ~15–20%, typically much less (*see* **Note 12**). Mean values ± standard error for that sample should be reported. Interassay variability (the same samples titrated in an independent assay on another day) should be explicitly determined for a proportion of the samples to confirm reliability of the data/operator/assay. Sensitivity is defined in each assay as the beginning of the linear portion of the titration curve (*see* **Note 8**).

Unless statistical normality is demonstrated, a condition that usually requires large numbers of human subjects, the resulting population data should be analyzed by nonparametric statistics.

3.3. Optimized Conditions for Analysis of Human Cytokine Levels

3.3.1. IFNγ

1. Using the protocol for ultrasensitive ELISA (*see* **Section 3.2.**), use the capture antibody, mouse anti-human IFNγ, at 0.5 µg/mL.
2. For the standard, use human recombinant gamma interferon and titrate from 20 to 0.15 U/mL.
3. Dilute antigen-driven samples from 1:4. Titrate polyclonally stimulated cultures from 1:10.
4. Use the detecting antibody, biotinylated mouse anti-human IFNγ monoclonal, at 0.05 µg/mL.
5. Read the plate after 4 h with substrate for useful sensitivity of 0.15–0.3 U/mL.

3.3.2. IL-2

1. Using the protocol for ultrasensitive ELISA (*see* **Section 3.2.**), use the capture antibody, rat anti-human IL-2, at 2 µg/mL.
2. Use standard IL-2 and titrate from 10 to 0.078 U/mL.
3. Antigen-driven samples are diluted 1:2, whereas polyclonally stimulated cultures are diluted 1:10.
4. Use the detection antibody, biotinylated mouse anti-human IL-2, at 1 µg/mL.
5. Read plate after 5–6 h with substrate for sensitivity of 0.078–0.15 U/mL.

3.3.3. IL-4

1. Using the protocol for ultrasensitive ELISA (*see* **Section 3.2.**), use capture antibody mouse anti-human IL-4 monoclonal at 0.4 µg/mL.
2. Use standard recombinant IL-4 titrated from 125 to 0.98 pg/mL.
3. Use antigen-driven samples either neat or at 1:2 dilution and polyclonally stimulated samples at 1:3 dilution.
4. Use detection antibody, biotinylated rat anti-human IL-4 monoclonal, at 0.06 µg/mL.
5. Read plate after 4–6 h with substrate to obtain sensitivity of 0.98 pg/mL or ~0.006 U/mL of WHO standard 88/656.

3.3.4. IL-5

1. Using the protocol for ultrasensitive ELISA (*see* **Section 3.2.**), use capture antibody, rat anti-mouse/human IL-5, at 0.5 µg/mL.

2. Use standard human recombinant IL-5 between 1000 and 7.8 pg/mL.
3. Use antigen and polyclonally driven samples from 1:3 dilution.
4. Use detecting antibody, biotinylated rat anti-human IL-5, at 0.04 µg/mL.
5. Read plate after 2 h with substrate for sensitivity of 7.8 pg/mL or ~0.025 U/mL.

3.3.5. IL-6

1. Using the protocol for ultrasensitive ELISA (*see* **Section 3.2.**), use the capture antibody, mouse anti-human IL-6, at 2.5 µg/mL.
2. Use standard IL-6 and titrate from 2000 to 15.6 pg/mL.
3. Antigen-driven samples are diluted from 1:4, whereas polyclonally stimulated cultures are diluted from 1:10.
4. Use the detection antibody, biotinylated mouse anti-human IL-6, at 0.175 µg/mL.
5. Read plate after 2–3 h with substrate for sensitivity of 62.5 pg/mL.

3.3.6. IL-10

1. Using the protocol for ultrasensitive ELISA (*see* **Section 3.2.**), use capture antibody, rat anti-human IL-10, at 2.5 µg/mL.
2. Use standard human recombinant IL-10 from 1000 to 7.8 pg/mL.
3. Use antigen-driven samples from 1:4 dilution and polyclonally stimulated cultures at 1:10 dilution.
4. Use detecting antibody at 1 µg/mL.
5. Read plate after 2 h with substrate for sensitivity of 7.8 pg/mL or ~0.01 WHO Reference Reagent 93/722 units.

3.3.7. IL-11

1. Using the protocol for ultrasensitive ELISA (*see* **Section 3.2.**), use the capture antibody, mouse anti-human IL-11, at 1.5 µg/mL.
2. Use standard IL-11 and titrate from 500 to 3.9 pg/mL.
3. Antigen-driven samples are diluted from 1:2.
4. Use the detection antibody, biotinylated mouse anti-human IL-11, at 0.08 µg/mL.
5. Read plate after 3–4 h with substrate for sensitivity of 7.8 pg/mL.

3.3.8. IL-13

1. Using the protocol for ultrasensitive ELISA (*see* **Section 3.2.**), use capture antibody, rat anti-human IL-13, at 0.4 µg/mL.
2. Use standard human recombinant IL-13 from 1000 to 15.6 pg/mL.
3. Use antigen-driven samples at a dilution of 1:4 whereas use polyclonally stimulated cultures at 1:10 dilution.
4. Use detecting antibody, biotinylated mouse anti-human IL-13, at 0.2 µg/mL.
5. Read plate after 4–6 h with substrate for sensitivity of ~15 pg/mL.

3.3.9. IL-13 Ultra High Sensitivity Assay

Typical food antigen-driven responses (i.e., peanut-specific) fall between 10 and 200 pg/mL and altered ELISA conditions may be used to yield an assay with higher sensitivity.

1. Using the protocol for ultrasensitive ELISA (*see* **Section 3.2.**), use capture antibody, rat anti-human IL-13, at 1 µg/mL.
2. Use standard recombinant IL-13 from 200 to 1.56 pg/mL.
3. Use detecting antibody, mouse anti-human IL-13, at 0.2 µg/mL.
4. Read plate after 6 h with substrate for sensitivity of 0.78 pg/mL.

3.3.10. TGFβ

1. Using the protocol for ultrasensitive ELISA (*see* **Section 3.2.**), use capture antibody, rat anti-mouse/human/pig TGFβ1, at 1 µg/mL.
2. Use standard recombinant human TGFβ1 from 2000 to 15.6 pg/mL.
3. Prior to assay, serum/culture samples are acidified to convert TGFβ1 from latent to active form for recognition in this assay. Incubate 50 µL of sample with 2 µL 1 N HCl for 15 min at room temperature; then add 2 µL 1 N NaOH. Carry out dilutions from 1:5 (which should be later calculated based on an actual dilution of 1:5.4, allowing for the addition of acid and base above).
4. Use detecting antibody, biotinylated rat anti-mouse/human/pig TGFβ1, at 250 ng/mL.
5. Read plate after 5 h with substrate for sensitivity of ~ rDNA TGFβ1 standard 89/514 U/mL.

3.3.11. TNFα

1. Using the protocol for ultrasensitive ELISA (*see* **Section 3.2.**), use the capture antibody, mouse anti-human TNFα, at 1.0 µg/mL.
2. Use standard TNFα and titrate from 2000 to 15.6 pg/mL.
3. Antigen-driven samples are diluted from 1:4, whereas polyclonally stimulated cultures are diluted from 1:10.
4. Use the detection antibody, biotinylated mouse anti-human TNFα, at 0.5 µg/mL.
5. Read plate after 3 h with substrate for sensitivity of 60 pg/mL.

4. Notes

1. All solutions are kept in a cold room and are stable for a minimum of 6 mo.
2. In initially developing an ELISA, it needs to be remembered that arbitrarily pairing two cytokine-specific monoclonal antibodies or a monoclonal and polyclonal antibody will not necessarily yield a useful assay. This is a largely empirical process that may require testing of several different antibody combinations to obtain an assay with high sensitivity.
3. Routinely, most ELISA reagents are reconstituted in saline as recommended by the manufacturer, then diluted with an equal volume of high-quality glycerol and stored at −20°C where they are stable for at least 1 yr. Addition of glycerol allows the Ag, Ab, and enzyme conjugates to be stored at this temperature and used without undergoing multiple freeze thaw cycles.
4. A variety of high-binding EIA plates are commercially available. We have found substantial differences in their ability to bind capture antibody or Ag. Costar 3369 plates work effectively in our assays.
5. "Edge" effects, most commonly values that are too high, result from evaporation of edge wells. The solution is to ensure plates are kept tightly wrapped in a humidified

chamber (plastic box with wet paper towels) for all incubations. Also, if samples are allowed to sit in plate for an extended period prior to carrying out the dilutions, assay reproducibility is reduced.

6. A broad variety of blocking reagents (skimmed milk, bovine serum albumin (BSA) or gelatin) can be used. Recommended wash buffers sometimes utilize very high concentrations of BSA and Tween-20. In our experience, BSA at 0.17% (1.7 g/L) in PBS with 0.05% Tween-20 is sufficient to minimize backgrounds with less cost and pollution of the environment than buffers containing up to 5% BSA and 2% Tween-20.

7. Biological standards are calibrated in units of biological activity which are established by consensus following exhaustive collaborative studies involving many laboratories. They have the advantage of allowing ready comparison of cytokine levels between different laboratories using a common standard. There is a hierarchy of standards, with the WHO International Standard being the primary standard. These standards are calibrated in arbitrary units, usually based on an initial functional bioassay, to provide a common standard that can be used to compare data internationally. It is vital for international harmonization that secondary standards are calibrated against these primary standards. Secondary standards may be national or regional standards or working reference materials used in the laboratories of manufacturers, regulators, or others. WHO reference standards are available for most cytokines. There are only 4 "official" custodian laboratories for WHO International Standards and these are NIBSC, CLB in the Netherlands, CDC, and NIH. NIBSC is a multidisciplinary scientific establishment located in the UK which has a national and international role in the standardization and control of biological substances used in medicine. As a WHO International Laboratory for biological standards it prepares, evaluates, and distributes ampouled biological reference substances which serve the pharmaceutical, regulatory, and research communities as International Standards. Similarly, the BRB Preclinical Repository is a (US) NCI-sponsored facility which contains bulk cytokines, monoclonal antibodies, and cytokine standards. Its purpose is to maintain a constant and uniform supply of high-quality reagents for scientists at nonprofit as well as commercial establishments. Information on free distribution (other than a nominal shipping charge) of these standards is available from the NIBSC at http://www.nibsc.ac.uk/catalog/standards or the US NCI at http://www.ncifcrf.gov/brb/preclin.

Many laboratories choose to utilize recombinant standards from well-known manufacturers (i.e., BD Pharmingen, Peprotech, R&D Systems) and instead express their data in mass units based on that commercial preparation and lot. Because such standards vary widely in specific activity, some manufacturers have calibrated the specific activity of their standards against the WHO standard. Others utilize the bioassay of their choice to obtain specific activities. It should be recognized that 10^6 U/mL in one assay is not necessarily equivalent to 10^6 U/mL in a different assay. Comparison between, for instance, two IL-4 preparations from different sources can easily be 100-fold different in terms of specific activity. In practice, many investigators use polyclonal activators to generate 30–100 mL of bulk tissue culture supernatant containing high concentrations of natural cytokine that can then be calibrated against WHO standards for routine usage as a laboratory standard. If this approach is selected, one should be aware that different polyclonal activators are optimal for inducing intense Th1 (i.e., soluble anti-CD3 at 30 ng/mL, Pharmingen; TSST-1 at 10 ng/mL, Sigma), Th2 (i.e., PHA at 10 µg/mL, Sigma), or monokine (SAC, formalin-fixed *Staphylococcus aureas* from Sigma at 0.01–0.1 µg/mL) associated cytokine production.

8. When assay sensitivity is not sufficient for a given application, the first step is to compare the sensitivity of the standard curve generated with those found in the literature or detailed above. Assuming you obtain similar sensitivity to others, you need an estimate of the cytokine levels expected. Some cytokines are produced at substantial levels (i.e., IL-5, IL-13) whereas others, notably IL-4, are very tightly regulated and present at pg/mL levels in antigen-stimulated cultures.

9. If experimental values do not agree throughout the titration range, it is possible that the dilution range selected is not within the linear range of the assay. The titration of the samples needs to be adjusted so that more of the points lie on the linear component of the standard curve.

10. When a trainee is first gaining experience with ELISA, we provide coded samples of known concentration that fall within the range of values typically obtained in experimental work. These are titrated in duplicate until the accurate concentration (±10–15%) is reproducibly determined.

11. Development antibodies directly conjugated with enzyme are rarely used in ultra-sensitive ELISA as they do not provide adequate signal. Biotinylated reagents yield at least a 10-fold increase in sensitivity. Avidin/streptavidin enzyme conjugates generally utilize alkaline phosphatase or horse radish peroxidase. The methods presented above use alkaline phosphatase with PNPP substrate as it is inexpensive, stable, and generates a robust signal that increases linearly over many hours.

12. The most common reason for duplicates which do not agree is poor titration precision/operator error.

11

Quantification of Human Chemokine Production in TLR-Stimulated and Antigen-Specific Recall Responses

Monique Stinson, Renee Douville, Yuriy Lissitsyn, Melanie Blanchard, William Stefura, Estelle Simons, Allan Becker, Peter Nickerson, Kevin Coombs, and Kent HayGlass

Abstract

Chemokines are primarily low molecular mass proteins that are produced and usually released by a wide variety of cell types. Differential chemokine responses can be excellent early markers of immune dysfunction, allowing clinical intervention prior to expression of full blown undesirable effector responses. Thus, assessment of the nature and intensity of Ag-dependent chemokine production provides a valuable tool for probing human immune regulation.

Here, we provide detailed instructions on approaches we have developed to assess the nature and intensity of recall responses to a wide variety of exogenous and endogenous antigens capable of consistently stimulating chemokine responses by PBMC from adult and pediatric populations. This chapter is divided into two sections. The first is focused on culture techniques for eliciting antigen-driven chemokine responses for a panel of chemokines that are relevant to immune function. The second section details assay systems for their quantitative analysis.

Key Words: Chemokine; quantitation; chemoattractant; human; immunoassay; ELISA; primary culture.

1. Introduction

During the 1970s, culture supernatants from a wide variety of stimulated leukocytes were shown to contain factors that acted as selective chemoattractants for monocytes, granulocytes, or lymphocytes. The cloning of these chemoattractants and their receptors now reveals in excess of 50 chemokines and 20 receptors. Through the late 1990s, our initial understanding of the activity of chemokines – selective leukocyte recruitment – was expanded as it became recognized that chemokines, like classical cytokines, play many other roles in

From: *Methods in Molecular Medicine: Allergy Methods and Protocols*
Edited by: M. G. Jones and P. Lympany © Humana Press Inc., Totowa, NJ

biology. Thus, chemokines are primarily low molecular mass proteins that are produced and usually released by a wide variety of cell types during ontogeny, homeostasis, the initial phase of host response to injury, allergens, antigens, or invading microorganisms, and during ongoing maintenance of immune responses.

One area in which study of chemokine production and responsiveness has made major contributions has been in understanding immune regulation. Much as certain patterns of cytokine gene expression are frequently associated with particular effector responses and subsequent clinical outcomes (i.e., increased IL-4, IL-5, IL-13 synthesis with allergen-specific IgE responses and immediate hypersensitivity), there is much interest in how differential chemokine production or receptor expression relates to immune regulation. Differential chemokine responses can provide excellent early markers of immune dysfunction (i.e., in chronic renal allograft rejection), allowing clinical intervention prior to expression of full blown undesirable effector responses. Thus, assessment of the nature and intensity of *Ag-dependent* chemokine production provides a valuable tool for probing human immune regulation.

A major advantage of examining chemokine production for analysis of human immune responses is that they are usually expressed at levels one to several orders of magnitude more intense than is seen with typical (Th1, Th2, Treg) cytokines. This greatly simplifies the demands on the assays used, improves the ability to obtain detectable responses in virtually every individual examined, and strengthens assay-to-assay reproducibility as the responses seen are usually well above detection limits.

The great majority of studies of human chemokine responses have utilized potent pharmacologic stimuli (i.e., PMA plus calcium ionophore) or polyclonal activators (i.e., LPS, anti-CD3). These stimulate intense production of many chemokines but the relationship between this response and the response elicited on antigen or allergen exposure remains speculative. Here, we provide detailed instructions on approaches we have developed to assess the nature and intensity of recall responses to a wide variety of exogenous (i.e., grass pollen, streptokinase, cat Ag) and endogenous (reovirus) antigens capable of consistently stimulating chemokine responses by PBMC from adult and pediatric populations.

This chapter is divided into two sections. The first is focused on culture techniques for eliciting antigen-driven chemokine responses for a panel of chemokines that are relevant to immune function. The second section details assay systems for their quantitative analysis.

2. Materials

2.1. Primary Culture of Fresh Human PBMC

Following study approval by the local Ethics Committee and written informed consent from each individual, 10–50 mL fresh peripheral blood is taken into

EDTA- or citrate-containing tubes (typically 2 mL of 2.5% EDTA for 40–50 mL blood) by venipuncture.

1. Polyclonal activators: anti-CD3 (30 ng/mL, BD Pharmingen) or TSST-1 (100 ng/mL, Sigma) provides excellent positive controls to assess the global capacity of an individual to generate the chemokine in question.
2. TLR ligands: TLR ligands act as excellent stimuli of chemokine production. Maximal responses by freshly obtained PBMC in primary culture are found using peptidoglycan (TLR2L) at 25 ng/mL, poly(I:C) (TLR3L) at 5 µg/mL, LPS (TLR4L) at 500 pg/ml, or TLR7 ligand 3M-011 at 50 ng/mL. In response to these stimuli, some chemokines are expressed at very high levels (i.e., MCP-1/CCL2, >500 ng/mL) whereas others are found at much lower levels (i.e., IP-10/CXCL10, ~2 ng/mL).
3. Antigen: In general we find that any antigen that elicits a detectable cytokine response in primary culture also elicits strong chemokine production. Relevant Ags we have used include streptokinase (Streptase; Aventis Behring), grass pollen (Bayer), and reovirus (American Type Culture Collection; atcc.org catalog # VR-824).
4. Miscellaneous reagents: Azide-free, low endotoxin anti-CD4, anti-CD8, anti-MHC class I or MHC class II, CTLA4-Ig fusion protein for cell culture can be obtained from multiple sources including BD Pharmingen.

2.2. Quantitation of Human Chemokine Responses

For antibodies and standards, we list three examples of suppliers below. Peprotech has a complete line, R&D and BD Pharmingen have many excellent reagents. We have obtained excellent results with several companies that supply similar materials. These reagents are available via the WWW from multiple sources including Peprotech (http://www.peprotech.com); BD Pharmingen (http://www.bdbiosciences.com), R&D Systems (http://www.rndsystems.com), and Serotec (http://www.serotec.co.uk). Prices vary considerably for products with very similar performance. Bear in mind that with polyclonal sources, the conditions we found to be optimal for these lots may vary somewhat from year to year as different animal pools are used. If you seek greater sensitivity (or lower cost), titrate the capture and development Abs twofold more concentrated/more dilute and extend the length of the color development phase to customize the assay for your purposes.

In some cases, hybridomas producing these Abs are available from the ATCC (http://www.atcc.org) providing a more cost-effective approach for labs which will make use of particular assays at high frequency. Here, we list combinations of clones and conditions that provide highly sensitive assays in our hands.

Establishing, validating, and optimizing one's own ELISA using commercial reagents takes a few days and is approximately 10 to 30-fold less expensive than buying kits. This is an important consideration if this technique is going to be commonly used in your laboratory.

Buffers: Coating, blocking, wash, and *p*-nitrophenyl phosphatase (PNPP) substrate buffers are prepared as detailed in Chapter 10.

2.2.1. Measurement of Human CCL2 (MCP-1) Levels

1. Capture antibody: mouse anti-human MCP-1 monoclonal (BD Pharmingen 23231D, clone 10F7.2, or Peprotech monoclonal or polyclonal).
2. Standard: recombinant human MCP-1 (BD Pharmingen or Peprotech).
3. Detection antibody: biotinylated mouse anti-human MCP-1 polyclonal (BD Pharmingen or Peprotech).

2.2.2. Measurement of Human CCL3 (MIP-1α) Levels

1. Capture antibody: mouse anti-human MIP-1α monoclonal (R&D Systems MAB670, clone 14215.41) or Peprotech monoclonal or polyclonal.
2. Standard: recombinant human MIP-1α (PeproTech #300-08).
3. Detection antibody: biotinylated goat anti-human MIP-1α polyclonal (R&D Systems BAF270 or Peprotech polyclonal).

2.2.3. Measurement of Human CCL17 (TARC) Levels

1. Capture antibody: mouse anti-human TARC monoclonal (R&D Systems MAB364, clone 54026.11) or Peprotech polyclonal.
2. Standard: recombinant human TARC (PeproTech #300-30).
3. Detection antibody: biotinylated goat anti-human TARC polyclonal (R&D Systems BAF364 or Peprotech polyclonal).

2.2.4. Measurement of Human CCL22 (MDC) Levels

1. Capture antibody: mouse anti-human MDC (R&D Systems MAB336, clone 57226.11) or Peprotech monoclonal or polyclonal.
2. Standard: recombinant human MDC (R&D Systems #336-MD).
3. Detection antibody: biotinylated chicken anti-human MDC polyclonal (R&D Systems BAF336 or Peprotech polyclonal).

2.2.5. Measurement of Human CXCL9 (MIG) Levels

1. Capture antibody: mouse anti-human MIG monoclonal (R&D Systems MAB392, clone 49106.11, or Peprotech monoclonal or polyclonal).
2. Standard: recombinant human MIG (PeproTech #300-26).
3. Detection antibody: biotinylated goat anti-human MIG polyclonal (R&D Systems BAF392 or Peprotech polyclonal).

2.2.6. Measurement of Human CXCL10 (IP-10) Levels

1. Capture antibody: mouse anti-human IP-10 monoclonal (R&D Systems MAB266, clone 33036.211, or Peprotech polyclonal).
2. Standard: recombinant human IP-10 (PeproTech #300-12).
3. Detection antibody: biotinylated goat anti-human IP-10 polyclonal (R&D Systems BAF266 or Peprotech polyclonal).

2.2.7. Measurement of Human CCL11 (Eotaxin) Levels

1. Capture antibody: mouse anti-human Eotaxin monoclonal (R&D Systems MAB320, clone 43911.11).
2. Standard: recombinant human Eotaxin (PeproTech #300-21).
3. Detection antibody: biotinylated goat anti-human Eotaxin polyclonal (R&D Systems BAF320).

3. Methods

3.1. Culture Conditions for Generation of Antigen or TLR-Driven Chemokine Responses

Peripheral blood is collected by venipuncture into a tube containing 2 mL of 2.7% EDTA, mixed immediately, and diluted by 1:2 (i.e., by adding 20 mL saline to 40 mL blood to increase the yield of PBMC recovered for culture), then mixed immediately by inverting the tube. PBMC are isolated by standard Ficoll procedures (Sigma).

After washing isolated PBMC twice with saline, the cells are resuspended in complete media, typically at 3×10^6 cells/mL. A total of 300,000 cells/well (96-well FB culture plate) are cultured with optimized antigen concentrations (predetermined by the investigator in preliminary experiments), to yield a final volume of 200 µL in round bottom plates. Cells are cultured for 16 h to 7 d depending on the chemokine analyzed and stimulus used. Typically, CCL2 has rapid kinetics, with peak polyclonal or Ag-driven responses evident at 12–18 h. CXCL9, CXCL10, CCL17, and CCL22 exhibit maximal polyclonally stimulated responses at 1–3 d and Ag-specific responses at ~5 d of culture (*see* **Note 1**).

Supernatants are harvested and stored at −20°C until chemokine concentrations are quantified as described below.

3.2. Analysis of Human Chemokine Levels

1. The ELISA plate is coated with 50 µL/well capture antibody in a high pH coating buffer at a predetermined optimal concentration. This is generally between 50 ng/mL and 2 µg/mL (*see* **Note 2**). For maximum sensitivity, this incubation is carried out overnight at 4°C in tightly wrapped plates that are kept in a plastic box lined with wet paper towels, to minimize evaporation that would lead to variability in edge wells (*see* **Note 3**).
2. Blocking, using 75 µL/well, is carried out at 37°C for 1–3 h (*see* **Note 4**). We find no difference in background between these times. This time period is used to prepare samples for the next step. Wash four times manually or using plate washer. Afterwards, bang plate dry three times on paper towels.
3. The standard curve is generated on each assay plate using recombinant chemokine standard in dilution buffer (*see* **Note 5**). The titration range is determined by the anticipated intensity of one's experimental values. Commonly, titration curves run from 2000 to 15 pg/mL.

4. Each experimental sample should be titrated in dilution buffer from an empirically determined starting dilution (typically between 1:5 and 1:20) for a series of four twofold 50-μL dilutions running down the plate (i.e., 1:2, 1:4, 1:8, 1:16) (*see* **Note 6**). This allows ~20 samples per plate. The initial dilutions should not sit in the starting well for more than 5 min before carrying out this titration or the resulting curves will not be linear.

5. Sample incubation can be 3 h at 37°C or overnight at 4°C. Maximal sensitivity is obtained following overnight incubation. Wash four times, then bang plates dry on paper towels.

6. Biotinylated development antibody in dilution buffer is added at a predetermined optimal concentration, generally between 50 ng/mL and 2 μg/mL, using 50 μL/well. Incubation can be 3 h at 37°C or overnight at 4°C. Maximal sensitivity is obtained following overnight incubation. Wash plates four times, then bang dry on paper towels.

7. Following washing, streptavidin–enzyme conjugate is added at a predetermined optimal concentration to maximize signal while minimizing background. In our experience, streptavidin-alkaline phosphatase used at 1:1000 to 1:5000 with 50 μL/well is useful. This incubation (45 min at 37°C) is followed by washing four times, banging dry, then adding 50 μL/well PNPP solution. This should be prepared no more than 30 min before use by adding one PNPP tablet to 5 mL of substrate buffer at room temperature (Sigma #S0942-200TAB).

8. Progress of the assay is monitored visually, with readings (405–690 nm) taken at intervals between 45 min and 6 h of assay development, depending on the sensitivity required. Running this phase of the assay at 37°C accelerates color development by ~40%. The standard curve should have an absorbance beginning from approximately 3.0 OD to obtain maximal sensitivity and precision.

9. A standard curve is prepared using the data obtained by serial dilution of the standard, with the chemokine concentration on the x axis (log) and the absorbance on the y axis (linear) to generate a sigmoidal curve.

When carrying out sample data analysis, the mean of at least two points (and generally three or four) falling on the linear component of the standard curve of that plate is required. These calculated values should not differ from one another by more than ~15–20%, typically much less. Mean values + standard error should be reported. Interassay variability (the same samples titrated in an independent assay on another day) should be explicitly determined for a proportion of the samples to confirm reliability of the data/operator/assay. Sensitivity is defined in each assay as the beginning of the linear portion of the titration curve (*see* **Note 7**).

The relationship between expression of the chemokines discussed below and specific immune responses is a rapidly developing field and should be considered in light of recent literature. At present, CXCL9 and CXCL10 are considered associated with expression of Th1-like immunity (along with receptors CCR5 and CXCR3); CCL17 and CCL22 with Th2-like responses (along with receptors CCR3, CCR4, CCR8); and CCL2, CCL17, and CCR21 with cells exhibiting regulatory T-cell-like activity. This list is not exhaustive, nor is expression of these ligands solely restricted to expression of that specific form of immunity.

Sample data for representative antigen-dependent chemokine responses to exogenous and endogenous Ags are provided in Fig. 1A,B respectively.

3.3. Detailed ELISA Protocols

3.3.1. CCL2 (MCP-1)

1. Following the protocol for ultrasensitive ELISA (*see* **Section 3.2.**), use the capture antibody, polyclonal anti-human MCP-1, at 1 µg/mL (either Peprotech or BD).
2. For the standard, use human rMCP-1 and titrate in eight twofold dilutions from 4000 to 31.3 pg/mL.
   Carry out a titration curve of antigen or polyclonally stimulated samples four times starting from 1/50 (i.e., 1/50, 1/100, 1/200, 1/400).
3. Use the detection antibody, biotinylated mouse polyclonal anti-human MCP-1, 50 ng/mL (Peprotech) or 250 ng/mL (BD).
4. Read plate after 3 h with development substrate. Sensitivity should be at least 31 pg/mL.

3.3.2. CCL3 (MIP-1α)

1. Following the protocol for ultrasensitive ELISA (*see* **Section 3.2.**), use the capture antibody, polyclonal anti-human MIP-1α, at 350 ng/mL.
2. For the standard, use human recombinant MIP-1α and titrate from 4000 to 31.25 pg/mL.
3. Dilute antigen and polyclonally driven samples 1/10.
4. Use the detection antibody, biotinylated goat anti-human MIP-1α, at 15 ng/mL.
5. Read plate after 5–6 h with substrate for sensitivity of 31.3 pg/mL.

3.3.3. CCL17 (TARC)

1. Following the protocol for ultrasensitive ELISA (*see* **Section 3.2.**), use the capture antibody, polyclonal anti-human TARC, at 250 ng/mL (Peprotech or R&D Systems).
2. For the standard, use human recombinant TARC and titrate from 500 to 3.9 pg/mL.
3. Dilute antigen and polyclonally driven samples 1/10.
4. Use the detection antibody, biotinylated goat anti-human TARC, at 50 ng/mL (R&D Systems or Peprotech).
5. Read plate after 3 h with substrate for sensitivity of 3.9 pg/mL.

3.3.4. CCL22 (MDC)

1. Following the protocol for ultrasensitive ELISA (*see* **Section 3.2.**), use the capture antibody, polyclonal anti-human MDC, at 0.1 µg/mL (Peprotech) or 0.5 µg/mL (R&D Systems).

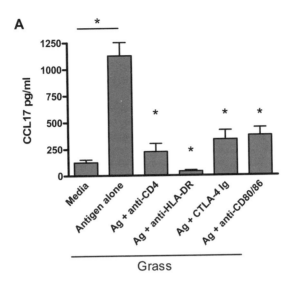

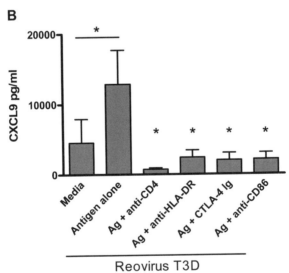

Fig. 1. (A) Antigen-driven chemokine production is CD4 T-cell dependent, requires CD28:CD80/86 costimulation and MHC class II dependent Ag-presentation. Freshly derived PBMC from 10 and **(B)** 5 adult volunteers were cultured 5 d as described, with grass pollen Ag at 50 μg/mL **(A)** or reovirus T3D (2×10^6 pfu/well) either alone, or in the presence of anti-CD4 (BD Pharmingen 2 μg/mL), anti-HLA-DR(2 μg/mL), anti-CD80 or anti-CD86 (1 μg/mL) or CTLA4-Ig (5 μg/mL). Chemokine responses were assessed by ELISA as described above. Significance was determined using a paired t-test (*$p < 0.01$).

2. For the standard, use human recombinant MDC and titrate from 1000 to 7.8 pg/mL.
3. Dilute antigen and polyclonally driven samples 1/10.
4. Use the detection antibody, biotinylated chicken anti-human MDC, at 20 ng/mL (R&D Systems or Peprotech).
5. Read plate after 1 h with substrate for sensitivity of 7.8 pg/mL.

3.3.5. CXCL9 (MIG)

1. Following the protocol for ultrasensitive ELISA (*see* **Section 3.2.**), use the capture antibody, polyclonal anti-human MIG, at 200 ng/mL (Peprotech) or 0.350 ng/mL (R&D Systems).
2. For the standard, use human recombinant MIG and titrate from 4000 to 31.25 pg/mL.
3. Dilute antigen and polyclonally driven samples 1/10.
4. Use the detection antibody, biotinylated goat anti-human MIG, at 15 ng/mL (R&D Systems or Peprotech).
5. Read plate after 3–5 h with substrate for sensitivity of 31.25 pg/mL.

3.3.6. CXCL10 (IP-10)

1. Following the protocol for ultrasensitive ELISA (*see* **Section 3.2.**), use the capture antibody, mouse anti-human IP-10, at 50 ng/mL (Peprotech) or 400 ng/mL (BD).
2. For the standard, use human recombinant IP-10 and titrate from 1000 to 7.8 pg/mL.
3. Dilute antigen and polyclonally driven samples 1/10.
4. Use the detection antibody, biotinylated goat anti-human IP-10, at 25 ng/mL (Peprotech) or 50 ng/mL (BD).
5. Read plate after 3–4 h with substrate for sensitivity of 7.8 pg/mL.

3.3.7. CCL11 (Eotaxin)

1. Following the protocol for ultrasensitive ELISA (*see* **Section 3.2.**), use the capture antibody, mouse anti-human Eotaxin, at 350 ng/mL.
2. For the standard, use human recombinant Eotaxin and titrate from 500 to 3.9 pg/mL.
3. Dilute plasma samples 1/4.
4. Use the detection antibody, biotinylated goat anti-human Eotaxin, at 50 ng/mL.
5. Read plate after 3 h with substrate for sensitivity of 3.9 pg/mL.

4. Notes

1. It is important to assess the levels of endotoxin contamination in the antigen preparation used. Some have very low levels whereas others (i.e., some commercial preparations used clinically for skin testing) have levels sufficient to elicit strong Ag-nonspecific chemokine production from mononuclear cells. To determine the extent to which chemokine production reflects Ag-specific induction, parallel cultures should be carried out incorporating validated inhibitors of classical T-cell activation (i.e., anti-CD4, anti-CD8 mAb, CTLA4-Ig). In our hands, use of these reagents reduces chemokine production to <10% of that seen in Ag-stimulated controls, indicating that the chemokine production quantified is truly Ag dependent.

2. A variety of high-binding EIA plates are commercially available. We have found substantial differences in their ability to bind capture antibody or Ag. Costar 3369 plates work effectively.

3. Spurious values that are too high and do not agree with the rest of the titration curve result from evaporation in wells at the edge of the plate. The solution is to ensure that plates are kept tightly wrapped in a humidified chamber (plastic box with wet paper towels) for all incubations. Also, if samples are allowed to sit in plate for an extended period prior to carrying out the dilutions, substantial chemokine will be bound, resulting in a nonlinear titration curve.

4. A broad variety of blocking reagents (skimmed milk, bovine serum albumin (BSA), or gelatin) can be used. Recommended wash buffers sometimes utilize very high concentrations of BSA and Tween-20. In our experience, BSA at 0.17% (1.7 g/L) in PBS with 0.05% Tween-20 is sufficient to minimize backgrounds with less cost and pollution of the environment than buffers containing up to 5% BSA and 2% Tween-20.

5. Biological standards are calibrated in units of biological activity and usually established by consensus following exhaustive collaborative studies involving many laboratories. For cytokines, international standards should be used to provide a common currency against which all results can be evaluated. When estimating the biological activity of different preparations with different specific activities by bioassay, mass units are not useful as different commercial preparations vary widely in specific activity. Unfortunately, there are currently no international standards available for chemokines, so most laboratories report their data in mass units. Many laboratories choose to utilize recombinant standards from well-known manufacturers (i.e., Peprotech, BD Pharmingen, R&D Systems) and express their data in mass units as measured against that commercial preparation (and that lot). This makes possible comparison between experimental groups, but greatly complicates comparisons between laboratories.

6. If experimental values for a given sample do not agree throughout the titration range, it is possible that the dilution series selected does not fall within the linear range of the assay. The starting titration of the samples needs to be adjusted so that more of the points lie on the linear component of the standard curve. The most common reason for duplicates which do not agree is poor titration precision/ operator error.

7. When assay sensitivity is not sufficient, the first step is to compare the sensitivity of the standard curve generated with those seen in the literature or those listed above. Assuming one obtains similar sensitivity, an estimate of the levels expected in your samples is required. Most chemokines are produced at substantial levels but some (i.e., Eotaxin) are not seen on stimulation of PBMC. A few additional strategies are useful to further enhance sensitivity. The assays described above are configured using minimum concentrations of these reagents in order to minimize cost. Use of higher concentrations of capture and development reagents often increases sensitivity by one or twofold. Similarly, there is a linear relationship between how long an ELISA is allowed to develop and the sensitivity of that assay.

Thus, chemokines such as CCL2 are rapidly produced at high concentrations (ng/mL levels) following stimulation with recall antigens, whereas chemokines such as CXCL10 or CCL17 are more tightly regulated. For chemokines produced at levels where sensitivity is a major issue, the assay is allowed to develop for up to 6 h. In all cases, the greater the difference between the absorbance of the maximum concentration of the standard and the background (all reagents except the recombinant chemokine standard), the better the precision of the assay.

12

Standardization of Allergen Extracts

Jørgen Nedergaard Larsen and Sten Dreborg

Abstract

Allergens are molecules with the capacity to elicit IgE responses in humans. When stimulated with allergens, most allergic patients respond with production of IgE specific for several proteins/allergens in the source material. The standardization of allergen extracts is essential in order to control variability and to achieve consistency and reproducibility in a clinical setting.

Because the IgE binding capacity of an allergen extract is related to the content of one or a few major allergens, it is important that the standardization procedure ensures consistency, not only in the overall IgE binding potency, but also in the content and ratio of individual major allergens. Owing to the complexity of allergen extracts, a key element in standardization of allergen extracts is the use of standards.

This chapter describes the principles for standardization of allergen extracts to be used by research laboratories. Other chapters in this volume describe methods in detail.

Key Words: Allergen; extracts; standardization; in vitro; in vivo.

1. Introduction

Allergen extracts are used for diagnosis and treatment of allergic diseases. In the manufacture of allergen extracts, it is essential to apply standardization in order to control the variability in naturally occurring source materials and achieve consistency and reproducibility for optimal safety and efficacy in clinical use. In the widest sense, standardization includes controlling the entire production chain of processes including qualifications of collectors of raw materials, establishment of robust and reproducible manufacturing procedures in compliance with 'good manufacturing practice' (GMP) regulations, and formulation of allergen extracts intended for clinical use in allergy diagnosis, in vivo as well as in vitro, and in allergen immunotherapy/vaccination. Standardization, however, is not a precisely defined term, as different qualities of

From: *Methods in Molecular Medicine: Allergy Methods and Protocols*
Edited by: M. G. Jones and P. Lympany © Humana Press Inc., Totowa, NJ

standardization are in current use by various laboratories and manufacturers of allergen extracts.

Allergens are molecules with the capacity to elicit IgE responses in humans. Inhalant allergens are proteins, readily soluble in water, and present in airborne particles. The particles carrying allergens are inhaled and deposited on the mucosal surfaces stimulating immunocompetent cells associated with the airway mucosa. When stimulated with low doses of allergens, most allergic patients respond with production of IgE specific for several proteins/allergens in the source material. A limited number of allergens, 'major' allergens *(1)*, stimulate IgE production in a majority of patients; however, any antigen in a given source material has the potential to elicit an IgE response. It is therefore important to ensure that all protein antigens/allergens in the allergenic source material, to which humans are exposed, are contained in the raw material. Because the IgE binding capacity of an allergen extract is related to the content of one or a few major allergens, it is also important that the standardization procedure ensures consistency, not only in the overall IgE binding potency, but also in the content and ratio of individual major allergens.

Owing to the complexity of allergen extracts, a key element in standardization of allergen extracts is the use of standards *(2)*. In Europe, each laboratory and manufacturer establishes In-House Reference (IHR) preparations for each source material. The IHR must be thoroughly characterized by in vitro methods as a basis for equilibration of subsequent batches, and the biological activity in humans should also be determined by in vivo methods. The IHR eliminates the need for in vivo methods in batch-to-batch standardization, which can be performed by comparing each and every new batch to the IHR using in vitro methods exclusively. Comparison of individual activities of different IHR preparations can be performed by use of International Standards (IS).

This chapter describes the principles for standardization of allergen extracts to be used by research laboratories. Other chapters in this volume describe methods in detail.

2. Materials

2.1. Selection of Source Materials

Inhalant allergens are present in airborne particles derived from natural allergen sources. These particles constitute the material to which humans are exposed, and the aim of raw material selection is to provide materials containing the same active allergens in a manageable form. In most cases, the optimal source material is rather obvious, but in some cases the allergen source is still debated (e.g., cat saliva/pelt/dander or mouse urine/dander).

The source materials should be selected with attention to the need for specificity and for inclusion of all relevant allergens in sufficient amounts *(2)*.

The collection of the source materials should be performed by qualified persons, and reasonable measures must be employed to assure that collector qualifications and collection procedures are appropriate to verify the identity and quality of the source materials. This means that only specifically identified allergenic source materials that do not contain avoidable foreign substances should be used in the manufacture of allergenic extracts. Means of identification and limits of foreign materials should meet established acceptance criteria for each source material. Where identity and purity cannot be determined by direct examination of the source materials, other appropriate methods should be applied to trace the materials from their origin. This includes complete identity labeling and certification from competent collectors. The processing and storage of source materials should be performed to ensure that no unintended substances, including microbial organisms, are introduced into the materials. When possible, source materials should be fresh or stored in a manner that minimizes or prevents decomposition. Records should describe source materials in as much detail as possible, including the particulars of collection, pretreatment, and storage.

2.2. Specific Aspects of Source Materials

Specific aspects of the most important raw material categories are briefly discussed below.

2.2.1. Pollens

The natural sources of inhalant allergens from plants are the pollens. Pollen may be obtained either by collection in nature or from cultivated fields or greenhouses. The collection may be performed by several methods, such as vacuuming or drying flower heads followed by grinding. The pollen may be cleaned either by passing through sieves of different mesh sizes or by flotation. Finally, pollens are dried under controlled conditions and stored in sealed containers at −20°C. The maximum level of accepted contamination with pollen from other species is 1% by number. Pollen should be devoid of flower and plant debris, with a limit of 5% by weight. Pollens may show large variation in quantitative composition depending on season and location of growth, and in order to achieve a relatively constant composition, harvests from different years and sites of collection should, after thorough characterization in vitro, be pooled for the production of allergen extracts.

2.2.2. Acarids

House dust mites are grown in pure cultures. Source materials are either pure mite bodies (PMB) or whole mite cultures (WMC). Extracts based on WMC include material from mite bodies, eggs, larvae, and fecal particles as well as mite decomposition material and contain all the material to which a mite-allergic patient is exposed under natural conditions. The culture medium should ideally be antigen free, or contaminants from the culture medium should be shown not to be allergenic. The PMB extract avoids extensive contamination with debris from the culture medium. Clinical trials comparing vaccines based on WMC and PMB extracts have shown similar clinical efficacy in specific allergy vaccination *(3)*.

2.2.3. Mammals

Allergens of mammalian origin may be present in various sources (e.g., dander, serum, saliva, or urine). The allergens to which humans are exposed depend on the normal behavior of the animal and, therefore, cannot be generalized. In each case, the optimal source or mix of sources of allergens from mammals should be thoroughly investigated using a large panel of sera from allergic patients. Whether derived from dander or deposited from body fluids, most allergens are present in the pelt. Source materials should be collected only from animals that are declared healthy by a veterinarian at the time of collection. When animals that are killed are used, the conditions for storing should minimize postmortem decomposition until the source materials can be collected. The optimal source materials are often dander, because hair proteins are insoluble. Use of whole pelt would increase the proportion of serum proteins, which are generally of low allergenic activity.

Because of the quantitative differences in the yield of the various allergens from different dog breeds *(4)*, a mixture of material from different breeds should be selected representing a balanced content of the major allergens *(5)*.

2.2.4. Insects

The optimal source for insect allergens is dependent on the natural route of exposure (i.e., inhalation, bite, or sting). Where whole insects or insect debris are inhaled, the whole insect body is selected as allergen source. In the case of biting or stinging insects, saliva or venom, respectively, is the proper allergen source.

2.2.5. Fungi

Moulds should be grown under controlled conditions. The harvested raw materials should consist of mycelia and spores. Owing to difficulties in maintaining a constant composition of fungal cultures, it is recommended that extracts should be derived from several independent cultures of the same species. The primary inoculum should be obtained from established fungal culture banks, i.e., American Type Culture Collection (ATCC, http://www.atcc.org/) or Central Bureau Schimmelcultures (CBS, http://www.cbs.knaw.nl/), and the following batches should be derived from the same strain to secure a constant composition, which may vary even under seemingly similar growth conditions *(6,7)*. The cultivation medium should be synthetic or at least devoid of allergenic constituents (i.e., proteins). Culturing should be conducted under aseptic conditions to reduce the risk of contamination by micro-organisms or other fungi, and controls must include tests for suspected toxins.

2.2.6. Foods

Foods constitute a diversified area, and the supply of standardized allergen extracts is scarce. Foods are often derived from various subspecies, grown under a broad variety of conditions reflecting geographical variation. In addition, foods are often cooked prior to ingestion, and the cooking procedures may differ geographically. Consequently, the source of allergen exposure, qualitative as well as quantitative, is highly variable *(8)*.

Ideally, source materials for food allergen extracts should reflect local subspecies, conditions, and habits for the cultivation, harvesting, storing, and cooking of the foods. However, ingested foods are increasingly derived from distant parts of the world. The best solution to these problems may be to combine materials from as many sources as possible, reflecting variation in as many parameters as possible.

The difficulties in producing consistent and reproducible food allergen extracts have resulted in many clinicians using untreated foods from retail trade for diagnosis by the prick–prick method *(9)*. Examples are fresh fruit, cow's milk, and hen's egg. Undiluted cow's milk and hen's egg have the best documented diagnostic properties *(10)*.

A further problem in food allergen extract production is the presence in many foods of natural or microbial toxins, pesticides, antibiotics, preservatives, and other additives that may be concentrated in the manufacturing process. The use of organic source material should therefore be preferred.

3. Methods

3.1. Preparation of Allergen Extracts

Allergen–IgE binding involves the interaction of molecular surfaces of allergens and IgE antibodies having contours exactly fitting each other *(11)*. Because the structure of the molecular surface of the allergen and thus the IgE binding epitopes are vulnerable to protein denaturation, procedures used for the preparation and storage of allergen extracts/vaccines should avoid organic solvents, elevated temperatures, and extreme pH and ionic conditions. The extraction should be performed under conditions resembling the physiological conditions in the human airways (i.e., pH and ionic strength) and suppressing possible proteolytic degradation and microbial growth *(12)*. The optimal extraction time is always a compromise between yield and degradation/denaturation of the allergens, and special attention should be drawn to the fact that different allergens are released with different kinetics *(13)*. In general, processing time should be minimized and extraction performed at low temperatures.

Low molecular weight, i.e., below 5000 Da, non-antigenic material should be removed from the extract by dialysis, ultra-filtration, or size exclusion chromatography. Any substance excluded from the final product should be shown to be nonallergenic. The production procedure should include procedures to measure and exclude below-defined thresholds for known toxins, viral particles, and free histamine or other physiologically active substances.

The final extract should be stored under conditions that impede deterioration of the allergenic activity either by lyophilizing the extract or by storage at low temperatures (i.e., $-20°C$ to $-80°C$), possibly in the presence of stabilizing agents, such as 50% glycerol, non-allergenic proteins (e.g., certified human serum albumin), or other stabilizers.

3.2. IHR Preparations and Standards

3.2.1. IHR Preparations

A particularly important aspect of the standardization procedure is the IHR. In Europe, the IHR is prepared by the individual laboratory or manufacturer, whereas in the United States, the US Food and Drug Administration (FDA) authorizes general standards of some common allergens for the purpose. The IHR is used by manufacturers/laboratories for equilibration of the potency and composition of each batch of manufactured extract *(14,15)*. By this procedure the batch-to-batch standardization can be performed by comparison to the IHR using in vitro techniques exclusively, and unethical use of in vivo methods can be avoided. The establishment of an IHR and subsequent production of new batches related to the IHR is illustrated in **Fig. 1**.

When a robust extraction procedure has been defined, three batches of the extract should be produced in order to verify consistency and reproducibility of the production processes. The three batches are compared, and if consistency is achieved one is selected to represent the new IHR, which is subsequently dispended into freeze-dried aliquots of suitable size. The IHR should be carefully defined including assessment of dry weight, protein content and composition, major allergen content, and total allergenic activity by in vivo and in vitro methods (**Fig. 1**). The dispensing into aliquots can be based on dry weight, as other methods are less precise, e.g., protein by Lowry, or too expensive for routine use, e.g., automated amino acid analysis.

The determination of total allergenic activity by in vivo methods, most often by skin prick testing (SPT) *(16)*, is not only laborious but also unethical to perform more than occasionally. Because the biological activity has been shown to correlate with the major allergen content *(17)*, the use of major allergen determination with a validated assay is sufficient in combination with a specific

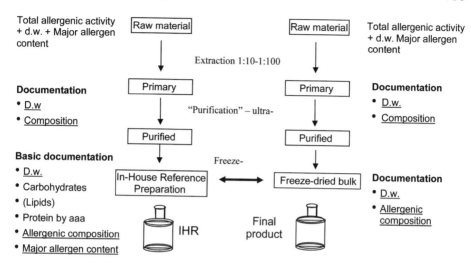

Fig. 1. Standardization of allergen extracts. The principle for establishment of an In House Reference (IHR) preparation to the left and standardization of subsequent batches, calibrated against the IHR. Different methods can be applied to determine the total allergenic activity in vitro and in vivo, major allergen content, and the allergenic composition.

IgE potency assay. If in vitro methods alone are used for the establishment of the potency of the IHR, comparison is best made with the IS.

3.2.2. International Standards

Allergen extract standardization ideally requires use of two types of standards for each source material, an IHR preparation as described above and an IS. IS of allergen extracts are obtainable from the National Institute of Biological Science and Control, NIBSC, London, United Kingdom, and were produced under the auspices of the WHO according to guidelines established by the Allergen Standardization Sub-Committee under the International Union of Immunological Societies (IUIS). IS enable comparison of specific activities of products from different manufacturers and can be used as calibrators by new producers and laboratories.

IS are available for the following allergen extracts: *Ambrosia artemisiifolia* (short ragweed) *(18)*, *Phleum pratense* (timothy grass) *(19)*, the house dust mite *Dermatophagoides pteronyssinus (20)*, *Betula verrucosa* (birch) *(21)*, and *Canis familiaris* (dog) *(22)*. Additional standards were planned for the mould *Alternaria alternata (23)*, for the grasses *Cynodon dactylon* (Bermuda grass) *(24)*, and *Lolium perenne* (rye grass) *(25)*, *Felis domesticus* (cat), and the house dust mite *Dermatophagoides farinae*, but unfortunately this initiative has stopped prematurely because of lack of general acceptance.

3.3. Units and Measure

The strength or potency of an allergen extract relies on the magnitude of the response it will elicit in human allergic subjects. Allergic patients respond individually to allergen extracts because they are sensitized to different allergens and the degree of sensitivity differs from patient to patient as well as for each allergen in the extract. Because allergen extracts from different producers differ in composition there is no straightforward relationship between potency and response when considering allergen extracts from different manufacturers. This paradox poses an inherent problem in the labeling of allergen extracts, as the potency of different extracts cannot be compared in a meaningful manner.

Direct skin testing of human allergic subjects is the predominant in vivo method for the assessment of allergen extract potency *(26)* and also constitutes the principle underlying the establishment of biological units of allergen extract potency. Patient selection criteria are obviously important, as all potency measures will be dependent on the patient panel. Several units are in use.

In Europe, SPT has been used for estimating the biological activity of allergen extracts. The aim is to equilibrate the potency between extracts of different inhalant allergen extracts *(27)*. At least 20 consecutive patients attending a specialist clinic should be included. The concentration inducing a weal of the same size as that of histamine dihydrochloride, 10 mg/mL, is estimated by parallel line bioassay. The median concentration constitutes 10,000 biological units (BU) *(28)*. This method was adopted by the Nordic Council on Medicines as the Nordic Biological Unit, HEP *(29)*. With proper patient selection the unit has been shown to be reproducible between different regions of Europe *(28)*. European manufacturers use their own company-specific units, most of which are based on the same method *(30)*.

In the United States, the FDA uses a unit based on intradermal testing with the allergen extract and subsequent measurement of the flare rather than the weal size. The 'intradermal end point' is expressed as the number of threefold dilutions producing a summed erythema diameter of 50 mm. The mean value of 15 individuals defines the potency of the allergen extract, which is expressed in 'allergy units' (AU). More recently the CBER in the United States proposed the 'bioequivalent allergy unit' (BAU). The method for assigning BAU is named the ID50EAL method, i.e., 'intradermal dilution for 50 mm sum of erythema diameters determines bioequivalent allergy units' *(31)*.

Labeling of the potency of allergen extracts based on the microgram amount or, more correctly, the millimolar concentration of major allergen has been proposed, as the major allergen content correlates with the biological activity *(17)*. Using the same antibodies, IHR and methodology, and with similar extract composition, determination of major allergen content can replace other methods for potency declaration. However, in most cases the composition of test materials and the specificity of anti-allergen antibodies vary between laboratories and the content of a single major allergen does not allow comparison of overall potency between marketed allergen extracts from different companies.

3.4. Stability Testing

Criteria, methods, and limits for stability should be established. In Europe, a total allergenic activity in the interval between 30 and 300% of the IHR is accepted, whereas the US authorities use limits of 50–200% of the labeled activity. Methods used to assess the potency should have a demonstrated higher precision, which is not always trivial. The reference should be the IHR stored at −70°C or lower. For stability assessment the extract should be stored at several different temperatures to assure safe storage at room temperature, in a refrigerator, and at −20°C. Accelerated degradation studies designed to measure the kinetics of breakdown of the allergen extract can be performed by incubation at multiple high temperatures.

3.5. Batch-to-Batch Control

Having established an IHR preparation, batch-to-batch standardization is performed by calibrating new freeze-dried batches in bulk with the IHR before dispensing into vials for distribution. Batch-to-batch standardization includes, apart from determination of dry weight, three steps:

1. Assessment of allergenic composition to ensure the presence in the final product of all allergens present in the source material. Techniques used include crossed (radio)-immunoelectrophoresis (CIE/CRIE)*(32)*, sodium dodecyl-sulfate polyacrylamide gel electrophoresis (SDS-PAGE)*(33)*, and immunoblotting *(34)*, as well as isoelectric focusing (IEF)*(35)*. CIE has the advantage of being a semiquantitative technique, and a reproducible precipitation pattern will ensure constant ratios between all major antigenic components.
2. Quantification of specific major allergens to ensure that essential allergens are present in constant ratios. Techniques used include quantitative immunoelectro-phoresis (QIE)*(32)* and enzyme-linked immunosorbent assay (ELISA)*(36)*.
3. Quantification of the total allergenic activity to ensure that the overall potency of the extract is constant. Techniques used include several variations of the radio-allergosorbent test (RAST)*(37)* and RAST inhibition assays.

In batch-to-batch standardization, in vitro laboratory techniques are used to compare individual batches to the IHR, which should be matched in every aspect, *see* **Fig. 2**.

3.6. Conclusion

Allergen extracts are complex mixtures derived from natural source materials and as such prone to natural variation. Standardization is necessary to control

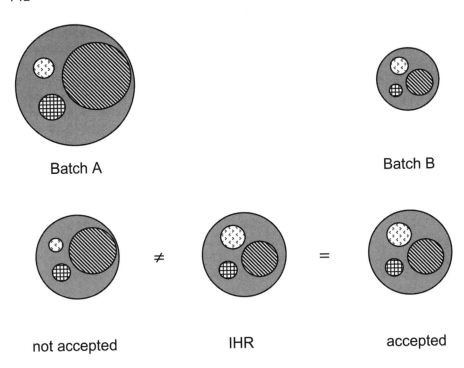

Fig. 2. Complexity of allergen extracts represented by a model with three major allergens. The area of shaded circles represents the relative potency of individual components. The area of outer circles represents the total allergenic potency of the extracts. The total allergenic potency of batches A and B may be adjusted by dilution or concentration, but still the composition of the extracts may vary stressing the importance of the measurement of individual components.

variation and ensure consistency and reproducibility for the safety and efficacy of specific allergy disease management. Batch-to-batch standardization is performed by comparison of new batches to established standards assessing complexity, major allergen content, and IgE binding.

3.7. Checklist for Standardization of Allergen Extracts

1. **Establish criteria for raw material quality**
   Criteria should define standard procedures for collection and storage of raw materials and thresholds for contamination with bacteria, viruses, and suspected toxins.
2. **Select supplier of raw materials**
   Suppliers of raw materials should document qualifications of experts, e.g., mycologists, acarocologists, and palynologists, and collection procedures to ensure optimal quality and absence of infectious particles.

3. **Select relevant raw materials**

   Source materials from different suppliers and different origin should ideally be included in initial screenings.

4. **Perform test extractions**

   Allergenic raw materials are complex. Empirical testing of the following parameters is essential: extraction buffer composition, time, and temperature.

5. **Remove low molecular weight components by dialysis or filtration**

   Excluded material should be verified to be non-allergenic in IgE binding assays.

6. **Establish criteria for batch-to-batch variability**

   Assess the robustness of the extraction procedure by performing three batches, and verify that the variability is below predefined limits.

7. **Define the IHR**

   The IHR should be characterized with respect to dry weight, allergen complexity, major allergen content, and IgE binding potency. Biologic activity should ideally be determined by skin testing.

8. **Assess stability of the IHR**

   Methods to be used and criteria for the precision of assays used for stability assessment should be established.

9. **Batch control**

   Production batches should be produced according to the established production processes, and the freeze-dried product should be calibrated to the IHR assessing complexity, major allergen content, and IgE binding.

References

1. King, T. P., Hoffman, D., Løwenstein, H., et al. (1994) Allergen nomenclature. WHO/IUIS Allergen Nomenclature Subcommittee. *Int. Arch. Allergy Immunol.* **105,** 224–233.

2. Løwenstein, H. (1987) Selection of reference preparation. IUIS reference preparation criteria. *Arb. Paul Ehrlich Inst.* **80,** 75–78.

3. Wahn, U., Schweter, C., Lind, P., and Løwenstein, H. (1988) Prospective study on immunologic changes induced by two different Dermatophagoides pteronyssinus extracts prepared from whole mite culture and mite bodies. *J. Allergy Clin. Immunol.* **82,** 360–370.

4. Lindgren, S., Belin, L., Dreborg, S., Einarsson, R., and Pahlman, I. (1988) Breed-specific dog-dandruff allergens. *J. Allergy Clin. Immunol.* **82,** 196–204.

5. Uhlin, T., Reuterby, J., and Einarsson, R. (1984) Antigenic/allergenic composition of Poodle/Alsatian dandruff extract. *Allergy* **39,** 125–133.

6. Steringer, I., Aukrust, L., and Einarsson, R. (1987) Variability of antigenicity/allergenicity in different strains of *Alternaria alternata*. *Int. Arch. Allergy Appl. Immunol.* **84,** 190–197.

7. Wallenbeck, I., Aukrust, L., and Einarsson, R. (1984) Antigenic variability of different strains of *Aspergillus fumigatus*. *Int. Arch. Allergy Appl. Immunol.* **73,** 166–172.

8. Lemanske, R. F. and Taylor, S. L. (1987) Standardized extracts, foods. *Clin. Rev. Allergy* **5,** 23–36.

9. Dreborg, S. and Foucard, T. (1983) Allergy to apple, carrot and potato in children with birch pollen allergy. *Allergy* **38,** 167–172.

10. Verstege, A., Mehl, A., Rolinck-Werninghaus, C., et al. (2005) The predictive value of the skin prick test weal size for the outcome of oral food challenges. *Clin. Exp. Allergy* **35,** 1220–1226.

11. Davies, D. R., Padlan, E. A., and Sheriff, S. (1990) Antibody–antigen complexes. *Annu. Rev. Biochem.* **59,** 439–473.

12. Løwenstein, H. and Marsh, D. G. (1981) Antigens of *Ambrosia elatior* (short ragweed) pollen. I. Crossed immunoelectrophoretic analyses. *J. Immunol.* **126,** 943–948.

13. Kauffman, H. F., van der Heide, S., van der Laan, S., Hovenga, H., Beaumont, F., and de Vries, K. (1985) Standardization of allergenic extracts of *Aspergillus fumigatus.* Liberation of IgE-binding components during cultivation. *Int. Arch. Allergy Appl. Immunol.* **76,** 168–173.

14. Løwenstein, H. (1980) Physico-chemical and immunochemical methods for the control of potency and quality of allergenic extracts. *Arb. Paul Ehrlich Inst.* **75,** 122–132.

15. Løwenstein, H. (1994) Methods used to develop standards. *Arb. Paul Ehrlich Inst.* **87,** 49–57.

16. Platts-Mills, T. A. and Chapman, M. D. (1991) Allergen standardization. *J. Allergy Clin. Immunol.* **87,** 621–625.

17. Dreborg, S. and Einarsson, R. (1992) The major allergen content of allergenic preparations reflect their biological activity. *Allergy* **47,** 418–423.

18. Helm, R. M., Gauerke, M. B., Baer, H., et al. (1984) Production and testing of an international reference standard of short ragweed pollen extract. *J. Allergy Clin. Immunol.* **73,** 790–800.

19. Gjesing, B., Jäger, L., Marsh, D. G., and Løwenstein, H. (1985) The international collaborative study establishing the first international standard for timothy (*Phleum pratense*) grass pollen allergenic extract. *J. Allergy Clin. Immunol.* **75,** 258–267.

20. Ford, A., Seagroatt, V., Platts-Mills, T. A. E., and Løwenstein, H. (1985) A collaborative study on the first international standard of *Dermatophagoides pteronyssinus* (house dust mite) extract. *J. Allergy Clin. Immunol.* **75,** 676–686.

21. Arntzen, F. C., Wilhelmsen, T. W., Løwenstein, H., et al. (1989) The international collaborative study on the first international standard of birch (*Betula verrucosa*) pollen extract. *J. Allergy Clin. Immunol.* **83,** 66–82.

22. Larsen, J. N., Ford, A., Gjesing, B., et al. (1988) The collaborative study of the international standard of dog, *Canis domesticus*, hair/dander extract. *J. Allergy Clin. Immunol.* **82,** 318–330.

23. Helm, R. M., Squillace, D. L., Yunginger, J. W., and members of the International Collaborative Trial (1988) Production of a proposed international reference standard *Alternaria* extract II. Results of a collaborative trial. *J. Allergy Clin. Immunol.* **81,** 651–663.

24. Baer, H., Anderson, M. C., Helm, R. M., et al. (1986) The preparation and testing of the proposed international reference (IRP) Bermuda grass (*Cynodon dactylon*)-pollen extract. *J. Allergy Clin. Immunol.* **78,** 624–631.

25. Stewart, G. A., Turner, K. J., Baldo, B. A., et al. (1988) Standardization of rye-grass pollen (*Lolium perenne*) extract. An immunochemical and physicochemical assessment of six candidate international reference preparations. *Int. Arch. Allergy Appl. Immunol.* **86,** 9–18.

26. Platts-Mills, T. A. E. and Chapman, M. D. (1991) Allergen standardization. *J. Allergy Clin. Immunol.* **87,** 621–625.

27. Aas, K., Backman, A., Belin, L., and Weeke, B. (1978) Standardization of allergen extracts with appropriate methods. The combined use of skin prick testing and radio-allergosorbent tests. *Allergy* **33,** 130–137.

28. Dreborg, S., Basomba, A., Belin, L., et al. (1987) Biological equilibration of allergen preparations: methodological aspects and reproducibility. *Clin. Allergy* **17,** 537–550.

29. Nordic Council on Medicines. (1989) Guidelines for registration and standardization of allergenic extracts. *NLN Publication* No **23,** 1–48.

30. Dreborg, S. and Frew, A. (1993) Standardization of allergenic preparations by *in vitro* and *in vivo* methods. *Allergy* **47**(Suppl. 14), 48–82.

31. Turkeltaub, P. C. (1987) Biological standardization based on quantitative skin testing – the ID50EAL method (intradermal dilution for 50 mm sum of erythema diameters determines the allergy unit). *Arb. Paul Ehrlich Inst.* **80,** 169–173.

32. Løwenstein, H. (1978) Quantitative immunoelectrophoretic methods as a tool for the analysis and isolation of allergens. *Prog. Allergy* **25,** 1.

33. Laemmli, U. K. (1970) Cleavage of structural proteins during the assembly of the head of bacteriophage T4. *Nature* **227,** 680–685.

34. Kyhse-Andersen, J. (1984) Electroblotting of multiple gels: a simple apparatus without buffer tank for rapid transfer of proteins from polyacrylamide to nitrocellulose. *J. Biochem. Biophys. Methods* **10,** 203–209.

35. Brighton, W. D. (1975) Profiles of allergen extract components by isoelectric focussing and radioimmunoassay. *Dev. Biol. Stand.* **29,** 362–369.

36. Engvall, E. and Perlmann, P. (1972) Enzyme-linked immunosorbent assay, ELISA. III. Quantitation of specific antibodies by enzyme-labelled anti-immunoglobulin in antigen-coated tubes. *J. Immunol.* **109,** 129–135.

37. Ceska, M., Eriksson, R., and Varga, J. M. (1972) Radioimmunosorbent assay of allergens. *J. Allergy Clin. Immunol.* **49,** 1–9.

13

Immunoelectrophoresis for the Characterization of Allergen Extracts

Gitte Nordskov Hansen and Jørgen Nedergaard Larsen

Abstract

Immunoelectrophoresis can be used for analysis of individual proteins in complex mixtures. The conditions involved in immunoelectrophoresis are mild, avoiding the risk of denaturation, and it is possible to perform relative quantification of individual components. The principle disadvantage is the dependence on rabbit antisera as reagents. The usefulness of immunoelectrophoresis in allergy research is greatly enhanced by the possibility of identification of allergens to which the individual in question has IgE.

The common principle is characterized by two independent electrophoreses having direction of current perpendicular to each other, i.e., crossed immunoelectrophoresis (CIE). This ultimately results in the formation of characteristic bell-shaped precipitates, each precipitate representing one antigen. There is a linear relationship between the amount of antigen and size of precipitate for a given antibody concentration for each precipitate and so relative quantification can be performed. The sensitivity and resolution power of CIE is very high and there are multiple variations of the technique, some of which will be illustrated in this chapter.

Key Words: Immunoelectrophoresis; crossed immunoelectrophoresis (CIE); allergen; IgE.

1. Introduction

Immunoelectrophoresis is the common name for a versatile family of electrophoretic precipitation-in-gel techniques which can be used for analysis of individual proteins in complex mixtures (1,2). Compared to similar techniques, the major advantages of immunoelectrophoresis are first that experimental conditions are mild avoiding the risk of denaturation, and secondly, the possibility of performing relative quantification of individual components. A disadvantage is the dependence on rabbit antisera as reagents.

From: *Methods in Molecular Medicine: Allergy Methods and Protocols*
Edited by: M. G. Jones and P. Lympany © Humana Press Inc., Totowa, NJ

The common principle is characterized by two independent electrophoreses having direction of current perpendicular to each other, i.e., crossed immuno-electrophoresis (CIE) (**Fig. 1a**). The first dimension electrophoresis is performed in an agarose gel at pH 8.6. Protein mixtures are separated into sharp bands according to a complex relation between mass and charge. In the second dimension electrophoresis, performed perpendicular to the first, the gel on both sides of the track of proteins resulting from the first dimension electrophoresis is replaced by a gel containing polyclonal rabbit antiserum. Again, the electrophoresis is performed at pH 8.6, at which pH the average charge of the antibody molecules is zero resulting in minimal mobility of the antibody molecules during electrophoresis. Formation of antigen–antibody complexes during second dimension electrophoresis will result in the formation of characteristic bell-shaped precipitates, each precipitate representing one antigen. The size of the precipitate will depend on the ratio between antigen and antibody as well as the average affinity of the interaction and is not a direct measure of antigen concentration. Relative quantification, however, can be performed, as there is a linear relationship between amount of antigen and size of precipitate for a given antibody concentration for each precipitate. This is a major advantage when applied in allergen extract standardization. Furthermore, the usefulness of immunoelectrophoresis in allergy research is greatly enhanced by the possibility of incubating the electrophoretic plate with allergic patients' serum IgE for simple and reliable identification of allergens to which the individual in question has IgE.

A major advantage of immunoelectrophoresis is the providing of a range of possibilities for immunochemical analyses of individual proteins directly in a complex protein mixture. Experiments are performed under mild conditions without increased risk of protein denaturation, an important aspect when studying allergen–IgE interactions. The sensitivity and resolution power of CIE is very high; at optimal conditions about 50 antigens may be distinguished on one immunoplate, and at least 20 antigens may be quantified. Furthermore, the ease of preparation and stability of immunoglobulins make rabbit antisera useful as reference reagents for the characterization of complex allergen extracts. The dependence on antiserum, however, may also represent a drawback. When used for assessment of allergen extract complexity and for identification of allergic reactivities, it is essential to perform additional experiments to verify that all relevant allergens are precipitated by the antiserum. A limitation of the technique is that protein antigens with p*I* near 8.6 are difficult to analyze. The buffer pH 8.6 cannot be changed without chemical modifications of the immunoglobulins (e.g., carbamylation).

Multiple variations of immunoelectrophoresis may be designed, some of which will be illustrated in this chapter.

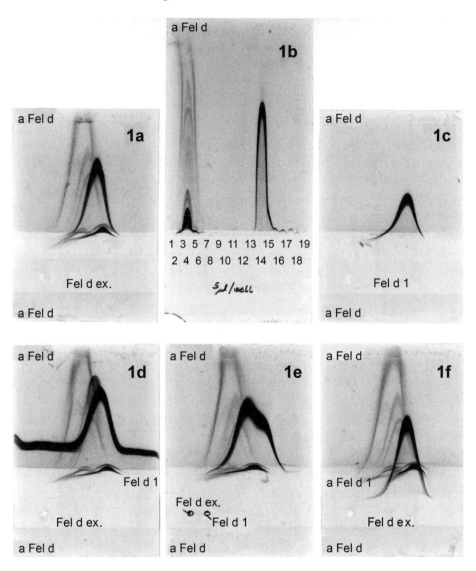

Fig. 1. Different types of immunoelectrophoresis of cat hair extract (Fel d) using a polyclonal rabbit antibody raised against the same extract (a Fel d). (**a**) CIE of Fel d extract, (**b**) FRIE following a purification (immunoabsorption) of the major allergen Fel d 1, (**c**) CIE of purified Fel d 1 against a Fel d, (**d**) CLIE with Fel d 1 in intermediate gel for identification of the allergen, (**e**) TCIE with Fel d extract and Fel d 1 showing a double peak, (**f**) CIIE with monospecific a Fel d 1 in intermediate gel.

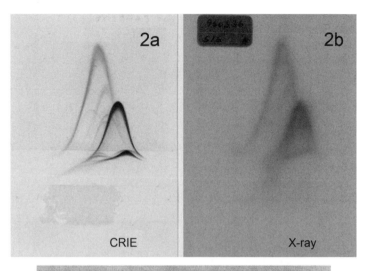

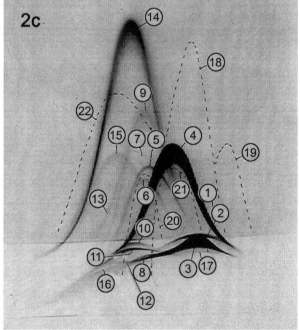

Fig. 2. (*Continued*)

Crossed radio-immunoelectrophoresis (CRIE, **Fig. 2a,b**) is used for the identification of allergens. The cold dried CIE plate is incubated with allergic patients' IgE and developed using radiolabeled anti-IgE and autoradiography. CRIE analyses of serum samples from several allergic patients may be used to

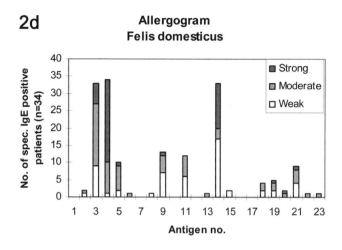

Fig. 2. CRIE and allergogram on Fel d extract. (**a** and **b**) Stained CRIE plate and corresponding X-ray print from a cat-allergic patient, (**c**) reference picture with numbered precipitates, (**d**) allergogram from CRIE investigation of 34 cat-allergic patients' sera.

construct an allergogram (**Fig. 2d**), a graphic representation of the relative importance of individual allergens.

Under carefully controlled experimental conditions the area delimited by the precipitate is proportional to the amount of antigen applied. Thus, quantitative immunoelectrophoresis (QIE, **Fig. 3c**) can be used for quantification of individual components in complex mixtures, for example, in batch-to-batch standardization. QIE is a method to quantify antigens without the need for monospecific antibodies.

A unique application is the use of fused rocket immunoelectrophoresis (FRIE, **Fig. 1b**) for the monitoring of a protein purification procedure. Aliquots of each fraction following a biochemical fractionation (e.g., a chromatographic step) are applied in wells in an agarose gel containing polyspecific rabbit antibody, and electrophoresis is performed in only fixed dimension. The wells are placed close together resulting in one large fused precipitate. Precipitates on the FRIE plate can be identified using crossed line immunoelectrophoresis (CLIE, **Fig. 1d**), in which an aliquot from the relevant fraction is added to an intermediate gel in a CIE design (**Fig. 1a**).

If only limited amount of material is available tandem crossed immuno-electrophoresis (TCIE, **Fig. 1e**) can be used as an alternative for this purpose. In TCIE, two wells about 0.75 cm apart are placed alongside in the first dimension gel; one well is filled with the reference extract and the other well with the sample to be analyzed. The precipitate formed by the antigen in the sample will make

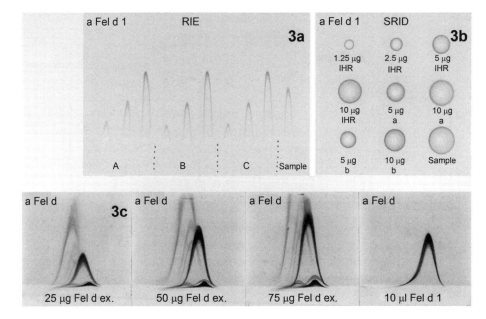

Fig. 3. Quantification methods using monospecific and polyspecific antibodies raised against Fel d 1 (**a** and **b**) and Fel d extract (c). (**a**) RIE of three dilutions of three Fel d batches and a sample, (**b**) SRID of four dilutions of in-house reference and different samples, (**c**) QIE of three concentrations of Fel d extract and a sample (Fel d 1).

a perfect fusion with the precipitate formed by the identical antigen in the reference extract resulting in a double peak. In addition, TCIE is ideal for the study of partial cross reactivity from which partially fused precipitates will result.

Having purified the protein antigen of interest, (**Fig. 1c**) enables the production of monospecific, polyclonal rabbit antibodies by repeated immunization using the purified antigen. The specificity of the monospecific antiserum can be analyzed in crossed intermediate gel immunoelectrophoresis (CIIE, **Fig. 1f**) in which the monospecific antiserum is placed in an intermediate gel in a CIE design. The precipitate resulting from the monospecific antiserum will precipitate in the intermediate gel.

The monospecific antiserum can furthermore be used for identification of the antigen in an unknown mixture by CIIE or for quantification by rocket immunoelectrophoresis (RIE, **Fig. 3a**) or single radial immunodiffusion (SRID, **Fig. 3b**). In RIE multiple samples can be quantified on the same plate, as only fixed dimension is performed, as mentioned for FRIE. In RIE, however, the wells are placed further apart so that individual samples can be analyzed separately. If the antigen has a high p*I* and the electrophoretic mobility is toward the cathode, quantification can be performed using passive diffusion, as in SRID. In both RIE and SRID the quantification is performed relative to an internal standard reference preparation applied as a dilution series on the same plate.

2. Materials
2.1. Equipment

Heated thermostat-controlled water bath 56–60°C.
Cooled thermostat-controlled water bath 15°C.
Electrophoresis apparatus (two buffer vessels, two electrodes, cooled surface, chamber).
Power supply.
Glass plates (std sizes, e.g., 5 ×5, 5 ×7, 10 ×7 cm).
Paper wicks: Whatman no. 1 filter paper, standard size: 21 ×10 cm.

2.2. Buffers and Solutions
2.2.1. Buffer for Electrode Vessels and Agarose Gel

5,5-Diethylbarbituric acid (Veronal)	Mw 184.20	112.1 g.
Tris (Sigma 7–9)	Mw 121.14	221.5 g.
Calcium lactate (purum)	Mw 308.30	2.7 g.

Milli Q H_2O to 5 L.
Dissolve overnight by stirring. Store at +5°C.
Dilute 1+4 before use to obtain ionic strength 0.02, pH 8.6.

2.2.2. Agarose Gel

1% (w/v) Litex Agarose type HSA ($M_r = -0.13$) in the above-mentioned buffer. The agarose is heated under stirring and boiled for 2 min and kept fluid in a water bath at +56°C.

2.2.3. Staining Solution

Coomassie Brilliant Blue R-250	5 g.
Ethanol 96%	450 mL.
Milli Q water	500 mL.
Glacial acidic acid	50 mL.

Dissolve overnight by stirring. After filtration the solution is ready for use.

2.2.4. Destaining Solution

Ethanol 96%	450 mL.
Milli Q water	500 mL.
Glacial acidic acid	50 mL.

2.2.5. Buffer for Incubation with Serum (CRIE)

1/15 M phosphate buffer pH 7.5.

Na$_2$HPO$_4$·12 H$_2$O   Mw 358.14   27.93 g.
KH$_2$PO$_4$ Mw 136.06   10.61 g.
NaN$_3$ Mw 65.02   2.0 g.
Milli Q H$_2$O to 2000 mL. Store at +5°C.

2.2.6. Buffer for Incubation with Isotope (CRIE)

1/15 M phosphate buffer pH 7.5, 1% (v/v) Tween 20.
Same as above with 1% (v/v) Tween 20 added.

2.2.7. Isotope for CRIE (αIgE*)

^{125}I-labeled anti-IgE: Blast Tracer from Bio-Line s.a., Brussels, Belgium.

2.2.8. Standard Developing and Fixing Solutions for Medical X-Ray Film Processing (e.g., AGFA G150 Developer and AGFA G354 Fixing Bath)

2.2.9. X-Ray Film (Kodak MXG) and X-Ray Cassette

3. Methods (see Notes 1 and 2)

3.1. CIE (Crossed Immunoelectrophoresis) (see Note 3)

3.1.1. First Dimension Electrophoresis (Fixed 1. Dimension)

1. Mark a 5 × 7 cm glass plate with identification numbers (e.g., year, month, and no.). Turn the plate upside down and clean with ethanol. Place it on a leveled surface and apply 5.3 mL of hot agarose.
2. After thorough setting, punch a well as indicated on the template (**Fig. 4a**) and apply antigen.
3. Place the glass plate on the cooled surface (approx. 15°C) of the electrophoresis apparatus, oriented as indicated in **Fig. 4a**. Connecting bridges of eight layers of paper wicks moistened with electrode buffer are established. The wicks should overlap the gel plate by approx. 0.5 cm.
4. Switch on the current and adjust the voltage across the gel to 10 V/cm. Continue electrophoresis for 25–30 min.

3.1.2. Second Dimension Electrophoresis

1. Cut away gel according to the template (**Fig. 4b**). Place the plate on the leveled surface.
2. Pour 1 mL agarose mixed thoroughly with the antibodies on the cathodic side of the first dimensional gel.
3. Pour 2 mL agarose mixed with antibodies on the anodic side of the first dimensional gel.
4. After thorough setting place the plate on the cooled surface of the electrophoresis apparatus and connect it to buffer reservoirs with five layers of paper wicks. The wicks should overlap the gel by approx. 0.5 cm.
5. Adjust the voltage to 2 V/cm. Place a glass plate on top of the wicks to avoid water to condense on the gel and perform electrophoresis overnight.

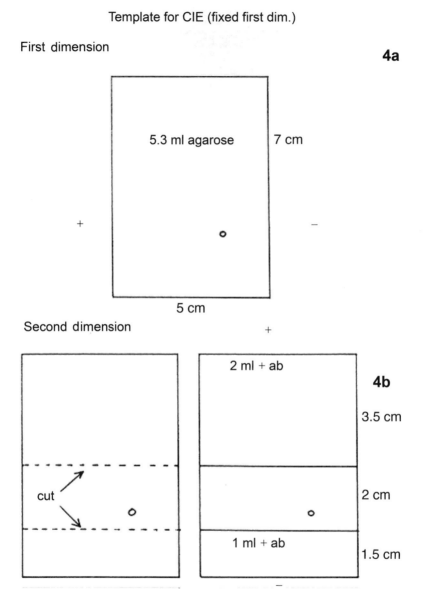

Fig. 4. Template for standard CIE indicating position of well, anode (+), and cathode (−) for the first dimension (**4a**) and dimensions of antibody containing gels for the second dimension (**4b**).

3.1.3. Pressing and Washing of the Plates (see **Note 4**)

1. Place the glass plates on a filter paper and fill all wells with distilled water (avoid air bubbles, which may cause rupture of the gel). Cover the gel with a wet filter paper (paper wick) and press the plates under several layers of filter paper (use large sheets, which can be air dried and reused), a thick glass plate, and a load of 3–4 kg.
2. Renew the upper layers of filter paper after 10 min and press again.
3. Transfer the plates to a container with excess 0.1 M NaCl for 15–30 min (washing) and press again as above.
4. Dry the plates in a stream of hot air.

3.1.4. Staining and Destaining (see **Note 5**)

1. Stain the plates for approx. 5 min in Commassie Brilliant Blue staining solution.
2. Immerse the plates for a few seconds in distilled water to remove a great deal of the surplus stain.
3. Destain the plates twice in successive baths until the optimal destaining is reached (approx. 15 min).
4. Dry the plate in hot air.
5. Turn gel-side down and write sample numbers and other information on the plate. Only write on the glass side.

3.2. Variations of CIE (see **Note 6**)

3.2.1. CLIE (Crossed Line Immunoelectrophoresis)

1. Run the one-dimensional electrophoresis as described in **Section 3.1.1**.
2. Cut and remove the intermediate gel (**Fig. 5**).
3. Pipet a sample of the protein to be investigated into a test tube and heat it in the water bath. Apply agarose to a total volume of 0.9 mL. Mix the gel and sample and pour it in the slit between the first dimension strip and the upper gel.
4. Allow the newly cast gel to settle before cutting and removing the anodic part of the gel. Apply the antibody-containing gels and run the electrophoresis as described in **Section 3.1.2**.

3.2.2. CIIE (Crossed Intermediate Gel Electrophoresis)

1. Run the one-dimensional electrophoresis as described in **Section 3.1.1**.
2. Cut and remove the intermediate gel (**Fig. 5**).
3. Pipet an antibody (polyclonal) into a test tube and heat it in the water bath. Apply agarose to a total volume of 0.9 mL. Mix the gel and antibody and pour it in the slit between the first dimension strip and the upper gel.
4. Allow the newly cast gel to settle before cutting and removing the anodic part of the gel. Apply the antibody-containing gels and run the electrophoresis as described in **Section 3.1.2**.

3.2.3. TCIE (Tandem Crossed Immunoelectrophoresis)

1. Cast a plate for the first dimension electrophoresis as described in **Section 3.1.1**.

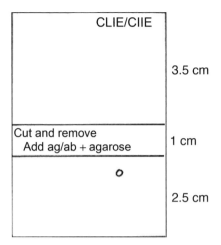

Fig. 5. Template for CLIE and CIIE indicating the position of the intermediate gel during second dimension electrophoresis.

2. Punch two wells alongside each other in the first dimension gel according to the template in **Fig. 6**.
3. Follow the instructions for CIE as described in **Section 3.1**.

3.3. Crossed Radio-Immunoelectrophoresis and Allergogram

3.3.1. CRIE (see **Note 7**)

1. Choose the optimized CIE standard conditions for the extract in question and perform one CIE for each serum sample to be tested.
2. After pressing and washing (*see* **Section 3.1.3.**) the plates are dried in a stream of *cold air*. This is important, as heat can denature the proteins, which may lead to loss of their biological activity.
3. To make reproducible results run all plates before serum incubation.

3.3.2. Incubations and Autoradiography

1. The plates are placed in small plastic boxes, which fit the size of the plate (5.3×7.3 cm) gel-side up, and incubated with a mixture of serum (200–500 µL) and 1/15 M phosphate buffer. Each plate should be totally submerged in a total volume of 8 mL. Before incubation each box is labeled with serum- or plate number. Incubate overnight at room temperature (RT) without stirring.
2. Wash each plate directly in the incubation box for 4×10 min with approx. 4×10 mL 0.9% NaCl.
3. Incubate with ^{125}I-labeled IgE overnight at RT. Use labeled IgE from Bio-Line s.a., 300,000 c.p.m./plate in a total volume of 8 mL 1/15 M phosphate buffer, 1% (v/v) Tween 20.

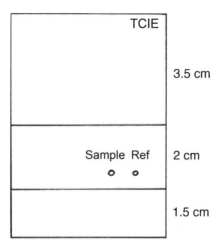

Fig. 6. Template for TCIE indication position of the two parallel wells for the first dimension electrophoresis.

4. Repeat the washing procedure (3×10 min. with NaCl, 1×10 min with distilled H_2O). Remove the plates from the individual boxes and dry them. Clean the glass side with ethanol and place in an X-ray cassette gel-side up. In a dark room place an X-ray film (Kodak MXB) on top of the plates and expose at $-80°C$ for 1, 3 and 10 days (a total of 14 days).

5. Following autoradiography all CIE plates are washed for approx. 10 min in distilled water, dried and stained (*see* **Section 3.1.4.**). Mark the position of the CRIE plates on the X-ray film with a pencil and label each autoradiography (well to the left) with plate no., serum ID, and exposure time, and cut the individual X-rays apart with scissors.

3.3.3. Standard Picture, Scoring and Allergogram

1. Choose one of the stained CIE plates and use it as the reference plate. Draw a standard picture. The precipitates are then numbered from right to left according to the peak of each precipitate (**Fig. 2c**).

2. A table with patient numbers and precipitate numbers are used to record the scorings. The stained CIE plate and the three corresponding autoradiograms from each patient are then, in sequence, compared to the standard picture, and the IgE binding precipitates visible on the X-ray film are identified.

3. When a precipitate is visible after 1 d score 3 (strong) is given, after 3 d score 2 (moderate), and after 10 d score 1 (weak).

4. Finally the allergogram is constructed as a histogram using the precipitate numbers from the standard picture and the number of patients reacting to each precipitate. On each column the number of patients reacting with the three different scores (1, 2, or 3) are indicated (**Fig. 2d**).

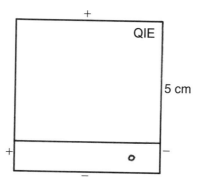

Fig. 7. Template for QIE indicating anode (+) and cathode (−) for both first and second dimension electrophoresis.

5. An allergen is classified as a *major allergen* if at least 50% of the patients show strong or moderate IgE binding. Other clearly specific IgE binding allergens are classified as *minor allergens*.

3.4. Quantification of Antigens (see Note 8)

3.4.1. QIE (Quantitative Immunoelectrophoresis)

1. Label four 5 ×5 cm glass plates in the upper right-hand corner with identification numbers. Turn the plates upside down and place them on a leveled surface. Clean with ethanol.
2. Pipet 3.5 mL agarose in each plate.
3. After thorough setting, punch wells according to the template (**Fig. 7**).
4. Apply, e.g., three concentrations of the standard and one concentration of the sample.
5. Perform the electrophoresis as described in **Sections 3.1.1.–3.1.4**.

3.4.2. RIE (Rocked Immunoelectrophoresis)

1. Label the glass plate (e.g., 10 ×7 cm) in the upper right-hand corner with identification number. Turn the plate upside down and place it on a leveled surface. Clean the plate with ethanol.
2. Pipet antibody into a test tube and heat it in the water bath (56°C). Pipet 11 mL of agarose into the tube and mix the gel and the antibody (seal the tube with Parafilm and invert four times). Pour the antibody-containing agarose onto the glass plate (avoid air bubbles).
3. After thorough setting, punch wells 1.5 cm from the lower edge of the plate, **Fig. 8a**. Well size adjusted to the volume to be applied.
4. Place the plate on the cooled surface on the electrophoresis apparatus as indicated in the template. Connecting bridges of five layers of filter paper are established. Switch on the current and adjust the voltage across the gel to 2 V/cm.

8a

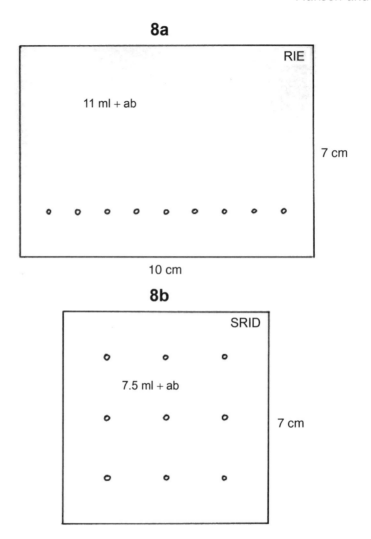

Fig. 8. Template for RIE (**a**) and SRID (**b**).

5. Apply the same volume of all samples. Place a glass plate on top of the wicks to avoid water to condense on the gel. Continue electrophoresis overnight.
6. Press and stain the plate as described in **Section 3.1.3.** and **3.1.4.**

3.4.3. SRID (Single Radial Immunodiffusion)

Prepare the gel as described in **Section 3.4.2.** Punch the wells equally spread on the plate (**Fig. 8b**), and apply the samples. Place the plate in a humid chamber for approx. 40 h. Press and stain the gel as described in **Sections 3.1.3.** and **3.1.4.**

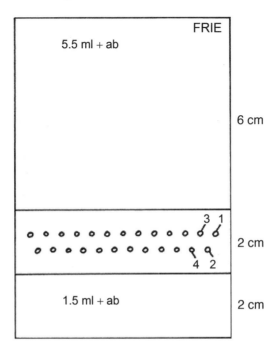

Fig. 9. Template for FRIE indicating position of wells and succession of the fractions applied.

3.4.4. Calculation of Results

RIE and SRID: Measure the area of each precipitate. Draw a standard curve and read each sample.

QIE: Measure the area limited by the precipitate to be quantified on the four plates. Use the line between the first dimension gel and the antibody-containing gel as a baseline for the precipitate. Draw a standard curve and read the sample.

3.5. Fused Rocket Immunoelectrophoresis (FRIE)

1. Mark and clean a glass plate (e.g., 7×10 cm). Pour 11 mL agarose onto the plate.
2. After thorough setting cut away the upper and lower parts of the gel according to the template (**Fig. 9**).
3. Pipet antibody into two test tubes and heat them in the water bath. Pipet 5.5 mL agarose into the tube for the anodic gel and 1.5 mL agarose for the cathodic gel. Mix the gel and the antibody and pour the mixture on the glass plate.
4. Punch wells in the middle section (not containing antibody) according to the template (**Fig. 9**) and apply samples from each fraction (from a fractionation experiment) starting as indicated on the template.

5. Place the plate on the cooled surface of the electrophoresis apparatus and connect it to buffer reservoirs with five layers of paper wicks. The wicks should overlap the gel by approx. 0.5 cm.
6. Adjust the voltage to 2 V/cm. Place a glass plate on top of the wicks and continue electrophoresis overnight.
7. Press and stain the gel as described in **Section 3.1.3.** and **3.1.4**.

4. Notes

1. When starting to work with an unknown antigen/antibody (ag/ab) system, several parameters have to be established before the final conditions for the standard CIE picture are selected. Plates sized 5×7 cm have been found convenient to work with. *Ag migration in the first dimension*: Make sure no ags run further than 3.5 cm toward the anode or 1.5 cm toward the cathode. As a control run the first dimension for, e.g., 10 and 30 min.
   Ag and ab concentrations: Adjust empirically the ratio between antigen and antibody so that a majority of the precipitates have a suitable size.
   Adjustments of the pattern: Initial examination of the CIE system may lead to adjustment of the gel dimensions. Positioning of the well is dependent on the mobility of the antigens in question. The size of the intermediate gel may be adjusted or a second ab may be included in this. If no antigens run toward the cathode, the antibody-containing cathodic gel can be spared and the first dimension gel moved to the edge of the glass plate.
   Agarose: The type of agarose can be changed. Usually agarose-type HSA with electroendosmosis ($M_r = -0.13$) is used. In rare occasions, agarose-type HSB ($M_r = -0.07$) or HSC ($M_r = -0.02$) may be more suitable.
2. Instead of glass plates, coated plastic sheets cut in suitable sizes can be used.
   Disposable plastic tubes can replace glass test tubes, but they are difficult to incubate in a rack in the water bath.
   Use a (rotating) diamond pen to scratch the labels into the glass plate for identification.
   After use the agarose gel may be stored at 5°C and used again after boiling.
   Heat the pipet to 56°C before pipeting the agarose. When not used, store the pipet in a tall cylinder glass placed in the water bath to keep the pipet hot. Work fast! The agarose will set quite quickly.
   The size of the well must correspond to the sample volume. Use a gel puncher (e.g., 5, 10, or 15-µL size) connected to a vacuum pump (water jet stream or mechanical pump).
   Always keep the anode to the same side in the apparatus.
   Cut the paper wicks to fit the size of the glass plates to cover.
   The current is measured in V/cm. Use a probe with a fixed distance between the electrodes connected to a voltmeter for the calculation of V/cm.
   Place a glass plate on top of the wicks during the overnight electrophoresis. Moisture from the air will condense on top of the upper glass plate instead of on the gel, which may cause fluffy precipitates.

The buffer in the electrophoresis vessels can be used for approximately six runs before renewal is necessary (first and second dimensions included in one run).

All volumes of agarose gel are calculated from the area in cm² and the thickness of the gel. The thickness is adjusted so that the first cast gel on a plate is a little higher than the next. *First dimension gel*: 1.5 mm. *Intermediate gel*: 1.4 mm. *Ab gel (anode)*: 1.3 mm.

Pipet the antibody into a test tube and heat the tube for approx. 10 sec in the water bath before applying the agarose. Let the agarose run along the side of the test tube. Avoid air bobbles when agarose and antibody are mixed. Pay attention to the temperature in the water bath; temperatures above 60°C will denature the antibodies. If air bobbles are present in the newly cast gel they may be removed (punctured) immediately with a clean pipet tip.

In order to reduce background staining, nonprecipitated proteins are removed by repeated pressing and washing. The use of purified immunoglobulins instead of crude antisera also reduces background staining.

3. The method described above uses a fixed first dimension directly on the glass plate, on which the antibody subsequently is applied. If several plates have to be performed in parallel a transferred fixed dimension may be preferred. In that case, several fixed dimension strips can be performed side by side on a larger plate, separated (with a long razor blade), and transferred to the final plates where intermediate gel and antibody-containing gels are cast. Care should be taken comparing plates run under the two different conditions (transferred and fixed first dimension).

   Check and adjust the voltage once during electrophoresis, e.g., after 15 min. Beware of the shock hazard.

4. The paper wick directly on the plates may stick to the gel. In that case, moisten the paper with distilled water and remove it carefully starting in one corner. Check with a touch of a fingertip that the gels are still on the glass plates. Pour on more water if the gel sticks to the paper.

   Put saline in a suitable box, place a paper wick in the bottom (easier to get the plates up again!), and carefully place the plates in the box. Do not move the box. The gels might slide off the plates.

   Dry in cold air if the proteins should retain their biological activity for subsequent incubation with, e.g., serum (CRIE).

5. Stain with gel-side up. Use a special rack accommodating several plates.

   Keep the staining and destaining solutions in tight plastic boxes for reuse.

   The destaining solution can be regenerated passing through a filter with activated charcoal and can be reused several times.

   If the gels by accident are destained too excessively, they can be restained. The best result is obtained if the plates are not dried before restaining.

6. Make a 2% agarose gel if more than 400 µL must be applied in the intermediate gel.

7. The dried plates can be stored at +5°C for several months in a sealed plastic box or wrapped in tinfoil. Place a piece of filter paper or a soft tissue between the plates to avoid scratching of the dried agarose gels.

For construction of an allergogram, include at least 15–20 patient sera (RAST class ≥2) and also remember to include a control serum (e.g., IgE-stripped serum).

Cover the plates with a lid during incubation to avoid evaporation.

If a gamma counter is not available the dilution of the isotope is calculated from the expiry date of the labeled αIgE* according to the following table (for Bio-Line αIgE*):

Weeks to exp.	µl for 300,000 c.p.m.
7	100
6	120
5	130
4	140
3	150
2	165
1	175
0	190
−1	205
−2	245
−3	260
−4	285
−5	305

Note: Usual precautions when working with radiolabeled reagents!

The washed and dried plates are placed edge by edge in the cassette not leaving any space between them. This will ease the cutting of the film later. Start in the upper right-hand corner. Make sure the plates do not slide in the cassette; keep it horizontal at all times.

Label the film in one edge with a pencil with date and cassette number. Expose the film in the freezer; the low-exposure temperature (−80°C, alternatively −20°C) will lead to stronger X-ray staining.

Before each film is developed remove the cassette from the freezer in ample time to allow complete equilibration at RT; otherwise condensed water will damage the X-ray film. Standard develop- and fixing solutions for medical X-ray film processing and procedures from the manufacturer are used.

The standard CIE picture is either drawn during projecting a stained CRIE plate in a photo magnifier or printed from a digitally scanned plate. Check the picture carefully with the stained CRIE plates to ensure that all precipitates are visible on the standard picture.

If it is difficult to recognize a CRIE precipitate on the X-ray film when individual patients are scored, it may help also to look at the stained CIE plate from which the standard picture was drawn.

Very often particular precipitates are visible only on the autoradiogram and not on the Coomassie stained plates. This is because of lower sensitivity in the Coomassie staining. These precipitates are drawn on the standard picture with dotted lines and numbered.

All autoradiograms should be scored by two individuals. In case of discrepancies, the scoring is re-evaluated.

The CRIE technique can also be performed with biotin-labeled αIgE followed by avidin-AP (alkaline phosphatase-conjugated avidin) and substrate. This method is much faster because autoradiography is avoided; however, the relative intensity in staining is lost. Furthermore, unspecific binding is more pronounced by using this method. The method is, however, useful if a fast analysis of an individual serum or a serum pool is wanted or when monitoring, e.g., an allergen purification.

8. The humid chamber for diffusion of the SRID plate is made by placing paper napkins or filter paper moistened with distilled water in a tight box. Leave at room temperature and beware of one-sided heat from, e.g., laboratory equipment, which will disturb the shape of the precipitates.

The height of the rockets (RIE) and $d \times d$ (diameters perpendicular to each other) of the SRID correlate with the area limited by the precipitates.

A more precise method to work out the area is to determine it electronically or place the plate in a photo magnifier, draw the precipitates on paper, cut them out, and weigh.

References

1. Løwenstein, H. (1978) Quantitative immunoelectrophoretic methods as a tool for the analysis and isolation of allergens. *Prog. Allergy* **25,** 1.
2. Axelsen, N. H., Krøll, J., and Weeke B. (eds.) (1973) A manual of quantitative immunoelectrophoresis. Methods and applications. *Scand. J. Immunol.* **2**(Suppl. 1)**,** 1.

14

Conjugation of Haptens

Ranulfo Lemus and Meryl H. Karol

Abstract

Many naturally occurring proteins, peptides, carbohydrates, nucleic acids, and lipids, as well as synthetic peptides, are successful immunogens. To elicit an immune response, a compound must contain an *antigenic determinant* or *epitope* and must be of sufficient size to initiate lymphocyte activation necessary for an antibody response. In practice, small chemical compounds (haptens) are generally not good immunogens. However, when attached to macromolecules (carriers), they can become immunogenic. An immunogen must have epitopes that can be recognized by antigen-presenting cells and a T-cell receptor, and it must be degradable.

Haptens and corresponding hapten–carrier conjugates have been essential to the development of sensitive quantitative and qualitative immunoassays. In the design of hapten conjugates, consideration must be given to the hapten, the carrier, the coupling strategy, and the hapten density because the amount of hapten attached to the carrier influences the strength of the immune response directed toward the newly created antigenic determinant. Hence the haptenic density of the conjugate is also important in the development of immunoassays. The optimal epitope density of a conjugate to elicit either a strong immune response or provide the best immunoassay is dependent on the structure of the epitope and the nature of the immunoassay.

The aim of this chapter is to describe the diverse techniques used to couple haptens to carriers and provide guidance in the selection of the most appropriate procedure for a particular hapten.

Key Words: Epitope; hapten; carrier; immunogen.

1. Introduction

Many naturally occurring proteins, peptides, carbohydrates, nucleic acids, and lipids, as well as synthetic peptides, are successful immunogens. To elicit

From: *Methods in Molecular Medicine: Allergy Methods and Protocols*
Edited by: M. G. Jones and P. Lympany © Humana Press Inc., Totowa, NJ

an immune response, a compound must contain a distinct structural component referred to as an *antigenic determinant* or *epitope* and must be of sufficient size to initiate lymphocyte activation necessary for an antibody response. In practice, small chemical compounds 700–1500 Da are generally not good immunogens. However, when attached to macromolecules, they can become immunogenic. The small molecule is referred to as a *hapten* and the macromolecules that render haptens immunogenic are referred to as *carriers*. The hapten can be thought of as an exogenous epitope attached to a carrier. The essential features of an immunogen are (a) it must have epitopes that can be recognized by antigen-presenting cells and a T-cell receptor and (b) it must be degradable *(1)*.

Haptens have diverse uses in immunology. They have been employed to evaluate the structure of epitopes and the valence, specificity, affinity, and heterogeneity of antibodies. They have also been employed in antibody purification, production of specific monoclonal antibodies, and investigation of biological properties of antibodies. Haptens and corresponding hapten–carrier conjugates have been essential to the development of sensitive quantitative and qualitative immunoassays *(2–4)*.

In the design of hapten conjugates, consideration must be given to the hapten, the carrier, the coupling strategy, and the hapten density, i.e., the hapten:carrier molar ratio (*H/P*) *(5)*. The amount of hapten attached to the carrier influences the strength of the immune response directed toward the newly created antigenic determinant *(6)*. The haptenic density of the conjugate is also important in the development of immunoassays. The optimal epitope density of a conjugate to elicit either a strong immune response or provide the best immunoassay is dependent on the structure of the epitope and the nature of the immunoassay. For example, several conjugates of hexamethylene diisocyanate (HDI) with HSA were prepared in our laboratory. The molar ratio ranged from 4:1 (hapten:carrier) to 49:1. The 12:1 conjugate was found to be optimum for stimulating proliferation of lymphocytes from patients with HDI hypersensitivity *(7)*, whereas the 36:1 conjugate was best for use in ELISA to detect IgG antibodies *(8)*, and a 25:1 conjugate was ideal in RAST testing to detect anti-HDI IgE antibodies *(8)*. Others have found a conjugate with *H/P* of 25:1 to yield better binding to ELISA plates when compared with conjugates having *H/P* of 54:1 *(9)*. In our experience with diisocyanate haptens, we use conjugates with *H/P* of 30–40 to immunize animals *(10)*, conjugates with *H/P* of 20–30 for ELISA *(11)*, and *H/P* of 10–20 for RAST.

The aim of this chapter is to describe the diverse techniques used to couple haptens to carriers and provide guidance in the selection of the most appropriate procedure for a particular hapten.

2. Materials

2.1. Preparation of Conjugates

2.1.1. Hardware

1. Hot/stir plates.
2. Centrifuge.
3. Freeze-dryer.

2.1.2. Spontaneous Chemical Reactions

1. Hapten (isocyanates or anhydrides).
2. Carrier protein (*see* **Table 1**).
3. 0.05 M phosphate buffer (pH 7.4).
4. Monoethanolamine.
5. Whatman paper # 4.
6. 1 and 6 N HCl.
7. 0.1 M ammonium carbonate.
8. Dialysis tubing.
9. 0.15 M saline.

2.1.3. Chemicals that Require Activation

1. Hapten (bearing a carboxyl group).
2. Bovine serum albumin (BSA): 4.2 g in 220 mL 1:1 water–dioxane containing 4.2 mL of 1 M NaOH.
3. Tri-*n*-butylamine.
4. Dioxane.
5. Isobutylchlorocarbonate.
6. 1 M NaOH.

2.1.4. Use of Crosslinking Intermediary Molecules

2.1.4.1. CARBODIIMIDES

1. Hapten.
2. Carrier protein.
3. EDC (1-ethyl-3-[3-dimethylaminopropyl] carbodiimide hydrochloride).
4. Sodium acetate.
5. Phosphate-buffered saline (PBS) (1× conc).
6. Sodium azide.

2.1.4.2. GLUTARALDEHYDE

1. Hapten.
2. Carrier protein.
3. Glutaraldehyde.

4. PBS (1× conc).
5. Sodium borohydride.
6. Sodium azide.

2.2. Characterization of Conjugates

2.2.1. Hardware

1. Spectrophotometer.

2.2.2. Determination of the Extinction Coefficient of Conjugated Haptens (Methylene Diphenyl Diisocyanate)

1. Methylene diphenyl diisocyanate (MDI).
2. Acetone.
3. Glycine.
4. Phosphate buffer, 0.02 M (pH 7.5).

2.2.3. Spectral Analysis of Hapten Conjugates (Toluene Diisocyanate)

1. Toluene diisocyanate (TDI)–HSA conjugate.
2. Human serum albumin (HSA).
3. Phosphate buffer, 0.05 M (pH 7.4).

2.2.4. Chemical Determination of Hapten Adduction

1. Borate–KCl buffer, 0.05 M (pH 9.4). Dissolve 3.09 g boric acid and 3.73 g potassium chloride in 800 mL water, adjust pH to 9.4 with NaOH, and bring to 1 L with distilled water.
2. 0.03 M picryl sulfonic acid (2,4,6-trinitrobenzenesulfonic acid, TNBS).

3. Methods

3.1. Selection of a Carrier

A variety of carriers can be used for coupling with haptens. Selection of a carrier is based on; availability of reactive sites for hapten conjugation, size, solubility after derivatization, potential for immunogenicity, lack of in vivo toxicity, commercial availability, and cost *(4,18)*. Proteins are most frequently used, but liposomes *(4)*, polysaccharides (AECM-Ficoll, dextran, agar, carboxymethyl cellulose *[12–15]*) and synthetic polypeptides such as poly-L-lysine and poly-L-glutamic acid *(16,17)* have also been employed.

Numerous proteins have been employed as carrier molecules as indicated in **Table 1**. Those most frequently used include serum globulins and albumins *(6,19)*, keyhole limpet-hemocyanin (KLH) *(20)*, gelatin *(21)*, ovalbumin *(22)*, casein, hemocyanin *(23)*, thyroglobulin *(24)*, fibrinogen, and tetanus *(25)*, cholera *(26)*, or diphtheria toxoid *(2,27,28)*. The protein carrier should be immunogenic and have a sufficient number of amino acid residues with

Table 1
Protein Carriers Frequently Used for Conjugation with Haptens

Protein carrier	M_r (kDa)	ε-NH$_2$ from Lys	-SH from Cys	Phenol from Tyr	Imidazole from His
Keyhole Limpet Hemocyanin (KLH)	$4.5 \times 10^2 -$ 1.3×10^4	2000[a] 6.9[b]	700[a] 1.7[b]	1900[a] 7.0[b]	8.7[b]
Human Serum Albumin (HSA)	66.5	61	1	28	16
Bovine Serum Albumin (BSA)	67	59[c]	1	19	17
Tetanus Toxoid (TT)	150	106	10	81	14
Ovalbumin (OVA)	43	20	4	10	7

Adapted from S. Muller, 1999.
Abbreviations: Da, Daltons; Lys, lysine; Cys, cysteine; Tyr, tyrosine; His, histidine.
[a]The amino acid composition is expressed using a molecular weight average of 5,000 kDa (T. Hermanson, 1996).
[b]Amino acid groups are expressed in grams of amino acid containing this functional group/100 g.
[c]30–35 of the 59 lysine residues are available for coupling.

reactive side chains for conjugation to the hapten *(29)*. When used for production of antibodies, conjugates can be injected into any animal except the animal of origin for the carrier protein. For example, human, mouse, and rabbit serum albumins have been employed for preparation of conjugates for use in guinea pigs *(31)*.

Haptens may be reactive or activated to a reactive state. As indicated in **Table 2**, electrophilic haptens react primarily with amino and thiol moieties. The ε-amino group of lysine is a good nucleophile, forming stable bonds above pH 8.0. The α-NH$_2$ group of N-terminal amino acids are less basic and are reactive around pH 7.0. Thiols (cysteine or methionine) are the most reactive functional group at neutral pH. Under specified conditions, haptens will react with phenols

Table 2
Methods for Coupling Haptens to Proteins

Hapten	Modified amino acid	Notes	Reference
Direct hapten binding			
Diisocyanate[a]	α-NH$_2$, ε-NH$_2$Lys, α-COOH, SH-Cys		Karol, 1983
Acid anhydride[b]	α-NH$_2$, ε-NH$_2$Lys, α-COOH, SH-Cys		Welinder and Nielsen, 1991
2,4,6 Trinitrobenzene sulfonic acid (TNBS)	α-NH$_2$, ε-NH$_2$Lys	Also used to measure the free amino content of proteins	Makela and Seppala, 1986
Aromatic amino acid	Tyr	Aromatic amino acid converted to diazonium group	Makela and Seppala, 1986
Carbohydrate	α-NH$_2$, ε-NH$_2$Lys	Coupling can occur through: a) the reducing end, b) carboxyl groups of acidic carbohydrates, or c) via hydroxyl groups	Makela and Seppala, 1986
Cyanogen bromide (CnBr)	α-NH$_2$, ε-NH$_2$Lys	Carbohydrates activated by CnBr spontaneously couple with amino groups	Makela and Seppala, 1986
Mixed anhydride	α-NH$_2$, ε-NH$_2$Lys	R-COOH converted into anhydride with isobutylchloro-carbonate	Karol and Tanenbaum, 1967
Use of coupling agents			
Glutaraldehyde	α-NH$_2$, ε-NH$_2$Lys	Two compounds are linked through their amino groups	S. Muller, 1999

(Continued)

Table 2 (Continued*)***

Hapten	Modified amino acid	Notes	Reference
Carbodiimides	α-NH$_2$, ε-NH$_2$Lys	Carboxylic groups are changed into reactive sites for coupling with free amino groups	Harlowe and Lane, 1988

[a]HDI, TDI, IPDI, MDI.
[b]TMA, PA.
Abbreviations: HDI: hexamethylene diisocyanate, IPDI: isophorone diisocyanate, MDI: methylene diphenyl diisocyanate, PA: phthallic anhydride, TDI: toluene diisocyanate, TMA: trimellitic anhydride

(tyrosine), carboxylic acids (aspartic and glutamic acids), and other amino acid chains (arginine, histidine, and tryptophan) *(30)*.

3.2. Preparation of Hapten Conjugates

Selection of the method for coupling hapten to protein is dictated by the functional groups present on the hapten and the carrier, as well as the desired orientation of the hapten for presentation to the immune system. Hapten conjugation to carriers can be spontaneous when the hapten is a chemically reactive molecule such as isocyanates and anhydrides, or it can occur with the aid of a crosslinking agent, such as glutaraldehyde or a carbodiimide, that has at least two chemically reactive groups. Reagents frequently used to couple nonreactive haptens to proteins are listed in **Table 2**.

Nonreactive haptens may be coupled to carriers using reagents that are either incorporated into the final product or that can activate sites of the carrier protein for subsequent linkage (**Table 2**). When preparing conjugates, inter- and intra-molecular crosslinking can occur *(32)*. Several factors that influence the extent of crosslinking in the final conjugate are the ratio of carrier and/or hapten to coupling agent, carrier/hapten concentration, ionic strength of the solution, temperature, and pH *(12)*.

3.2.1. Spontaneous Chemical Reactions

When the hapten is chemically reactive (i.e., isocyanates and acid anhydrides), conjugation to carriers can be spontaneous reactions.

Procedure:
1. Warm 200 mL of 0.05 M phosphate buffer (pH 7.4) to 37°C in a water bath (using a hot/stir plate), add 1 g of carrier protein (*see* **Notes 1** and **2**).

2. To the middle of the rapidly stirred solution, add dropwise 110 μL of hapten.
3. Stir vigorously for 1 h, then moderately for 3 h (total time 4 h).
4. Place the flask at ambient temperature, add 420 μL of monoethanolamine, and stir moderately for 1 h.
5. Filter the solution using Whatman paper #4.
6. Adjust the pH to 4.0 using 6 N HCl initially. (The starting pH is around 10.0). As the pH nears 7, use 1 N HCl. The solution will come cloudy and protein will precipitate (*see* **Note 3**). Cover the flask and refrigerate overnight.
7. Centrifuge solution for 20 min at 4°C at 4000 rpm.
8. Retain the supernatant until the conjugate is analyzed, then discard.
9. Dissolve the precipitate in 15 mL of 0.1 M $(NH_4)_2CO_3$. Transfer the solution to dialysis tubing and dialyze against 1 L of 0.15 M NaCl (saline) 4 h at 4°C.
10. Dialyze against distilled water for 3–4 d with 3–4 changes of distilled water/d.
11. Lyophilize the solution. Record the yield of protein.
12. Analyze the product for the amount of hapten conjugated to protein (*H/P*).

3.2.2. Chemicals that Require Activation – Mixed Anhydride Reaction

The method has been used for coupling steroids *(33)* and nucleosides *(34)* to proteins.

1. Dissolve 3.05 mmol of hapten (bearing a carboxyl group) and 3.05 mmol of tri-*n*-butylamine in 30 mL dioxane.
2. Cool the solution to 10°C.
3. Add 3.05 mmol of isobutylchlorocarbonate and stir at 4°C for 20 min.
4. Add mixture to a cooled solution of BSA (4.2 g in 220 mL of 1:1 water–dioxane containing 4.2 mL of 1 M NaOH).
5. Stir the mixture for 1 h, add 2 mL NaOH, and stir for another 3 h.
6. The product should contain approximately 30 mol hapten per mol BSA *(35)*.

3.2.3. Use of Crosslinking Intermediary Molecules

3.2.3.1. CARBODIIMIDES

Carbodiimides have the general formula R–N=C=N–R', where R and R' are aliphatic (i.e., ethylcarbodiimide) or aromatic groups (i.e., diphenylcarbodiimide). Conjugation using carbodiimides requires the presence of α and ε-amino and carboxyl groups. For the most part, lysyl residues of the carrier protein and carboxyl groups donated by the hapten are involved in the reaction. Carbodiimides also react with sulfhydryl and phenolic residues. Although the reaction mechanism is not fully understood, it is proposed that (1) an intermediate product (IP) is formed that can react with an amine to give the desired peptide at low temperature by reaction between the IP and amino groups and (2) there is rearrangement to an acyl urea, which is a side product at elevated temperatures *(3,12)*.

The following method typically yields 50–70% conjugation of protein (*see* **Note 4**) *(1,4,12)*.

1. Dissolve the hapten (up to 4 mg/mL) in 1 mL water (*see* **Note 5**).
2. Add EDC to a final concentration of 10 mg/mL with constant mixing. Adjust the pH to 5 (*see* **Note 6**).
3. Incubate for 5 min at ambient temperature with gentle agitation.
4. Add an equal volume of carrier protein to yield a final hapten:carrier molar ratio of 20:1–40:1.
5. Stir at ambient temperature for 4 h.
6. Stop the reaction by addition of sodium acetate (pH 4.2) to a final concentration of 100 mM. Incubate at ambient temperature for 1 h.
7. Dialyze the product against 3–4 changes of PBS for 24 h to separate free hapten from the hapten–protein conjugate (*see* **Note 7**). Store at 4°C in the presence of sodium azide (0.02%) or in aliquots at −20°C.

3.2.3.2. GLUTARALDEHYDE

Glutaraldehyde is a bifunctional coupling reagent that can react with amine groups to create Schiff bases or Michael-type double bond addition products. In general, high pH favors formation of Schiff base intermediates and results in greater conjugation, but also in higher molecular weight conjugates. Varying the pH and the amount of glutaraldehyde added to the reaction allows some control of the yield and the molecular weight of the conjugate. The concentration of glutaraldehyde added generally varies from 0.2 to 2% with sporadic use of very dilute solutions (0.05%) *(4)*. The glutaraldehyde crosslink is very stable, but in most cases the glutaraldehyde bridge is recognized as an epitope by the immunized animal *(1,4,12)*.

Glutaraldehyde crosslinking can be performed in a one- or two-step conjugation protocol. Most frequently, the single step method is used. This method is recommended for haptens that do not contain internal lysine or cysteine residues *(12)*.

1. Prepare a 1 mg/mL solution of the carrier protein in PBS, pH 7.4.
2. Add the hapten to the carrier protein solution using a molar ratio of 20:1–40:1 hapten:carrier protein. Cool to 4°C.
3. Just before use, prepare a 2% (v/v) glutaraldehyde solution in water.
4. Add dropwise, with constant agitation, an equal volume of 2% glutaraldehyde to the hapten–protein carrier solution.
5. After 1 h at 4°C, stabilize the conjugate by addition of sodium borohydride ($NaBH_4$) to a final concentration of 10 mg/mL.
6. Incubate at 4°C for 1 h.
7. Dialyze against 3–4 changes of PBS for 24 h (*see* **Note 7**). Store at 4°C in the presence of 0.02% sodium azide (or in aliquots at −20°C).

3.3. Use of Spacers

Hapten-directed immunogenicity may be enhanced through the use of spacers. These molecules function to extend the distance of the hapten from the surface of the carrier. The length provided by the spacer may provide less steric hindrance to conjugation by the hapten. The nature of the spacer may also govern the hydrophilicity of the hapten. Generally the spacer is attached to the hapten prior to coupling, but may also be attached to the carrier. Spacers may be immunogenic. With small haptens, the actual epitope will include portions of the carrier. In this instance, the spacer will become part of the structurally known epitope, thus reducing the size of the structurally unknown portion. Glycine and alanine residues are the frequently used spacers *(12,35)*.

3.4. Analysis of Conjugates

The degree of haptenation of the conjugate can be determined using radioactive hapten tracers *(3)*, by measurement of UV or visible light-absorbing groups on the hapten, using non-denatured gel electrophoresis *(36)*, amino acid analysis *(37)*, fluorodensitometric methods *(38)*, gas chromatography *(39)*, HPLC *(40)*, or electrospray mass spectrometry *(41)*.

3.4.1. Spectral Analysis of Conjugates

The hapten may have an absorbance spectrum that allows it to be differentiated from the carrier protein. This procedure is especially useful when the hapten has a strong chromophore. The H/P determination by spectroscopy is accomplished by first dialyzing the preparation to remove unbound hapten. The absorption of the conjugate is measured at the λ_{max} for the hapten, then the protein concentration of the conjugate is determined from absorbance at 280 ηm. The result is corrected for the $A_{280\ nm}$ because of the hapten. The H/P is calculated using Beer's law: $A = \varepsilon Cl$, where ε is the extinction coefficient, A the molar absorbance, C the molar concentration, and l the path length *(6,30)*. It should be noted that inaccuracy might result if the spectral characteristics of the hapten change when conjugated to the protein *(30)*. The following assumptions are made when hapten conjugates are analyzed by UV absorbance: (1) the solution is free of noncovalently bound hapten, (2) conjugates are soluble in the matrix used for analysis, and (3) chromophores of the carrier protein and hapten do not change on conjugation *(6)*.

3.4.1.1. DETERMINATION OF THE EXTINCTION COEFFICIENT OF CONJUGATED MDI

The extinction coefficient of the free hapten and protein can be obtained from tables or handbooks. That of the conjugated form can be calculated using the following approach *(32)*:

1. MDI (Mondur M, Bayer USA, Pittsburgh, PA) was recrystallized, then dissolved in acetone at 2.1 mg/mL.
2. A total of 10 µL of the solution was added to 0.16–2.8 mM glycine in 0.02 M phosphate buffer, pH 7.5.

Table 3
Determination of the Extinction Coefficient of MDI Following Carbamoylation of the Nucleophile

Glycine (mg)	MDI (µg)	λ_{max} (nm)	Absorbance at λ_{max}	Molar extinction coefficient
0.2	21	245.1	0.415	24714
2.0	21	246.8	0.480	28577
20	21	248.8	0.592	35238
200	21	248.8	0.615	36613

Adapted from Jin and Karol, 1988.

3. The absorbances of the solutions were determined at 200–350 nm. *See* **Table 3**.
4. The extinction coefficients were calculated from Beer's law: $A = \varepsilon Cl$ (*see* **Section 3.4.1.**).

3.4.1.2. SPECTRAL ANALYSIS OF TDI CONJUGATES

When there is overlap in the spectra of the hapten and the carrier, *H/P* can be determined from a "difference" spectrum (*see* **Fig. 1**). The hapten can be quantified by subtracting the absorbance of the uncoupled protein carrier at the haptenic λ_{max} from that of the conjugate *(42,43)*.

1. Separately dissolve 3 mg of the TDI–HSA conjugate and 3 mg of HSA in 0.05 M of phosphate buffer, pH 7.4 to a final concentration of 600 µg/mL.
2. Determine the absorbance from 600 to 190 nm of the following solutions:
   a. carrier protein vs buffer,
   b. conjugate vs buffer,
   c. conjugate vs carrier protein.

3. Calculate *H/P* using Beer's law with the absorbance value of the conjugate obtained from 2c.

3.4.2. Chemical Determination

When the hapten does not have absorbance in the UV or visible range, the extent of hapten coupling to protein can be estimated from the determination of the number of remaining amino groups on the carrier protein. 2,4,6-Trinitrobenzene sulfonic acid (TNBS) is frequently used for this estimation. Haptenic content of conjugates is determined from absorption of the trinitrophenyl derivative of the protein before and after conjugation *(3,37)*.

1. Separately prepare 1% solutions of the carrier protein and conjugate in 0.05 M borate–KCl buffer, pH 9.4.

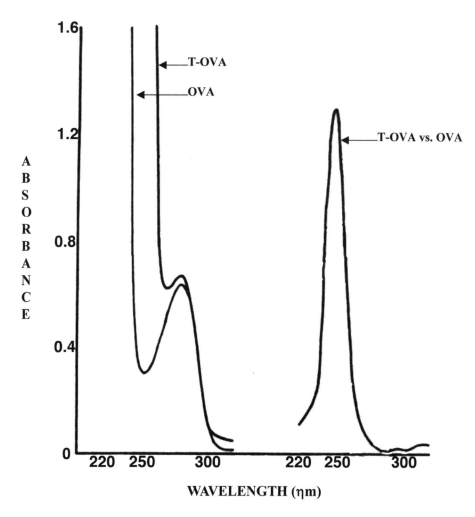

Fig. 1. Ultraviolet absorption spectra. **Left:** Ovalbumin (**OVA**) and p-tolylureido-ovalbumin (**T-OVA**) conjugate each 1 mg/ml, 0.05 M phosphate buffer, pH 7.0. **Right:** the difference spectrum of T-OVA versus OVA (**T-OVA vs. OVA**).

2. Prepare assay tubes according to **Table 4**.
3. Prepare 0.03 M picryl-sulfonic acid (TNBS; Sigma, Cat # p-2297) in distilled water using a glass beaker.
4. Add 50 µL of TNBS to each tube.
5. Vortex, let sit at ambient temperature for 30 min.
6. Immediately thereafter, read absorbance 420 nm (do not use quartz cuvettes) (*see* **Note 8**).

Table 4
Set Up for Conjugate Analysis by TNBS

Volume of borate buffer (ml)	Volume of conjugate solution (μl)	Volume of protein solution (μl)
2*	—	—
2*	—	—
1.95	50 (500 μg)	—
1.90	100 (1 mg)	—
1.85	150 (1.5 mg)	—
1.95	—	50 (500 μg)
1.90	—	100 (1 mg)
1.85	—	150 (1.5 mg)

   * Blanks.

7. Read blanks vs H_2O, then samples against the lowest blank.
8. Calculate the hapten substitution using the following formula:

9.
$$\% \, \text{Substitution} = 100 - \frac{[100(\text{Absorbance conjugate})]}{(\text{Absorbance carrier protein})}$$

4. Notes

1. In general, conjugates of serum albumin are more soluble than those of globulins or ovalbumin. Because of its large size, KLH is more likely to precipitate during crosslinking conjugation. To preserve the solubility and stability of the conjugate, coupling reactions using KLH should be performed under conditions of high salt (at least 0.9 M NaCl) *(4)*.
2. The haptenic content (*H/P*) of the final conjugate will vary with (1) the amount of hapten added, (2) pH of the solution with higher pH usually favoring greater substitution, (3) incubation temperature (higher temperatures favor higher substitution).
3. Conjugates having low hapten substitution will usually not precipitate at pH 4. Adjust the pH to 7 before starting dialysis.
4. Adding 5 mM *N*-hydroxysulfosuccinimide may enhance the efficiency *(12)*.
5. To avoid amino acid modification in the hapten, you may block it with citraconic anhydride (CA). For this, dissolve the hapten in water to 10 mg/mL. Adjust the pH to 8.5 and stir at room temperature. Prepare a 10 mg/mL solution of CA in water and slowly add an equal volume to the hapten solution and incubate for 1 h. Following the reaction with ECD, the citraconylated amino groups are deprotected by dialysis against 5% acetic acid. Finally, dialyze the conjugate against PBS *(1,12)*.
6. Adding *N*-methyl-imidazole to the coupling mixture may decrease the formation of acylurea adducts *(12)*.

7. Larger haptens may not dialyze efficiently. Gel filtration can be used to separate the free hapten from the conjugate.
8. If the absorbance of the conjugate is equal to that of the carrier protein, H/P is very low. A more sensitive method of analysis is needed (such as electrospray mass spectrometry).

Acknowledgment

This work was supported by grant # ES 05651 from the National Institute of Environmental Health Sciences, USA.

References

1. Harlow, E. and Lane, D. (eds) (1988) *Antibodies. A Laboratory Manual*, Cold Spring Harbor Laboratory, New York.
2. Makela, O., Mattila, P., Rautonen, N., et al. (1987) Isotype concentrations of human antibodies to haemophilus influenzae type B polysaccharide (Hib) in young adults immunized with the polysaccharide as such or conjugated to a protein (diphtheria toxoid). *J. Immunol.* **139**, 1999–2004.
3. Erlanger, B. F. (1980) The preparation of antigenic hapten–carrier conjugates: a survey, in *Immunochemical Techniques. Part A* (Vunakis, H. V. and Langone, J., eds), Academic Press, New York, **70**, pp. 525.
4. Hermanson, G. T. (ed.) (1996) *Bioconjugate Techniques*. Academic Press, San Diego.
5. Sarlo, K. and Karol, M. (1994) Guinea pig tests for respiratory allergy, in *Immunotoxicology and Immunopharmacology* (Dean, J. H., Luster, M. I., Munson, A. E., and Kimber, I., eds) Raven Press, New York, **2**, pp. 703–720.
6. Adamczyk, M., Buko, A., Chen, Y. Y., et al. (1994) Characterization of protein–hapten conjugates. 1. Matrix-assisted laser desorption ionization mass spectrometry of immuno BSA–hapten conjugates and comparison with other characterization methods. *Bioconjug. Chem.* **5**, 631–635.
7. Wisnewski, A. V., Lemus, R., Karol, M. H., and Redlich, C. A. (1999) Isocyanate-conjugated human lung epithelial cell proteins: A link between exposure and asthma. *J. Allergy Clin. Immunol.* **104**, 341–347.
8. Redlich, C. A., Karol, M. H., Graham, C., et al. (1997) Airway isocyanate-adducts in asthma induced by exposure to hexamethylene diisocyanate. *Scand. J. Work Environ. Health* **23**, 227–231.
9. Vyjayanthi, V., Capoor, A. K., and Sashidhar, R. B. (1995) Binding characteristics of bovine serum albumin–aflatoxin B1 to polysterene microtiter plates: importance to carrier protein molar ratio. *Ind. J. of Exp. Biol.* **33**, 329–332.
10. Jin, R., Day, B. W., and Karol, M. H. (1993) Toluene diisocyanate protein adducts in the bronchoalveolar lavage of guinea pigs exposed to vapors of the chemical. *Chem. Res. Toxicol.* **6**, 906–912.
11. Satoh, T., Kramarik, J. A., Tollerud, D. J., and Karol, M. (1995) A murine method for assessing the respiratory hypersensitivity potential of chemical allergens. *Toxicol. Lett.* **78**, 57–66.

12. Muller, S. (1999) Peptide-carrier conjugation, in *Synthetic Peptides as Antigens* (Van Regenmortel, M. H. V. and Muller, S., eds), Elsevier, Amsterdam, Netherlands, **28,** pp. 381.
13. Seppala, I. J. and Makela, O. (1984) Adjuvant effect of bacterial LPS and/or alum precipitation in responses to polysaccharide and protein antigens. *Immunology* **53,** 827–836.
14. Bocher, M., Giersch, T., and Schmid, R. (1992) Dextran, a hapten carrier in immunoassay for s-triazines. A comparison with ELISA based on hapten–protein conjugates. *J. Immunol. Methods* **151,** 1–8.
15. Seppala, I. and Makela, O. (1989) Antigenicity of dextran–protein conjugates in mice. Effect of molecular weight of the carbohydrate and comparison of two modes of coupling. *J. Immunol.* **143,** 1259–1264.
16. Diner, U. E., Kunimoto, D., and Diener, E. (1979) Carboxymethyl cellulose a nonimmunogenic hapten carrier with tolerogenic properties. *J. Immunol.* **122,** 1886–1891.
17. Pauillac, S., Naar, J., Branaa, P., and Chinain, M. (1998) An improved method for the production of antibodies to lipophilic carboxylic hapten using small amount of hapten–carrier conjugate. *J. Immunol. Methods* **220,** 105–114.
18. Hudecz, F. (1995) Alteration of immunogenicity and antibody recognition of B-cell epitopes by synthetic branched chain polypeptide carriers with poly[L-lysine] backbone. *Biomed. Pept. Proteins Nucleic Acids* **1,** 213–220.
19. Welinder, H. and Nielsen, J. (1991) Immunologic tests of specific antibodies to organic acid anhydrides. *Allergy* **46,** 601–609.
20. Gabor, F., Pittner, F., and Spiegl, P. (1995) Drug–protein conjugates: Preparation of triamcinolone–acetonide containing bovine serum albumin/keyhole limpet hemocyanin-conjugates and polyclonal antibodies. *Arch. Pharm.* **328,** 775–780.
21. Marini, S., Bannister, J., and Giardina, B. (1989) A simple method for increasing hapten immunogenicity by a specific structural modification of the carrier. *J. Immunol. Methods* **120,** 57–63.
22. De Ceaurriz, J., Ducos, P., Micillino, J. C., Gaudin, R., and Cavelier, C. (1987) Guinea pig pulmonary response to sensitization by five preformed monoisocyanate–ovalbumin conjugates. *Toxicology* **43,** 93–101.
23. Naar, J., Branaa, P., Chinain, M., and Pauillac, S. (1999) An improved method for the microscale preparation and characterization of hapten–protein conjugates: the use of cholesterol as a model for nonchromophore hydroxylated haptens. *Bioconjug. Chem.* **10,** 1143–1149.
24. Pandey, R. N., Davis, L. E., Anderson, B., and Hollenberg, P. F. (1986) Photochemical linking of primary aromatic amines to carrier proteins to elicit antibody response against the amine haptens. *J. Immunol. Methods* **94,** 237–246.
25. Peeters, C. C., Tenbergen-Meekes, A. M., Poolman, J. T., et al. (1991) Effect of carrier priming on immunogenicity of saccharide–protein conjugate vaccines. *Infect. Immun.* **59,** 3504–3510.
26. Azcona-Olivera, J. I., Abouzied, M. M., Plattner, R. D., Norred, W. P., and Pestka, J. J. (1992) Generation of antibodies reactive with fumonisins B1, B2, and B3 by using cholera toxin as the carrier-adjuvant. *Appl. Environ. Microbiol.* **58,** 169–173.

27. Maeji, N. J., Tribbick, G., Bray, A. M., and Geysen, H. M. (1992) Simultaneous multiple synthesis of peptide–carrier conjugates. *J. Immunol. Methods* **146,** 83–90.
28. Marcussen, J. and Poulsen, C. (1991) A nondestructive method for peptide bond conjugation of antigenic haptens to a diphtheria toxoid carrier, exemplified by two antisera specific to acetolactate synthase. *Anal. Biochem.* **198,** 318–323.
29. Coligan, J. E., Kruisbeek, A. M., Margulies, D. H., Shevach, E. M., and Strober, W. (1992) Peptides, in *Current Protocols in Immunology* (Coligan, J. E., Kruisbeek, A. M., Margulies, D. H., Shevach, E. M., and Strober, W., eds) John Wiley & Sons, New York. **2.**
30. Brinkley, M. (1992) A brief survey of methods for preparing protein conjugates with dyes, haptens, and cross-linking reagents. *Bioconjug. Chem.* **3,** 2–13.
31. Sarlo, K. and Karol, M. (1999) Animal models of occupational asthma, in *Asthma in the Workplace* (Bernstein, I. L., Chang-Yeung, M., Malo, J. L., and Bernstein, D., eds), Marcel Dekker, Inc., New York.
32. Jin, R. and Karol, M. H. (1988) Intra- and intermolecular reactions of 4,4'diisocyanatodiphenylmethane with human serum albumin. *Chem. Res. Toxicol.* **1,** 281–287.
33. Erlanger, B. F., Borek, F., Beiser, S. M., and Lieberman, S. (1957) Steroid–protein conjugates. (I) Preparation and characterization of conjugates of bovine serum albumin with testosterone and with cortisone. *J. Biol. Chem.* **288,** 713–727.
34. Karol, M. H. and Tanenbaum, S. W. (1967) Antibodies to hapten-conjugated proteins which cross-react with RNA. *Proc. Natl. Acad. Sci.* **57,** 713–720.
35. Makela, O. and Seppala, J. (1986) Haptens and Carriers, in *Immunochemistry* (Weir, D., ed.), Blackwell Scientific Publications, Oxford, **1,** pp. 3.1–3.13.
36. Kamps-Holzapple, C., Carlin, R. J., Sheffield, C., et al. (1993) Analysis of hapten–carrier protein conjugates by nondenaturing gel electrophoresis. *J. Immunol. Methods* **164,** 245–253.
37. Sashidhar, R. B., Capoor, A. K., and Ramana, D. (1994) Quantitation of epsilon-amino group using amino acids as reference standards by trinitrobenzene sulfonic acid. *J Immunol. Methods* **167,** 121–127.
38. Ragupathi, G., Prabhasankar, P., Sekharan, P. C., Annapoorani, K. S., and Damodaran, C. (1992) Novel-solid state fluorodensitometric method for the determination of haptens in protein–hapten conjugates. Demonstration with a toxic glycoside of Cleistanthus collinus. *J Chromatogr.* **574,** 267–271.
39. Tse, C. S. and Pesce, A. J. (1979) Chemical characterization of isocyanate–protein conjugates. *Toxicol. Appl. Pharmacol.* **51,** 39–46.
40. Hill, M., Lapcik, O., and Hampl, R. (1997) Evaluation and separation of steroid–bovine serum albumin conjugates by high-performance liquid chromatography. *J. Chromatogr. B. Biomed. Sci. Appl.* **691,** 187–191.
41. Adamczyk, M., Gebler, J. C., and Mattingly, P. G. (1996) Characterization of protein–hapten conjugates. 2. Electrospray mass spectrometry of bovine serum albumin–hapten conjugates. *Bioconjug. Chem.* **7,** 475–481.
42. Karol, M. H., Ioset, H. H., Riley, E. J., and Alarie, Y. C. (1978) Hapten-specific respiratory hypersensitivity in guinea pigs. *Am. Ind. Hyg. Assoc.* **39,** 546–556.
43. Karol, M. H. and Alarie, Y. (1980) Antigens which detect IgE antibodies in workers sensitive to toluene diisocyanate. *Clin. Allergy* **10,** 101–109.

15

Monoclonal Antibodies

Helga Kahlert and Oliver Cromwell

Abstract

Monoclonal antibodies (mabs) are powerful tools for the quantification, detection, and targeting of specific molecules. Allergen-specific mabs are important for the quantification of major allergens in allergen preparations used for allergen-specific immunotherapy and allergy diagnosis. Indeed, progress in the understanding of the mechanisms of the immunological responses underlying allergic disease would not have been possible without the use of mabs. Quantification assays are also important in the assessment of environmental allergen exposure and monitoring of avoidance procedures.

Mabs against human IgE provide the basis for various test systems for the detection of specific and nonspecific IgE. Mabs raised against IgE or defined cytokines or cytokine receptors have potential as neutralizing reagents in vivo for the treatment of allergic diseases.

Allergen-specific mabs are also valuable tools for the localization of allergens within their source material and the characterization of allergens derived from natural sources and by recombinant technologies. Furthermore they are often used for the isolation of allergens from complex extracts by affinity chromatography.

The procedure described in this chapter has been used successfully to produce mabs against numerous allergens from house dust mites, insect venoms, cat, hens egg white, tree-, grass-, and herb pollens, and fungi, with the ultimate aim of obtaining matched antibody pairs to establish two-site binding assays for the quantification of major allergens. The method has also been used successfully to generate mabs against human IgE.

Key Words: Monoclonal antibody; IgE; allergen.

1. Introduction

Monoclonal antibodies (mabs) are powerful tools for the quantification, detection, and targeting of specific molecules. Allergen-specific mabs are important for the quantification of major allergens in allergen preparations used for allergen-specific immunotherapy and allergy diagnosis. They allow the concentrations of major allergens to be defined in these preparations, thus contributing to better

From: *Methods in Molecular Medicine: Allergy Methods and Protocols*
Edited by: M. G. Jones and P. Lympany © Humana Press Inc., Totowa, NJ

standardized preparations. The quantification assays are also important in the assessment of environmental allergen exposure and monitoring of avoidance procedures.

Allergen-specific mabs are also valuable tools for the localization of allergens within their source material, e.g., pollen grains and mite bodies and the characterization of allergens derived from natural sources and by recombinant technologies. Furthermore they are often used for the isolation of allergens from complex extracts by affinity chromatography.

Mabs against human IgE provide the basis for various test systems for the detection of specific and nonspecific IgE. Humanized mabs raised against IgE or defined cytokines or cytokine receptors have potential as neutralizing reagents in vivo for the treatment of allergic diseases.

Progress in the understanding of the mechanisms of the immunological responses underlying allergic disease would not have been possible without the use of mabs. Fluorescence-activated cell analysis, immunohistochemical and cytochemical investigations, and in situ hybridization have been undertaken using a diverse range of labeled antibodies in order to identify cell types, specific activation markers, and the sources of various cytokines and chemokines.

Antibodies are a product of B cells. Immunoglobulin-producing B cells from the spleens of mice are not able to survive in culture in vitro, as they are only capable of dividing a few times. In order to render them immortal and capable of infinite reproduction, they are fused with cells of a permanent myeloma cell line. The resulting hybridoma cells combine the features of antibody production and perpetual reproduction. The progeny of a single antibody-producing hybridoma cell represent a cell clone which produces antibodies with a single specificity: mabs. The method of mab production was originally described by Köhler and Milstein *(1)*.

In order to ensure that only hybridoma cells but not the nonfused myeloma cells grow after fusion, mutated myeloma cells are used. The mutational defect imparts the inability to synthesize nucleic acids by salvage pathways. The *de novo* pathways of the nucleotide synthesis are inhibited by aminopterin. Only myeloma cells fused with B cells are able to maintain the nucleic acid synthesis by salvage pathways using compounds, e.g., hypoxanthine and thymidine, added to the medium for selection, and it is these cells that are able to survive and multiply in culture. The fusion of the two cell types is facilitated by the addition of polyethylene glycol. In order to obtain antibodies of a defined specificity, the mice are immunized with the desired antigen, and the respective antibody-producing B cells accumulate in the spleens of the mice.

The procedure described here is according to Köhler and Milstein *(1)* and Goding *(2)* and has been used successfully to produce mabs against numerous allergens from house dust mites, insect venoms, cat, hens egg white, tree-, grass-, and herb pollens, and fungi *(3–12)*, with the ultimate aim of obtaining matched antibody pairs to establish two-site binding assays for the quantification of major allergens. The method has also been used successfully to generate mabs against human IgE. Purification of the mabs is an important prerequisite for many applications. As most of the mabs belong to the IgG class this is easily done by protein A chromatography. With special exceptions *(12)* two-site binding assays for the quantification of allergens require mabs of different epitope specificity. Thus an epitope analysis using biotinylated mabs and unlabeled mabs is necessary. After selecting mabs of different epitope specificity the next step is to determine whether they are suitably matched for a two-site binding assay. For the quantification of allergens another important step is to provide a suitable standard. After development and validation, the assay is ready for use for the quantification of allergens in the samples.

2. Materials

For each step the general basic laboratory equipment for cell culture is needed: sterile working-bench with laminar flow hood, cell incubator (37°C, 5% CO_2, humidified atmosphere), centrifuge, microscope, autoclave, and for cryopreservation a −80°C freezer and storage container with liquid nitrogen.

2.1. Immunizing Mice

1. Use 6-wk-old female mice of the strain Balb/c (*see* **Note 1**).
2. Complete Freund's adjuvant (CFA) and incomplete Freund's adjuvant (IFA) (Sigma, Taufkirchen, Germany) (*see* **Note 2**).
3. Antigen against which mabs are to be generated.
4. Syringes (1–5 mL) and appropriate cannulas (23–25 gauge).

2.2. Preparation of Reagents for Cell Fusion

2.2.1. Myeloma Cell Line

Myeloma cell line P3X63Ag8U.1 (ATCC No. CRL 1597) according to Yelton et al. *(13)*.

2.2.2. Media

1. Equipment for sterile filtration of media.
2. Culture medium RPMI 1640 (PAA, Cölbe, Germany).
3. HAT-media supplement (Sigma) (*see* **Note 3**).
4. HT-media supplement (Sigma) (*see* **Note 3**).
5. L-Glutamine, 20 mM stock solution (PAA).
6. Penicillin/streptomycin stock solution with 10,000 IU/mL or 10,000 UG/mL (PAA).
7. Na-pyruvate, 100 mM stock solution (PAA).
8. Fetal calf serum (FCS) (supply is variable and depends on prior testing of the respective batch).

9. RPMI∅: RPMI 1640 medium without supplements. Shelf-life: 3 wk at 4°C.
10. RPMI⊕ = RPMI 1640 supplemented with 2 mM glutamine, 1 mM Na-pyruvate, penicillin/streptomycin (100 U/mL), and 5% heat-inactivated FCS. Add the supplements after sterile filtration using a vacuum filtration device. Shelf-life: 3 wk at 4°C.
11. HAT-medium: Same supplements as in RPMI⊕ and additionally HAT-supplement. Reconstitute two vials each with 10 mL sterile purified water and add 12 mL to the basic medium under sterile filtration. Shelf-life: 3 wk at 4°C.
12. Freezing medium: RPMI⊕ with 20% DMSO. Shelf-life: 1 wk at 4°C. Use as a 4°C cold solution.

2.2.3. Preparation of Instruments

1. Scissors and tweezers for the preparation of the spleen from the mouse.
2. Bags for sterilization and a special adhesive tape with sterile indicator.
3. Cell dissociation sieve CD-1 with mesh screen 40 and pestle (Sigma).

2.3. Cell Fusion

See **Section 2.2.** and additionally:

1. Polyethylene glycol (PEG 1500; Roche Diagnostics, Mannheim, Germany).
2. Petri dishes for cell culture, 20-mL volume (Greiner).
3. 96-Well flat bottom culture plates (Nunc, Wiesbaden, Germany).
4. Trypan blue solution (0.4%; Sigma).

2.4. Cultivation of Cells After Cell Fusion

1. 24-Well plates (Greiner).
2. Cryo vials, 2-mL volume (Greiner).
3. HAT-medium.

2.5. Screening for Antibody Production

1. 96-Well round bottom microtiter plates (Greiner).
2. Microplate washer/ELISA washer.
3. Microplate reader/ELISA photometer.
4. Multichannel pipete.
5. Mouse hyperimmunserum (serum taken on the day of the fusion).
6. Antigen to which mabs are desired.
7. Peroxidase (POD)-conjugated goat-anti-mouse IgG (FC-specific) (Dianova/Jackson Immuno Research 115-036-071, Hamburg, Germany) (*see* **Note 4**).
8. ABTS-substrate [2′,2-azino-bis(3-ethylbenzthiazolin-6-sulphonacid)] tablets (Sigma).
9. Citric acid (Merck, Darmstadt, Germany).
10. Hydrogen peroxide, 30% H_2O_2 (Merck).
11. Sodium azide, NaN_3 (Merck).
12. Carbonate buffer: 1.59 g Na_2CO_3 and 2.93 g $NaHCO_3$ (Merck), adjust with sterile purified water to 1 L. The pH should be 9.6 ± 0.1. Shelf-life: 4 wk at 4°C.

13. Phosphate-buffered saline/Tween 20 (PBS/TW): 6.845 mM NaCl, 0.135 mM KCl, 0.507 mM Na_2HPO_4, 0.073 mM KH_2PO_4, 0.05% Tween 20 (all chemicals from Merck), 0.01% Thimerosal (Sigma). pH 7.4. Shelf-life: 6 wk at RT.
14. PBS/TW/BSA: PBS/TW + 1% BSA (Merck). pH 7.4. Shelf-life: 4 wk at 4°C.
15. Citrate buffer: Dissolve 2.82 g citric acid and 1.5 g Na_2HPO_4 in 250 mL purified water each separately. Adjust the pH of the phosphate solution by adding the citric acid solution until a pH of 4.2 is reached. Bring the volume to 500 mL. Shelf-life: 4 wk at 4°C.
16. Substrate solution: Prepare the solution directly prior to use. Dissolve one tablet of ABTS-substrate in 12 mL citrate buffer and add 12 µL H_2O_2.
17. Stop solution: 0.002 M NaN_3.

2.6. Cloning of Selected Hybridomas

1. Trypan blue.
2. Hematocytometer.
3. HAT-medium.
4. Sterile 1-mL Eppendorf cups and 15-mL tubes.
5. 96-Well flat bottom culture plates.
6. 24-Well culture plates.

2.7. Cultivation of Selected Hybridomas

1. HT-medium: Same supplements as in RPMI⊕ and additionally HT-supplement. Reconstitute one vial HT-supplement with 10 mL purified water and add it to the basic medium under sterile filtration. Shelf-life: 4 wk at 4°C.
2. RPMI⊕: *See* **Section 2.2.2.**, No. 10.

2.8. Two-Site Binding Assay for the Quantification of Allergens

The material is similar to the ELISA equipment described under **Section 2.5**. The additional items needed are

1. POD-conjugated streptavidin (Sigma).
2. Biotin labeling kit (Roche Diagnostics).

3. Methods

For detailed descriptions of any variations of the procedure described here, refer to comprehensive books (*14,15*).

3.1. Immunizing Mice

1. Prime with 10–50 µg purified antigen or 100 µg antigen extract (*see* **Note 5**). Dissolve the antigen in 100 µL sterile PBS and make an emulsion by adding 100 µL CFA (*see* **Note 6**). Note that Freund's adjuvants are potentially harmful. Protect the eyes and be careful during the preparation of the emulsion and injection into mice. It is recommended to start the immunization procedure with more than one animal, take five to ten mice.

2. On day 28 after priming perform a boost with the same amount of antigen emulsi-fied in 100 µL IFA and 100 µL PBS per intraperitoneal injection (*see* **Note 7**).
3. After 7–10 d (on day 35–38) take blood from the mice and check for antigen-specific antibodies by ELISA (*see* **Section 3.5.**). Select the best responder for the planned fusion (*see* **Note 8**).
4. After 42–50 d boost the selected mouse with antigen in the same concentration as above in a total volume of 150 µL PBS without adjuvant via ip route. Boost the remaining mice as described under **Section 3.1.** ujsing IFA as adjuvant.
5. Take the selected mouse for fusion 3 d later.

3.2. Preparation of Fusion

1. 5–10 d before fusion thaw PU1 myeloma cells and expand in culture to obtain approximately 5×10^7 cells for fusion. Daily splitting of the cells in a 1:4 ratio ensures that they remain in the desired exponential growing phase.
2. Prepare HAT-medium 4 d prior to fusion. Perform a sterile control and a control with PU1 cells. The PU1 cells should not grow in this medium.
3. Boost the selected mouse 3 d prior to fusion (*see* **Section 3.1.**).
4. Prepare sufficient sterile scissors and tweezers. Sterilize the cell dissociation sieve CD-1 with mesh screen 40 and the pestle using the sterilization bags and indicator tape.

3.3. Cell Fusion

1. Prepare 2–3 petri dishes with 37°C warm RPMIØ.
2. Adjust HAT-medium and an aliquot of 500 µL PEG to 37°C in a water bath.

3.3.1.Preparation of the Spleen

1. Kill the mouse. When desired, take blood from the mouse prior to killing (*see* **Note 9**).
2. Disinfect the mouse by splashing with 70% ethanol and transfer it to a clean bench.
3. Fix the mouse on its back on a preparation board and open the peritoneum asepti-cally: Make a little cut in the skin over the gut. Separate the skin from the peri-toneal wall with the round end of a pair of tweezers and fix the skin on the preparation board with needles so that the peritoneum is accessible.
4. Open the peritoneum with a vertical cut, taking care not to damage the gut.
5. Put the gut carefully on the right side of the animal. The spleen is now exposed in the upper part of the abdomen (the spleen is smaller than the liver, elongated, and of a dark red color, whereas the liver is of red-brown color and is multilobed).
6. Remove the spleen carefully without damaging the gut and transfer it into a petri dish with prewarmed (37°C) RPMIØ.
7. Put the spleen into the cell sieve and use the pestle to isolate the cells from the tis-sue by rubbing them carefully through the mesh of the sieve. Rinse the mesh with medium and transfer the cell suspension to a 15-mL tube and adjust the volume to 10–14 mL with RPMIØ (*see* **Note 10**).
8. Centrifuge at 200*g* for 10 min.

9. Wash once with 10 mL RPMIØ.
10. Resuspend the spleen cells in 10 mL RPMIØ. Take an aliquot, dilute it 1:10 with Trypan blue solution, and count the cells using a hematocytometer.

3.3.2. Preparation of the Myeloma Cells

1. Check the myeloma cells for their morphology and possible contamination.
2. Pool the cells from several culture dishes in 50-mL tubes and centrifuge at 200g for 10 min.
3. Wash the cells once with RPMIØ and centrifuge again.
4. Resuspend the myeloma cells in 10 mL RPMIØ and count the cells using Trypan blue and a hematocytometer.

3.3.3. Fusion

1. Take a small volume (50 µL) of each cell suspension for sterile and HAT-control in 1 mL HAT-medium.
2. Put the cells in a ratio of 10 spleen cells to 1 myeloma cell together in one 50-mL tube and centrifuge at 200g for 10 min.
3. Decant the supernatant completely, loose the sedimented cells, and add 400 µL prewarmed PEG dropwise under slight agitation over a period of 30 s.
4. After addition of the PEG, agitate the tube slightly for another minute.
5. Dilute the cell–PEG suspension stepwise by slowly adding a defined volume of RPMIØ within a defined time:
   1st minute → 1 mL RPMIØ
   2nd minute → 1 mL RPMIØ
   3rd minute → 8 mL RPMIØ
   4th minute → 10 mL RPMIØ
6. Adjust to 50 mL with RPMIØ and centrifuge for 10 min at 200g.
7. Decant the supernatant and suspend the cells carefully in 1–2 mL HAT-medium.
8. Bring the cell suspension to the desired cell concentration (recommended concentration: 1×10^5 cells/well) with HAT-medium, mix carefully in order to obtain a homogenous suspension, and seed into 96-well flat bottom culture plates.
9. Incubate at 37°C, 5% CO_2, and humidified atmosphere.

3.4. Cultivation of Cells After Cell Fusion

1. Check the fusion plates daily for growing cells, any contamination, and the effectiveness of HAT-selection.
2. After 5–7 d evaluate the progress of the growth of the cells and feed with 50–100 µL HAT-medium (*see* **Note 11**).
3. After 2–4 further days remove the medium completely and add 100–200 µL fresh HAT-medium (*see* **Note 12**).
4. After 2–4 d check the growing hybridomas by ELISA (*see* **Section 3.5.**).
5. When the cells of a selected hybridoma cover more than half the bottom of the well, transfer them to a 24-well plate and clone (*see* **Section 3.8.**) as soon as possible (*see* **Note 13**).

6. Harvest the noncloned hybridoma cells from the 24-well culture at 3–5 time-points and freeze in order to save the cells of origin. One fully grown well will give 1 cryo vial (*see* **Note 14**).

3.5. Screening for Antibody Production

1. Coat a 96-well microtiter plate with antigen (1–10 μg/mL) in 100 μL carbonate buffer per well. Incubate overnight at 4°C (*see* **Note 15**).
2. Wash five times with PBS/TW using a microtiter plate washer.
3. Transfer 50 μL culture supernatant under sterile conditions from the 96-well culture plate to the test plate and add 50 μL PBS/TW/BSA per well. Use the hyperimmune serum from the donor mouse diluted 1:500 as a positive control and culture medium as negative control. Incubate for 2 h at room temperature (*see* **Note 16**).
4. Wash five times with PBS/TW.
5. Dilute the POD-conjugated goat-anti-mouse IgG (FC-specific) 1:10,000 with PBS/TW/BSA. Incubate 100 μL/well, 1.5 h at room temperature (*see* **Note 4**).
6. Wash five times with PBS/TW.
7. Incubate with 100 μL freshly prepared ABTS-substrate per well.
8. Positive wells develop a greenish color. Stop the reaction after 15 min – max. 60 min – by adding 100 μL 0.002 M Na-azide solution.
9. Read the optical density with a microplate reader at a wavelength of 414 nm.

3.6. Cloning of Selected Hybridomas

1. Suspend the cells of a selected hybridoma from a 24 well and count the cells diluted 1:1 with Trypan blue using a hematocytometer.
2. Prepare two sterile tubes with 6 mL HAT-medium, and two Eppendorf cups one with 500 μL and one with 950 μL HAT-medium.
3. Add as many cells as necessary to the 500-μL cup to achieve a final concentration of 12,000 cells/mL by exchanging an equal volume of medium for cell suspension. Mix thoroughly.
4. Add 50 μL of this suspension into the 950-μL cup. Mix thoroughly. The cell suspension of this cup is now 600 cells/mL.
5. Add volumes of this suspension, as indicated below, into 10 mL HAT-medium in order to achieve final concentrations of 2, 1, and 0.5 cells/well and seed 100 μL/well of each suspension into 96-well plates:
   333 μL for 2 cells/well
   167 μL for 1 cell/well
   83 μL for 0.5 cell/well

6. Check for growing clones daily.
7. Feed with 50–100 μL HAT-medium when the bottom of a growing well is approximately one-fourth covered with cells.
8. Perform a screening ELISA 2–4 d after feeding (*see* **Section 3.5.**).
9. Select three clones with the strongest positive reaction. Select the clones from the plates in the order 0.5, 1, 2 cells/well (*see* **Note 17**).

10. As soon as the cells are spread over more than half of the bottom of the plate, transfer them into wells of a 24-well plate, harvest cell samples at three successive time-points, and freeze in cryo vials.
11. Then transfer the cells into the wells of a 6-well plate and again freeze cells at different time-points (*see* **Note 18**).

3.7. Cultivation of Selected Positive Hybridoma Cells

1. After the first cloning, convert the cells to HT-medium. Perform this in a stepwise manner so that the HAT-medium is slowly replaced by HT-medium, for example, if the culture has to be divided between two wells adjust the total volume with HT-medium after splitting.
2. 1–2 wk after cultivating the cells in HT-medium, convert to RPMI⊕ medium.

3.8. Establishment of a Two-Site Binding Assay for the Quantification of Allergens

3.8.1. Purification and Biotinylation

1. Expand the selected and cloned hybridoma cells for sufficient mab-containing supernatant (*see* **Note 19**).
2. Purify the mab from the supernatant (*see* **Note 20**).
3. Determine the protein content of the purified mab.
4. Aliquot and lyophilize the purified mab.
5. Confirm its activity by a direct ELISA and its purity by SDS-PAGE.
6. Conjugate an aliquot of several mabs with biotin (*see* **Note 21**).
7. Check the activity of the biotinylated mabs by direct ELISA (*see* **Note 22**).
8. Store the biotinylated mabs in aliquots at –20°C.

3.8.2. Epitope Analysis

1. Coat a 96-well microtiter plate with antigen as described under **Section 3.5**.
2. Wash five times with PBS/TW.
3. The biotinylated mab should be used in a dilution referring to approximately 80% binding in the direct ELISA. Make a dilution which is twice concentrated to that and incubate it with an equal volume of unconjugated mab in 10 twofold serial dilutions, starting with 80 µg/mL in tubes. Preincubate for 30 min in the tubes and then transfer the mixture to the microtiter plate (100 µL/well) and incubate for 2½ h at room temperature.
4. Wash five times with PBS/TW.
5. Incubate with POD-conjugated streptavidin diluted 1:1000 with PBS/TW/BSA for 30 min at room temperature.
6. Wash five times with PBS/TW.
7. The substrate incubation is as described under **Section 3.5**.
8. Plot the optical density against the concentration of the unlabeled mab.
9. Mabs which inhibit the binding of the biotinylated mab to the allergen coated onto the microtiter well yield a sigmoid curve and recognize a similar epitope on the

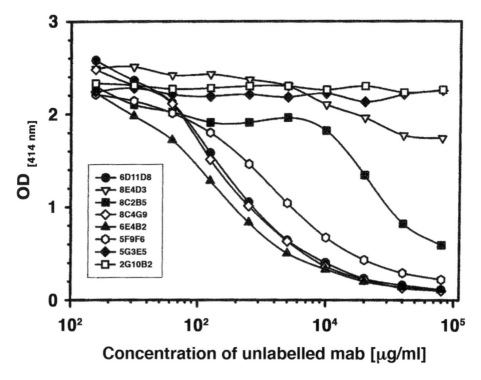

Fig. 1. Epitope analysis of monoclonal antibodies against the major hazel pollen allergen Cor a 1 with biotin-labeled 8C4G9. The mab 5G3E5, 2G10B2 and partly 8E4D3 do not inhibit the binding of biotin labelled mab 8C4G9 to solid phase bound Cor a 1 and are thus candidates for a two-site binding assay in combination with mab 8C4G9.

allergen as the biotinylated mab. These mabs are generally not suited for a two-site binding assay (*see* **Note 23**).

10. Mabs which do not inhibit the binding of the biotinylated mab recognize a different epitope and are candidates for matched antibody pairs in an ELISA (*see* **Fig. 1**).

3.8.3. Two-Site Binding Assay

1. Coat an unlabeled mab to a 96-well microtiter plate in a concentration of 1–10 µg/mL in carbonate buffer. Incubate overnight at 4°C.
2. Wash five times with PBS/TW.
3. Block free binding sites with 200 µL PBS/TW/BSA for 15 min. Then discard the blocking solution.
4. Apply purified allergen as a standard and the samples in which the allergen should be quantified in two- to threefold serial dilutions. Often the starting solution of the allergen standard is 1 µg protein/mL whereas the samples should be used in higher protein concentrations (*see* **Note 24**).

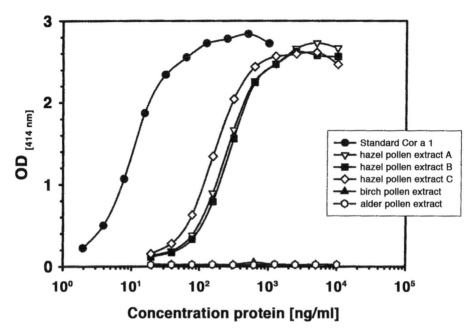

Fig. 2. Two-site binding assay for the major hazel pollen allergen Cor a 1 with mab combination 8C4G9-2G10B2:B using affinity purified Cor a 1 as a standard. Cor a 1 was detected in different batches of hazel pollen extract but not in birch or alder pollen extracts.

5. Incubate for 2 h at room temperature.
6. Wash five times with PBS/TW.
7. Apply the biotinylated mab in constant dilution. Incubate for 1 h at room temperature.
8. Wash five times with PBS/TW.
9. Apply POD-streptavidin diluted 1:1000 in PBS/TW/BSA.
10. Wash five times with PBS/TW.
11. Perform the substrate incubation as described under **Section 3.5**.
12. Calculate the amount of allergen in the samples from the linear part of the standard curve considering the dilution factor.

An example for a two-site binding assay is given in **Fig. 2**.

4. Notes

1. Other strains of mice may be useful for the production of mabs against particular antigens *(16)*. For example, we eventually obtained suitable mabs for the house dust mite allergens Der p 1 and partly for Der p 2 when using A/J mice instead of Balb/c mice.
2. Other adjuvants like aluminum hydroxide or new formulations like TiterMax (Vaxcel, Norcross, Georgia) may be used.

3. HAT/HT-medium supplements = hypoxanthine, aminopterin, thymidine. H and T are supplements for nucleotide synthesis salvage pathways; A is an inhibitor of the *de novo* nucleotide pathway for nucleotide synthesis.

4. This antibody enables the selection of hybridomas of the IgG isotype right from the beginning and avoids selection of IgM hybridomas, which are unstable and more difficult to purify.

5. The amount of antigen depends on the availability of purified antigen. For most purified allergens good results are generally obtained with immunization doses of 20 µg protein/mouse. When only allergen extracts are available, a dose of 100 µg protein/mouse should be used.

6. Prepare the emulsion by using two syringes connected by a valve and push the mixture between the two syringes until it becomes difficult to move. Transfer the emulsion in one of the syringes and connect an appropriate cannula (23–25 gauge). Remove any air from the syringe before injecting it intraperitoneally. Alternatively, when there is only a small volume of antigen solution it is possible to aspirate the two components with a syringe (with luer locks) and then push the mixture out into a small cup. Repeat this procedure several times until it becomes difficult. Then proceed as described above.

7. Other immunization intervals may be chosen, for example, a short immunization protocol with priming at day 1 and first boost at day 14, second boost at day 25, and fusion 3 d later. Sometimes the final boost is done by iv injections or by daily injections without adjuvants 3 d prior to fusion; for more possibilities, *see* **Refs**. *(14–17)*.

8. Dilute the mouse hyperimmune serum 1:100 and then make threefold serial dilutions over 8–10 steps. Good responders show a plateau of their titer with serum dilutions of 1:3,000–1:10,000.

9. This may be done, for example, by puncture of the retro-orbital plexus. For detailed descriptions on bleeding mice, *see* **Refs**. *(14,15)*.

10. Alternatively, the spleen cells may be released by fragmenting the spleen mechanically using scissors and repeated aspiration through a cannula followed by sedimentation (let the tube sit for 2 min) of remaining larger tissue pieces. Experience has shown that the method of using a cell sieve as described under **Section 3.3.1.** is faster and more elegant.

11. When the cells grow slowly, then it is recommended that the smaller volume of 50 µL is added. Stronger growing cells should receive 100 µL medium. Under certain conditions it might be necessary to transfer strongly growing cells to larger culture wells (24-well plate) prior to screening. Experience shows that in most cases strongly growing cells at this time-point of the fusion do not produce the desired antibodies.

12. This step is necessary because unfused B lymphocytes may still produce antibodies in the first hours after fusion before they die. Because these antibodies are not derived from hybridoma cells this may lead to false results in screening ELISA and thus useless work. Remove the medium using a pasteur pipet connected to a vacuum device and aspirate the supernatant by holding the pipet at an angle to the wall of the well. If this is done carefully the cells will remain in the well.

13. It is recommended to perform the cloning as soon as possible because hybridomas which produce no antibodies or antibodies of a different specificity may be present in the origin well and may overgrow the desired hybridoma cells.

14. Freezing procedure: Suspend the desired cells in the well and transfer them into a centrifuge tube. Spin them down 10 min at 200g. Discard the supernatant and suspend the cells in 0.5 mL cold (4°C) RPMI⊕ and then add 0.5 mL of freezing medium, mix, close the vial, and transfer it immediately into a styropor box and the box into a −80°C freezer. This procedure is especially recommended when cells of different hybridomas should be handled and frozen at the same time because a prolonged exposure to DMSO (final concentration 10%) should be avoided because of cell damage at higher temperatures.

15. The optimal concentration of antigen has to be determined individually. In general, 1 µg/mL of purified allergen is appropriate for plate coating and 10 µg protein/mL if only allergen extracts are available.

16. Choose a pipeting scheme that allows the positive and negative controls to be included in duplicate wells on each test plate. It is good practice to seed only the center 60 wells of a 96-well culture plate, leaving the peripheral wells empty. It is then possible to test 1½ fusion plates on one ELISA test plate with the indicated controls.

17. In order to achieve the highest probability of monoclonal cells it is best to select the hybridomas from the plate with a seeding concentration of 0.5 cells/well, but when growing clones are visible only in the plates with 1 or 2 cells/well, then these clones should be taken.

18. In order to obtain stable clones, a second cloning procedure is recommended.

19. For a first estimation of the suitability of the selected mab we usually take 500 mL supernatant of hybridoma culture. Harvesting of the supernatant is performed when more than 90% of the cells are dead.

20. Good results for mabs of the subclasses IgG1, IgG2a, and IgG2b are obtained using 50% saturated ammonium sulfate precipitation in the first step for enrichment and concentration of the antibody and protein A chromatography in the second step for purification.

21. For example, with the biotin labeling kit from Roche Diagnostics.

22. Most of the antiallergen antibodies keep their activity after biotin labeling, but it has to be considered that sometimes the labeling occurs in the antigen binding region of the antibody resulting in a loss of activity. It is also possible that the biotin-labeled antibody retains its reactivity to soluble allergen but loses it when the allergen is coated to microtiter plates. We experienced this with biotin-labeled mabs for Der p 1 which perform very well in two-site binding assays but fail to show reactivity to Der p 1 coated to microtiter plates.

23. For allergens which occur in the form of homodimers it is not necessary to obtain a pair of antibodies with different specificities because the same antibody may serve as both capture mab and detector. A two-site binding assay for Alt a 1 from *Alternaria alternata* has been established on this basis *(12)*.

24. The final concentrations of standard and samples have to be assessed individually.

196 Kahlert and Cromwell

References

1. Köhler, G. and Milstein, C. (1975) Continuous cultures of fused cells secreting antibody of predefined specificity. *Nature* **256**, 495–497.
2. Goding, J. W. (1980) Antibody production by hybridomas. *J. Immunol. Methods* **39**, 285–308.
3. Kahlert, H., Weber, B., Teppke, M., et al. (1996) Characterization of major allergens of *Parietaria officinalis*. *Int. Arch. Allergy Immunol.* **109**, 141–149.
4. Kahlert, H., Weber, B., Wahl, R., Fiebig, H., and Cromwell, O. (1994) Quantification of two major allergens from Parietaria extracts with monoclonal antibodies. *Allergy Clin. Immunol.* **308**, Suppl. 2, Abstr. 1101.
5. Suck, R., Weber, B., Kahlert, H., et al. (2000) Purification and immunobiochemical characterization of folding variants of the recombinant major wasp allergen Ves v 5 (antigen 5). *Int. Arch. Allergy Immunol.* **121**(4), 284–291.
6. Kahlert, H., Weber, B., Franke, D., Teppke, M., and Cromwell, O. (1993) Quantifizierung der Hauptallergens Bet v 1 in Birkenallergenextrakten mit monoklonalen Antikörpern. *Allergo J.* **2**, 36/16.
7. Bufe, A., Spangfort, M. D., Kahlert, H., Schlaak, M., and Becker, W.-M. (1995) The major birch pollen allergen, Bet v 1, shows ribonuclease activity. *Planta* **199**, 413–415.
8. Kahlert, H., Weber, B., Cromwell, O., and Fiebig, H. (1996) Quantification of the major allergen Pla l 1 from plantain extracts using monoclonal antibodies. *J. Allergy Clin. Immunol.* **97**, 212, Abstr. 118.
9. Kahlert, H., Petersen, A., Becker, W.-M., and Schlaak, M. (1992) Epitope analysis of the allergen ovalbumin (Gal d II) with monoclonal antibodies and patients' IgE. *Mol. Immunol.* **29**, 1191–1201.
10. Müller, W.-D., Diener, C., Jung, K., and Jäger, L. (1988) Antigens of timothy and other grass pollen extracts identified by monoclonal antibodies. *Allergol. Immunopathol.* **16**, 315–320.
11. Fahlbusch, B., Müller, W.-D., Diener, C., and Jäger, L. (1993) Detection of crossreactive determinants in grass pollen extracts using monoclonal antibodies against group IV and group V allergens. *Clin. Exp. Allergy* **23**, 51–60.
12. Aden, E., Weber, B., Bossert, J., et al. (1999) Standardization of *Alternaria alternata*: extraction and quantification of Alt a 1 by using an mAb-based 2-site binding assay. *J. Allergy Clin. Immunol.* **103**, 128–135.
13. Yelton, D. E., Diamond, B. A., Kwan, S.-P., and Scharff, M. D. (1978) Fusion of mouse myeloma and spleen cells. *Curr. Top. Microbiol. Immunol.* **81**, 1–7.
14. Harlow, E. and Lane, D. (1988) *Antibodies. A Laboratory Manual.* Cold Spring HarborLaboratory, New York.
15. Peters, J. H. and Baumgarten, H. (1990) Monoklonale Antikörper. Herstellung und Charakterisierung. 2. Auflage. Springer Verlag, Berlin.
16. Ovsyannikova, I. G., Vailes, L. D., Li, Y., Heymann, P. W., and Chapman, M. D. (1994) Monoclonal antibodies to group II Dermatophagoides spp. Allergens: murine immune response, epitope analysis, and development of a two-site ELISA. *J. Allergy Clin. Immunol.* **94**, 537–546.
17. Chapman, M. D. (1988) Allergen specific monoclonal antibodies: new tools for the management of allergic disease. *Allergy* **43**, 7–14.

16

Purification of Antibodies

Per H. Larsson

Abstract

Immunoglobulins are a heterogeneous group of proteins. It naturally follows that the strategies for purifying them are diverse and numerous. A good knowledge of their respective physiochemical properties will obviously make the task easier. The choice between using polyclonal and/or monoclonal antibodies will govern the basic approach. Each approach will present its own advantages/disadvantages including cost, ability to produce a high yield, quality, and a need for standardization. The context in which the antibodies will be used is another important aspect to consider. When the demand is for establishing "ultrasensitive" assays, optimal purity and specificity is obviously required.

This chapter will focus on the purification of mammalian IgG from polyclonal (i.e., rabbit) and monoclonal (i.e., mouse sources). IgG is the principal immunoglobulin constituent of mammalian sera. In older animals, it may well represent >80% of the total Ig concentration, because of its higher rate of synthesis and longer half-life.

Key Words: IgG; monoclonal antibody; polyclonal antibody; immunoglobulin.

1. Introduction

As immunoglobulins are a quite heterogeneous group of proteins it naturally follows that the strategies for purifying them are diverse and numerous. A good knowledge of their respective physiochemical properties will obviously make the task easier.

The choice between using polyclonal and/or monoclonal antibodies will govern the basic approach. Each approach will present its own advantages/disadvantages. For short-term projects (≤2 yr), especially those at small budgets, polyclonal antibodies would be the logical choice. These are much less expensive to produce relative to the cost of initiating monoclonal antibody technology. High yields of good-quality antibodies, within only 2–3 mo time, may be obtained from the serum of only one immunized animal (i.e., rabbit, goat, swine, chicken, etc.).

From: *Methods in Molecular Medicine: Allergy Methods and Protocols*
Edited by: M. G. Jones and P. Lympany © Humana Press Inc., Totowa, NJ

High-affinity antibodies are often easily isolated. However, long-term projects depending on a high degree of standardization and bulk production will benefit from the use of monoclonal antibodies.

The context in which the antibodies will be used is another important aspect to consider. For immunodiffusion, agglutination, and nephelometric methods, for instance, IgG-enriched fractions will most often suffice. When the demand is for establishing "ultrasensitive" assays, optimal purity and specificity are obviously required.

Perhaps, from an immunoassay technological point of view, the "ideal setup" would be the use of monoclonal antibodies for capturing antigens and high-affinity polyclonal antibodies for detecting them. Generally, any given immunoassay will not perform optimally if its antibody constituents are not optimally prepared.

Some useful techniques for antibody purification are listed in **Table 1**.

This chapter will focus on the purification of mammalian IgG from polyclonal (i.e., rabbit) and monoclonal (i.e., mouse sources). IgG is the principal immunoglobulin constituent of mammalian sera. In older animals, it may well represent >80% of the total Ig concentration, because of its higher rate of synthesis and longer half-life.

The main procedures of antibody purification are shown in **Fig. 1**.

Precipitation of immunoglobulins by salting-out is an inexpensive, rapid, and very effective method. It removes most of the nonspecific proteins and concentrates the IgG fraction. If high purity is required it is often chosen as the first step. The theory behind salting-out has been thoroughly described by Cohn and Edsall, Czok and Bücher, and Dixon and Webb *(1–3)*. It is very useful for enriching large amounts of, for instance, rabbit IgG antibody. Such preparations can be further IgG enriched by employing ion exchange chromatography.

Antigen affinity purification of polyclonal antibody preparations is the optimal way to achieve the highest specificity and immunoreactivity possible. It can be performed as consecutive steps starting with affinity binding to pure antigen, followed by passage(s) over unrelated antigen(s) matrice(s), i.e., solid phase adsorption *(4–6)*. The latter procedure removes background problems and is recommendable for sensitive assays.

Regarding the purification of monoclonal antibodies we advocate the use of culture media (if possible, serum free) as the antibody source. There are two good reasons for not recommending ascites fluid. The first and most important one is for laboratory animal ethical reasons, because of the highly invasive procedures involved. The second reason is that in ascites fluid approx. 90% of the total IgG fraction will be normal mouse IgG. Thus, only 10% will represent monoclonal antibody production. However, as it is still used for practical and

Table 1
Techniques for Antibody Purification

Technique	Agent(s)	Applicability
Salting-out	$NH_4(SO_4)_2$, Na_2SO_4	Starting step
Selective precipitation	Caprylic acid	Starting step
Ion exchange	DEAE, QAE	Starting to second step
Gel filtration	Sephacryl S-200, Superdex 200	Isolation of IgM
Affinity matrix	Protein A	Species?, Subclass?
	Protein G	If protein A is ruled out
	Protein L	If protein A/G is ruled out
	Anti-Ig	Species and class specific
	Antigen	High purity—high affinity

economical reasons, a method for purifying mouse ascites fluid will be described. Such a method is selective precipitation of contaminating proteins by caprylic acid *(7)* (which works nicely for rabbit, horse, and human sera too). Protein A or G purification of such a preparation will obviously bind normal mouse IgG too and can, thus, not yield pure monoclonal antibody. The optimal procedure for obtaining pure preparations of monoclonal antibody would be to use hybridoma cell serum-free medium as the source followed by affinity purification (e.g., Protein G). As protein G compared to protein A has a broader IgG-binding range regarding species and subclasses and also yields purer preparations we consider it to be the first choice *(8)*.

2. Materials

There are several useful protocols for antibody purification. The procedures described below have been used successfully for our own research purposes. Generally, all reagents should be of at least *pro analysi* (p.a.) quality and the water needed for reagent preparation should be of at least Milli-Q Plus (Millipore Corporation) or double-distilled quality.

2.1. Enrichment of Polyclonal IgG from Rabbit Serum by Salting-Out Using Sodium Sulfate

2.1.1. Equipment

1. Dialysis membrane (e.g., Spectra/Por®, Spectrum Laboratories Inc., 20-mm diameter membrane with a cutoff of 100 kDa).
2. Dialysis membrane seal.
3. Pipets.
4. 50-mL conical test tubes (polypropylene).

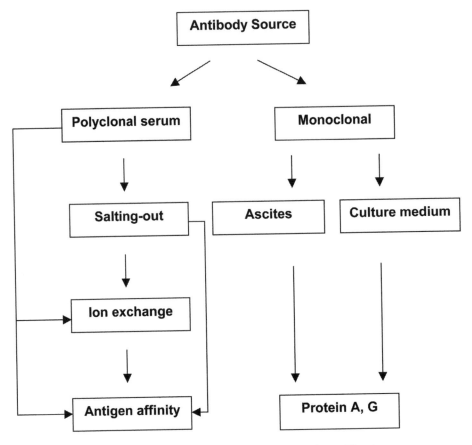

Fig. 1. Showing schematic steps for antibody purification.

5. 37°C incubator.
6. Beaker (100-mL size).
7. Centrifuge (capable of holding 50-mL tubes and deliver 1500g).
8. Magnetic stirrer.
9. Vortex mixer.
10. UV-spectrophotometer.

2.1.2. Buffers and Reagents

1. Phosphate-buffered saline (PBS), 10-fold concentrated (1.5 M). Dissolve 81.23 g of NaCl, 5.1 g KH_2PO_4, 20.06 g $Na_2HPO_4 \cdot 2H_2O$ in about 900 mL water in 1-L container using a magnetic stirrer. Adjust pH to 7.4 if necessary and add water to 1 L. Store at room temperature. For use, dilute 1 part PBS 10-fold concentrate + 9 parts water. Store ready to use PBS at 4–8°C.

2. Sodium sulfate (Na_2SO_4, e.g., Sigma S 6547).
3. 18% (w/v) sodium sulfate in water.

2.2. Preparation of Polyclonal Rabbit IgG from Salting-Out Enriched Fraction Using DEAE Sepharose; Batch Method

2.2.1. Equipment

1. Rotation mixer.
2. Glass filter funnel.
3. Pipets.
4. 50-mL conical test tubes (polypropylene).
5. Glass beaker (1000-mL size).
6. Stirred cell equipped with ultrafiltration membrane, molecular weight cutoff 100 kDa (e.g., Sigma S 2403 with membrane Sigma U 3005).
7. Magnetic stirrer.
8. UV-spectrophotometer.
9. Dialysis membrane (e.g., Spectra/Por® 20-mm diameter membrane with a cutoff of 100 kDa).
10. Dialysis membrane seal.
11. Nitrogen (N_2) source with pressure regulator for ultrafiltration step.

2.2.2. Buffers and Reagents

1. DEAE Sepharose CL 6B (e.g., Sigma DCL-6B-100).
2. 0.1 M Tris buffer, pH 8.0. Dissolve 12.1 g Tris base (tris[hydroxymethyl] amino-methane mw 121.1) in approx. 800 mL H_2O. Adjust pH to 8.0 by using conc. HCl. Add H_2O to 1000 mL final volume.
3. Ready-to-use PBS (above).

2.3. Preparation of Specific Polyclonal Rabbit IgG from Serum or Enriched Fraction Using Antigen Affinity

2.3.1. Equipment

1. Dialysis membrane (e.g., Spectra/Por® 20-mm diameter membrane with a cutoff of 100 kDa).
2. Dialysis membrane seal.
3. Pipets.
4. Minisorp™ (or similar low-protein binding type) 12-mL test tubes (Nunc cat. no. 468608).
5. Minisorp™ (or similar low-protein binding type) 5-mL test tubes (Nunc cat. no. 466982).
6. 37°C incubator.
7. Beaker (250-mL size).
8. Bench top centrifuge.

9. Magnetic stirrer.
10. UV-spectrophotometer.

2.3.2. Buffers and Reagents

1. AminoLink® Plus Immobilization Kit (Pierce, art. no. 4489).
2. Ready-to-use PBS-azide containing 0.1% (w/v) sodium azide or PBS-K containing 0.15% (v/v) Kathon CG® (Rohm and Haas).
3. Elution buffer 0.1 M glycine–HCl (pH 2.5) containing 0.5 M NaCl. Dissolve 7.51 g glycine (mw 75.05) and 29.22 g NaCl (mw 58.44) in approx. 800 mL H_2O. Adjust pH to 2.5 using conc. HCl. Add H_2O to 1000 mL final volume.
4. 1 M Tris, pH 9.5. Dissolve 121.1 g Tris base in approximately 800 mL H_2O. Adjust pH to 9.5 using conc. HCl. Add H_2O to 1000 mL final volume.

2.4. Enrichment of Mouse Monoclonal Antibodies from Ascites Using Selective Precipitation by Caprylic Acid

2.4.1. Equipment

1. Dialysis membrane (e.g., Spectra/Por® 20-mm diameter membrane with a cutoff of 100 kDa).
2. Dialysis membrane seal.
3. 50-mL conical test tubes (polypropylene).
4. Centrifuge (capable of holding 50-mL tubes and deliver 1500*g*).
5. Glass beaker (100-mL size).
6. pH-meter.
7. UV-spectrophotometer.

2.4.2. Buffers and Reagents

1. Caprylic acid (*n*-octanoic acid, e.g., Sigma C 2875).
2. Stock solutions for making acetate buffer: (A) 0.2 M acetic acid (glacial acetic acid 100%, mw 60.05, density 1.05 g/mL; 11.44 mL glacial acetic acid/1000 mL H_2O), (B) 0.2 M sodium acetate trihydrate (mw 136.08; 27.22 g/1000 mL H_2O).
3. 60 mM sodium acetate buffer, pH 4.0. Mix 246 mL of 0.2 M acetic acid with 54 mL 0.2 M sodium acetate and add H_2O to 1000 mL final volume.
4. Ready-to-use PBS (above).
5. 1 M NaOH (mw 40.0; 40 g/1000 mL H_2O).
6. Magnetic stirrer.

2.5. Preparation of Mouse Monoclonal Antibodies from Culture Media (Supernatant) Using Protein G Sepharose

2.5.1. Equipment

1. Column (e.g., Sigma C 3794).
2. Dialysis membrane (e.g., Spectra/Por® 4 membrane with a cutoff of 12–14 kDa).
3. 0.45-μm filter (e.g., Nalgene FastCap, Sigma Z37,743-0 ⌀ 90 mm).
4. 0.2-μm filter (e.g., Nalgene FastCap, Sigma Z37,742-2 ⌀ 90 mm).

5. UV-spectrophotometer.
6. Vacuum source.

2.5.2. Buffers and Reagents

1. Protein G Sepharose 4 Fast Flow (e.g., Amersham Pharmacia Biotech 17-0618-01).
2. PBS-azide; ready-to-use PBS (above) containing 0.1% (w/v) sodium azide (NaN_3).
3. 76 mM glycine–HCl buffer, pH 2.8. Dissolve 5.7 g glycine (mw 75.05) in approximately 800 mL H_2O. Adjust pH to 2.8 using conc. HCl. Add H_2O to 1000 mL final volume.
4. 1 M Tris buffer, pH 9. Dissolve 121.1 g Tris base in approximately 800 mL H_2O. Adjust pH to 9 using conc. HCl. Add H_2O to 1000 mL final volume.

3. Methods

3.1. Enrichment of Polyclonal IgG from Rabbit Serum by Salting-Out Using Sodium Sulfate

Add the calculated volume of the rabbit antiserum to the beaker.

1. Put the beaker on the magnetic stirrer for 60 min at 37°C.
2. During continuous stirring add *slowly* 0.18 g Na_2SO_4/mL serum (final conc. 18% w/v).
3. After the addition of the salt, let stirring continue for 30 min at 37°C.
4. Transfer the content of the beaker to 50-mL conical test tube(s).
5. Centrifuge at 1500g for 10 min at ambient temperature.
6. Discard supernatant and use vortex mixer to get the pellet loose.
7. Fill the tube with 18% Na_2SO_4 and mix.
8. Centrifuge as above (6).
9. Repeat 7–9 once.
10. Dissolve the precipitate using the initial serum volume of PBS.
11. Use rotational mixing for 60 min at ambient temperature.
12. Dialyze against proper buffer, e.g., PBS overnight at 4°C. If further purification is desired, use 0.1 M Tris, pH 8.0, and proceed to **Section 3.2**. The total volume of dialysis buffer should be approximately 200× initial serum volume.
13. Read absorbance at 280 nm ($A_{280\ nm}$) of the dialyzed solution. Use the dialysis buffer as the blank.
14. Calculate protein concentration using the absorbance coefficient 1.4 equaling 1 mg IgG/mL (0.1% protein) (0.1%, $A_{280\ nm}$ = 1.4). Recovery is usually 10–15 mg/mL at ≥90% purity.

For storage of prepared antibodies *see* **Note 1**.

3.2. Preparation of Polyclonal Rabbit IgG from Salting-Out Enriched Fraction Using DEAE Sepharose; Batch Method

1. Use enriched fraction of rabbit IgG (**Section 3.1.**) in 0.1 M Tris at pH 8.0. Each milliliter of rabbit IgG requires 1 mL of DEAE Sepharose.

2. Using 20× the Sepharose volume of the Tris buffer, wash the Sepharose over a glass filter funnel in consecutive steps.
3. Transfer the Sepharose to test tube(s) and add rabbit IgG.
4. Use rotational mixing for 60 min at ambient temperature.
5. Pour the slurry into the glass filter funnel and save the passed-through fluid in the glass beaker.
6. Wash the Sepharose with 10 volumes of Tris buffer and save washes in beaker.
7. Read absorbance at 280 nm ($A_{280\ nm}$) of the pooled volumes. Use the Tris buffer as blank. Calculate concentration and recovery according to **Section 3.1.**, no. 14.
8. Prepare the stirred ultrafiltration cell and the filter membrane according to the manufacturers' specifications.
9. Transfer the content of the beaker to the ultrafiltration cell. Apply N_2-pressure not exceeding 70 psi. Concentrate the protein solution to its initial volume.
10. Dialyze against proper buffer, e.g., PBS overnight at 4°C.
11. Read absorbance at 280 nm ($A_{280\ nm}$) of concentrate. Use the PBS as blank. Calculate concentration and recovery according to **Section 3.1.**, no. 14.
12. For storage of prepared antibodies *see* **Note 1**.

3.3. Preparation of Specific Polyclonal Rabbit IgG from Serum or Enriched Fraction Using Antigen Affinity

General procedure; detailed protocols, necessary reagents, and columns are included in the kit (see **Note 2**).

Preparation of immunoaffinity matrix

1. Antigen/ligand to be coupled should be in the relevant coupling buffer at 1–20 mg/mL (pH 7.2 or pH 10, enhanced).
2. Bring reagents and columns to ambient temperature.
3. Allow the storage solution of the activated gel in column to drain but do not let the gel run dry.
4. Equilibrate the gel using proper coupling buffer.
5. Replace bottom cap after drainage of coupling buffer.
6. Add 2–4 mL of antigen.
7. Replace top cap and use rotational mixing for 4 h at ambient or 4°C temperature.
8. Drain column and wash with 5 mL pH 7.2 buffer. Pool and save drainage plus washing fluid for later calculation of coupling efficiency. Calculation of bound IgG can be done according to **Section 3.1.**, no. 14. For determining the concentration of other protein antigens we highly recommend the Pierce BCA Protein Assay (*see* **Note 5**).
9. In a fume hood add 2 mL pH 7.2 buffer plus 40 μL of the provided reducing agent (sodium cyanoborohydride, which is highly toxic!) to the gel.
10. Replace top cap and use rotational mixing for 4 h to overnight at ambient temperature or 4°C.
11. Remove top and bottom caps and drain column. Wash with 4 mL of quenching buffer (Tris). Replace bottom cap and add 2 mL quenching buffer plus 40 μL sodium cyanoborohydride. Replace top cap and use rotational mixing for 30 min to block any remaining reactive sites.

12. Wash the gel using 4×5 mL wash solution (1 M NaCl) and monitor $A_{280\,nm}$ for any ligand presence (should be ≈ 0). Wash with 2×5 mL PBS-azide or PBS-K. Position the top porous membrane which prevents the gel running dry besides filtering off any macroscopic contaminants. Remove the bottom cap and let 5 mL PBS run through the gel. The matrix is now ready for use.

Typical affinity purification protocol

1. Apply 1 mL of your sample (antibodies to be purified) and let it run into the gel. Add 200 µL sample buffer (PBS). Replace bottom cap and add 2 mL PBS. Replace top cap and incubate for 1 h at ambient temperature.
2. Remove top and bottom caps (in that order) and wash with 14 mL PBS. If a stronger selection of high-affinity binding antibodies is desired the use of PBS containing 1 M NaCl is recommended. Monitor $A_{280\,nm}$ to ensure that the washing procedure results in the complete removal of nonbinding components (e.g., $A_{280\,nm} \approx 0$).
3. Elute with 0.1 M glycine–HCl, pH 2.5, containing 0.5 M NaCl. Collect 1-mL fractions and monitor $A_{280\,nm}$ to locate protein peak. Neutralize each of the eluted fractions by adding 50 µL 1 M Tris, pH 9.5.
4. Pool protein-containing fractions and dialyze against PBS overnight at 4°C.
5. Regenerate column matrix by washing with 16 mL 1 M NaCl, followed by 8 mL PBS-azide or PBS-K. The column can now be stored or reused.
6. Calculate antibody concentration as in **Section 3.1.**, no. 14. Calculate recovery (*see* **Note 6**).
7. For storage of prepared antibodies *see* **Note 1**.
8. For alternative ligand immobilization strategy *see* **Note 3**.

3.4. Enrichment of Mouse Monoclonal Antibodies from Ascites Using Selective Precipitation by Caprylic Acid

1. To a magnet-stirred glass beaker add 1 part ascites fluid to 2 parts of 60 mM sodium acetate buffer, pH 4.0, yielding a final pH of 4.8.
2. 25 µL caprylic acid/mL diluted ascites is added dropwise during vigorous stirring.
3. Stirring is continued for 30 min at room temperature to prevent gelation.
4. Remove precipitate by centrifugation at 1500g for 10 min.
5. Raise pH in supernatant (containing IgG at approximately 90% purity) to 5.7 by dropwise addition of 1 M NaOH. Monitor pH by using pH-meter.
6. Dialyze supernatant against PBS overnight at 4°C.
7. Read absorbance at 280 nm ($A_{280\,nm}$) for the dialyzed solution. Use PBS as blank.
8. Calculate protein concentration as in **Section 3.1.**, no. 14.
9. For storage of prepared antibodies *see* **Note 1**.

3.5. Preparation of Mouse Monoclonal Antibodies from Culture Media (Supernatant) Using Protein G Sepharose

Preparation of a new column

1. Rinse the new column with water and make sure that there is no trapped air in the bottom filter.

2. Fill the column to one-third with degassed PBS-azide. Allow some buffer to pass through the bottom filter.
3. Add protein G Sepharose and let the slurry settle (for faster sedimentation keep outlet open).
4. Wash the column with the settled gel using 5–10 column volumes of PBS-azide.
5. Wash the column with 2–3 column volumes of 76 mM glycine buffer pH 2.8 (or 0.7% acetic acid).
6. Do a final wash using 1 column volume of PBS-azide.

Sample handling

1. Filter supernatant through the 0.45-µm filter using vacuum source.
2. Apply filtered supernatant to column.
3. Wash column using PBS-azide until $A_{280\text{ nm}}$ of effluent is ≈0.
4. Elute the bound antibodies using glycine buffer, pH 2.8. Save 1-mL fractions of the eluate. Check $A_{280\text{ nm}}$ for protein peak. (The column should be washed with an additional volume of elution buffer followed by on volume of PBS-azide before a rerun or storage).
5. Pool protein-containing fractions and neutralize by adding 50 µL 1 M Tris buffer, pH 9.
6. Dialyze overnight at 4°C against PBS-azide (3 × 1 L).
7. Filtrate dialyzed abs through the 0.22-µm filter using vacuum source and calculate protein concentration and recovery as in **Section 3.1.**, no. 14.
8. For storage of prepared antibodies *see* **Note 1**.
9. For fast, small-scale protein G purification of antibody *see* **Note 4**.

4. Notes

1. Prepared and purified solutions of antibodies can be stored frozen at −20 to −80°C for decades provided the cryo vials/tubes are air tight to prevent freeze drying effects. This is particularly relevant at higher temperature. Freezing–thawing denaturing effects will generally not be a problem if not exceeding four to five times. Storage of antibodies at 4–8°C will retain high functionality for several years but requires the addition of a proper antimicrobial agent such as sodium azide (0.1% w/v) or Kathon CG® (0.15% v/v). We prefer the latter because of its lower general toxicity. PBS or Tris buffers can generally be used.
2. The Pierce AminoLink® Plus Immobilization Kit contains all necessary reagents for coupling antigen to the aldehyde-activated agarose matrix. Binding of the ligand requires that it contains primary amino groups (e.g., *lysine residues*). Thus, for instance, Tris-, glycine-, or ethanol amine buffers will inhibit ligand binding and must be absent in the antigen preparation. The manufacturer provides detailed protocols for antigen binding at pH 10 (enhanced binding) or pH 7.2. Provided that the antigen is known to be stable at pH 10 for at least 4 h the enhanced protocol is recommended as it results in a higher binding efficiency and ligand density *(4)*. If the pH stability of the antigen is unknown or if it is sensitive to an alkaline environment the pH 7.2 protocol is advocated.
3. Site-specific coupling of ligands to a suitable matrix may sometimes be necessary or result in better functionality when preparing immunoaffinity matrices. Coupling

through antigen-oxidizable carbohydrate groups to a hydrazide-substituted matrix can thus make specific binding of the Fc portion of IgG possible. The methodology involved was initially described by O'Shanessy et al. *(9–11)*. Examples of such commercially available matrices are for instance, adipic acid hydrazide agarose (Amersham Pharmacia Biotech, prod. code 27-5496-02) and Carbolink™ Coupling Gel (Pierce, prod. # 20391ZZ).

4. Small-scale protein G purification of monoclonal and polyclonal antibodies can be done in a very rapid and convenient way using the Amersham Pharmacia Biotech *MabTrap G II* kit (prod. no. 17-1128-01). The 1 mL gel has the capacity of binding ≥25 mg IgG. The procedure of isolating that amount of IgG in a single run can be done within 15 min.

5. Two very convenient and reliable protein assays are the Coomassie® Plus Protein Assay (Pierce, prod. no. 23236) and the BCA Protein Assay (Pierce, prod. no. 23225).

6. Checking reasonable recoveries in immunoaffinity purification of polyclonal antibodies: Starting material (e.g., IgG-enriched fraction) holds 10–15 mg IgG/mL. 2–10% of this IgG will be specific antibodies. The eluted specific antibody fraction should hold at least 50–80% immunoreactivity.

References

1. Cohn, E. J. and Edsall, J. T. (eds.) (1943) *Proteins, Amino Acids and Peptides.* Reinhold, New York.
2. Czok, R. and Bücher, T. (1960) Crystallized enzymes from the myogen of rabbit skeletal muscle. *Adv. Protein Chem.* **15,** 315–415.
3. Dixon, M. and Webb, E. C. (1961) Enzyme fractionation by salting out; a theoretical note. *Adv. Protein Chem.* **16,** 197–219.
4. Hornsey, V. S., Prowse, C. V., and Pepper, D. S. (1986) Reductive amination for solid-phase coupling of protein. A practical alternative to cyanogen bromide. *J. Immunol. Methods* **93,** 83–88.
5. Domen, P., Nevens, J., Mallia, K., Hermanson, G., and Klenk, D. (1990) Site directed immobilization of proteins. *J. Chromatogr.* **510,** 293–302.
6. Hermanson, G. T., Mallia, K. A., and Smith, P. K. (1992) *Immobilized Affinity Ligand Techniques.* Academic Press, Inc. San Diego, CA.
7. Steinbuch, M. and Audran, R. (1969) The isolation of IgG from mammalian sera with the aid of caprylic acid. *Arch. Biochem. Biophys.* **134,** 279–284.
8. *Affinity Chromatography Handbook; Principles and Methods.* GE Healthcare, Product Code 18-1022-29, pp. 609.
9. O'Shanessy, D. J., Dobersen, M. J., and Quarles, R. H. (1984) A novel procedure for labeling immunoglobulins by conjugation to oligosaccharide moieties. *Immunol. Lett.* **8,** 273–277.
10. O'Shanessy, D. J. and Quarles, R. H. (1987) Labeling of the oligosaccharide moieties of immunoglobulins. *J. Immunol. Methods* **99,** 153–161.
11. Hoffman, W. L. and O'Shanessy, D. J. (1988) Site-specific immobilization of antibodies by their oligosaccharide moieties to new hydrazide derivatized supports. *J. Immunol. Methods* **112,** 113–120.

17

Collection of Air Samples to Quantify Exposure to Airborne Allergens

Susan Gordon

Abstract

Under normal conditions, airborne allergens are present at very low concentrations. Allergens may be carried on relatively large identifiable particles such as grains of pollen and mould spores or smaller amorphous particles or both.

The methods that have been applied to quantify animal airborne allergens will be described in this chapter. By careful selection of the air sampling equipment and conditions, samples can be collected which quantify, for example, the personal exposure of an individual when performing a specific task or changes in exposure when allergen control methods are implemented. If as with animal allergens, an airborne allergen is not comprised of identifiable microscopic fragments, it is necessary to extract the soluble allergen for quantification in a specific immunoassay. The basic methods used for the elution of animal allergen from polytetrafluoroethylene (PTFE) filters will be described. The optimization of this method to suit different allergens and the influence of the buffer on extraction efficiency and stability of the allergen during storage will also be discussed.

Key Words: Allergen; exposure; air sampling; quantification.

1. Introduction

Over the last decade of allergy research, interest has grown in quantifying the amount of airborne allergen inhaled by individuals. Research has focused on describing the factors that affect the intensity of exposure to airborne allergens in both domestic and occupational indoor environments and in assessing the efficacy of allergen avoidance measures. The quantification of airborne allergen has facilitated investigations of the exposure–response relationship to occupational respiratory sensitizers *(1)*. There is still very little information available about the intensity of exposure to allergens required to sensitize naïve subjects or provoke symptoms in susceptible individuals.

From: *Methods in Molecular Medicine: Allergy Methods and Protocols*
Edited by: M. G. Jones and P. Lympany © Humana Press Inc., Totowa, NJ

The techniques required to make these measurements were first described by Agarwal and co-workers in 1981 (2) and is an adaptation of traditional occupational hygiene practices (3,4). Under normal conditions, airborne allergens are present in very low concentrations (ng/m³ or less). The ambient level of an allergen is affected by the rate of production of the allergen and the rate of its removal. Factors that influence the rate of production will depend on the allergen under investigation, but current or recent disturbance of allergen-containing dust may raise airborne levels 10-fold or more. The airborne concentration of an allergen will be reduced if the allergen source is contained or if the local ventilation is increased.

Allergens may be carried on relatively large identifiable particles such as grains of pollen (10–15 µm) and mould spores (2–5 µm) or smaller amorphous particles or both. The size of the carrier particle will influence the site of deposition in the respiratory tract. The total inhalable (or inspirable fraction) is the fraction of dust which enters the nose or mouth. The respirable fraction is the fraction that enters the gas exchange region of the lung (3,4). After a period of disturbance, allergen-containing particles will settle out of the air; the sedimentation rate will be greater for larger particles. Conversely, allergen carried on small particles may remain airborne for long periods of time and get widely dispersed. It is not known for how long allergens retain their allergenic properties in contaminated dust.

The methods that have been applied to quantify animal airborne allergens will be described. Animal allergens are carried on amorphous particles with a wide aerodynamic range (>19 to <0.4 µm) and the adaptations of the method to enable accurate measurement of exposure under a wide range of conditions may be applied to the quantification of most airborne allergens. Air containing the aeroallergen is drawn through a filtration medium by means of a pump. The allergen-containing particles impact on the filter and may be eluted for quantification in an immunoassay. As the volume of the air sampled is known, the concentration of the allergen can be reported in ng/m³. By careful selection of the air sampling equipment and conditions, samples can be collected which quantify the personal exposure of an individual when performing a specific task or decrease in background or static exposure when allergen control methods are implemented.

If the airborne allergen of interest is not comprised of identifiable microscopic fragments (as is the case with animal allergens), it is necessary to extract the soluble allergen from the filter for quantification in a specific immunoassay. As there may be 1 ng of allergen or less impacted on each filter, the optimization of the elution step to maximize allergen recovery is important. Several variations of methods to extract or elute airborne allergens have been described (5), but all involve the wetting or soaking of the filter with an aqueous buffer. Various lengths of elution time and methods of agitating the filters have been employed. The basic methods used for the elution of animal allergen from polytetrafluoroethylene (PTFE) filters will be described *(6)*. The optimization of this method to suit different allergens and the influence of the buffer on extraction efficiency and stability of the allergen during storage will be discussed.

2. Materials
2.1. Collection of Air Samples

1. Air sample pumps (mains operated or battery operated, *see* **Notes 1** and **2**).
2. Flow meter.
3. Flexible plastic tubing (internal diameter 6 mm), length approximately 0.7 m.
4. Sampling heads (Institute of Occupational Medicine (IOM), seven-hole, *see* **Note 3**).
5. Filter media (e.g., PTFE, glass fiber, *see* **Note 4**).
6. Forceps.
7. Cassettes for storage of exposed filters (e.g., Millipore PetriSlides).

2.2. Elution of Air Samples

1. Two pairs of forceps.
2. Plastic tube (75 mm × 12 mm) and cap – 1 per filter.
3. Plastic screw cap vial – 2 per filter.
4. Extraction buffer made up fresh such as 0.1 M PBS or ammonium bicarbonate buffer: 1.58 g Ammonium hydrogen carbonate dissolved in 200 mL distilled water and pH adjusted to 7.0–7.5 using 6 M hydrochloric acid. One milliliter of Tween 20 is added after adjusting pH (*see* **Note 5**). Additional protein and preservatives can be added to the buffer (*see* **Note 6**).

3. Methods
3.1. Collection of Air Samples

1. Attach the pump to the sampling head using the tubing.
2. If the concentration of the airborne dust is required (gravimetric analysis), the filter must be weighed on a sensitive balance before and after sampling (*see* **Note 7**).
3. Using clean forceps, transfer filter to sampling head and secure by fastening to 'finger tightness' (*see* **Note 8**).
4. Switch on pump and leave running for approximately 1 min.
5. Adjust flow rate to desired level (e.g., 2 L/min) using flow meter for accurate calibration (*see* **Note 9**) or if level cannot be adjusted, record the flow rate (*see* **Note 10**).
6. Position air sampling unit equipment in situ (*see* **Note 11**) and record the time switched on and off (some pumps have integral timers). The flow rate should be checked and recorded at the beginning and end of each sampling period as a minimum. For prolonged sampling periods or if sampling in a dusty environment, more frequent checks of the flow rate are recommended.
7. At the end of the sampling period, transfer the exposed filter to its own individually labeled cassette and store at −20°C.

8. Appropriate blank samples should also be collected and analyzed in parallel. 'Media blanks' are filters that have been taken 'straight from the box' whereas 'field blanks' are filters that have been loaded into the sampling equipment and taken into the sampling area, but the pump has not been turned on. As a guide one 'field blank' should be collected for every 10 samples.
9. The volume of air sampled is calculated in m^3 (*see* **Note 12**).
10. Wash the sampling heads in warm soapy water, rinse, and leave to air dry.
11. Wipe over casing of the sampling pumps and recharge as required.

3.2. Elution of Air Samples

1. In a ventilated safety cabinet, remove filter from the sampling head or storage cassette using clean forceps. Fold the filter loosely in half, exposed side inwards, and transfer to a labeled tube (*see* **Note 13**).
2. Wash the forceps in distilled water and wipe dry (*see* **Note 14**).
3. Repeat steps 1 and 2 until all the filters have been transferred to appropriately labeled tubes for extraction.
4. Add 2 mL of extraction buffer to each tube and cap.
5. Agitate tubes, for example, vortex mix each tube for 3 × 1-s bursts and then leave to stand for 1 h at room temperature (*see* **Note 15**).
6. Repeat step 5 once more.
7. Vortex mix each tube for 3 × 1-s bursts.
8. With clean forceps, remove the filter from the extraction buffer by slowly drawing the filter up the side of the tube. Discard the filter and recap the tube.
9. Remove all the filters as described in step 8, making sure to wash and wipe the forceps in between each tube as described in step 2.
10. Centrifuge all tubes containing the eluate for 10 min at 1300*g*.
11. For each filter eluate, transfer 0.9 mL of the supernatant to each of the labeled screw cap vials, taking care not to disturb the pellet of dust debris.
12. Store all vials sealed at −70°C (*see* **Note 16**).

4. Notes

1. A wide range of pumps is available from manufacturers such as Casella (http://www.casella.co.uk), SKC Inc. (http://www.skcinc.com), etc. For measuring the exposure of an individual, a small portable pump is required which is battery operated and can sample air at a smooth flow rate of 2 L/min. For approved methods for quantifying personal exposure for compliance with exposure thresholds, please refer to published guidance such as in **refs.** *3* and *4*. These small pumps may also be used as 'static' or 'area' monitors if the aeroallergen concentration is expected to be high. Static samples collected may provide additional useful information for the clinician or researcher. If the intensity of exposure is expected to be low (e.g., appropriate control measures are being used or monitoring for contamination of 'clean' areas), larger mains-operated pumps can be purchased, which operate at flow rates of 15 L/min or more. Caution must be exercised when operating pumps at high flow rates in a confined area because if the rate of removal of allergen by

the pump exceeds the rate of production, a falsely low level of allergen will be recorded. Under such circumstances, a pump that operates at a lower flow rate should be employed and longer sampling times performed.

2. In some environments such as animal houses and food preparation areas, it is of paramount importance not to spread contamination. It is therefore good practice to ensure that all the air sampling equipment is cleaned with mild detergent, then alcohol. If sterilization is required, H_2O_2 may be used safely with some air sampling equipment but the manufacturer's instructions (both for the air sampling equipment and sterilization equipment) should be followed.

3. The main types of sampling heads which are available and most practical are: (a) open faced (25- and 37-mm diameter), (b) IOM head (25-mm diameter, has one orifice, measures 'inhalable' fraction), (c) the Seven-Hole sampling head (25-mm diameter, seven equally spaced 4-mm diameter holes, measures 'inhalable' fraction), (d) cyclone sampling head (25-mm diameter, measures 'respirable' fraction). Preloaded cassettes (which may be more practicable if sterile filters area required, for example, if measuring exposure to endotoxin) are also commercially available. Foams which selectively sample different particle sizes are also usefully and may be successfully used for size-selective allergen quantification *(7)*.

4. A wide variety of filters are available from companies such as Millipore (http://www.millipore.com), Sartorius (http://www.sartorius.com), etc. When selecting the filter type, consideration needs to be given to several factors. The diameter of the filter must be compatible with the diameter of the sampling head. The pore size of the filter will determine the size of particle captured, and a pore size of 1.0 µm is recommended for most applications. However, if the allergen of interest is carried on smaller particles, a smaller pore size may be required. The ability of the filter media to absorb moisture during the sampling period may influence the stability of the allergen and gravimetric analysis. Allergen has been shown to be more efficiently eluted from hydrophobic filter media such as PTFE.

5. The addition of a small amount of detergent such as Tween 20 (0.05–0.5% v/v) has been shown to increase the efficiency of a number of aeroallergens up to 10-fold *(6)*.

6. The addition of protein (e.g., human serum albumin 0.3% w/v), stabilizers (e.g., glycerine 50% v/v), preservatives (Kathon 0.15% v/v), or enzyme inhibitors should be considered if the allergen is unstable and/or the filter eluates are to be stored for prolonged periods. The compatibility of these additives with the immunoassay used to quantify the aeroallergen should be determined.

7. Gravimetric analysis: Before the filter is weighed prior to sampling, the filter should be 'conditioned'. This means that any moisture in the filter should be allowed to equilibrate with the atmosphere in the weighing room. This can be done by leaving the filter overnight in its individual, labeled container with the lid slightly ajar. The balance used to weigh the filters should measure to at least five decimal places. If the balance is to be transported to the location where the fieldwork is to be conducted, the instructions from the manufacturer should be followed with respect to a suitable surface for the balance to be sited, an adequate warm-up period, and calibration checks. After the sampling period, the filters should be 'conditioned'

again before being weighed. The mass of dust captured is obtained by subtracting the weight before sampling from that obtained after sampling. Corrections are then made for the volume of air sampled (*see* **Note 11**) and dust expressed as mg/m^3.

8. The front of the sampling head should not be overtightened as this may dislodge the filter underneath.

9. Some pumps have an integral flow meter but, if not, a variety of equipment are available to calibrate the flow rate of the pump. These range from basic flow meters to more sophisticated electronic devices. Contact the manufacturer (*see* **Note 1**) for further information about the best device to suit your needs.

10. If the resistance to the flow of air is high, the operating noise of the pump will increase and/or the pump may cut out. This can be reduced by one or more of the following: (a) operate the pump at a lower flow rate, (b) increase the pore size of the filter, (c) select a different filter media, (d) increase the diameter of the sampling head/filter.

11. The position of air sampling equipment is of paramount importance and will greatly influence the quality of the data obtained. If personal exposure of an individual is being measured, the sampling head must be situated within the breathing zone of the person, i.e., as close as possible (i.e., <30 cm) to their nose and mouth. In practice, it is most convenient to place the sampling head securely on the subject's lapel. For collection of static samples, attention must be paid to the airflow in the room; sampling close to the inlet or exhaust air supplies may decrease or increase the aeroallergen concentrations recorded. In practice, the collection of several samples may be needed. For static samples, the sampling head should be positioned at least 1 m from the ground and preferably at head height. The collection time is another factor that can influence the data obtained. The shorter is the sampling time, the more information will be available about the 'peaks' of exposure. However, in practice, this needs to be balanced against obtaining enough allergen on the filter for detection in the immunoassay.

12. The volume of air sampled is obtained by calculating the total sampling time in minutes, multiplying this by the average flow rate in L and then converting from L to m^3 (10,000 L = 1 m^3).
    Example: Pump switched on at 09.15 (2 L/min) and off at 10.45 (1.9 L/min).
    Total volume of air sampled $- 90 \times 1.95 \times 0.001 = 0.175$ m^3.

13. Under optimal conditions, the dust on the filter should not be excessive. If the filter is overloaded and the material falls off, then this can be quantitatively transferred to the elution tube (and any extra volume of buffer taken into account). Investigators who use disposable sample heads may elute the filter in situ *(7)*.

14. Cleanliness in the handling of the filters is essential. Crosscontamination between filters is very easy and immunoassays are very sensitive! Thorough cleaning of the forceps is required.

15. Methods of elution other than vortexing have been employed, namely 'end over end' rotation and sonication. For more details see reference *(8)*. All are satisfactory, provided the elution buffer contains Tween 20, although prolonged sonication should be avoided.

16. The concentration of aeroallergen in the filter eluate can be measured by immuno-assay directly or after storage at −20°C. If the concentration of the analyte is below the limit of detection of the assay, then the filter eluate can be concentrated by lyophilization and reconstituted in a smaller volume. However, it is advisable to check the stability of the analyte before using this method routinely. If the eluates are consistently below the level of detection of the immunoassay, then the sensitivity of the method can be increased by (a) increasing the volume of air sampled and (b) pooling extracts from several filters and concentrating prior to assay.

References

1. Heederik, D., Venables, K. M., Malmberg, P., et al. (1999) Exposure–response relationships for work-related sensitization in workers exposed to rat urinary allergens: results from a pooled study. *J. Allergy Clin. Immunol.* **103,** 678–684.
2. Agarwal, M. K., Yuninger, J. W., Swanson, M. C., and Reed, C. E. (1981) An immuno-chemical approach to measure atmospheric allergens. *J. Allergy Clin. Immunol.* **68,** 194–200.
3. Methods for the determination of hazardous substances (MDHS). 14/3. General methods for sampling and gravimetric analysis of respirable and inhalable dust. (2000) HSE books. ISBN 0-7176-1749-1.
4. Guidelines for air sampling and analytical method development and evaluation. (1995) DHHS (NIOSH) publication NO. 95–117.
5. Hollander, A., Gordon, S., Renström, A., et al. (1999) Comparison of methods to assess airborne rat and mouse allergen levels. I. Analysis of air samples. *Allergy* **54,** 142–149.
6. Gordon, S., Tee, R. D., Lowson, D., and Newman Taylor, A. J. (1992) Comparison and optimisation of filter elution methods for the measurement of airborne allergen. *Ann. Occup. Hyg.* **36,** 575–587.
7. Bogdanovic, J., de Pater, A. J., Doekes, G., Wouters, I. M., and Heederik, D. J. (2006) Application of porous foams for size-selective measurements of airborne wheat allergen. *Ann. Occup. Hyg.* **50,** 131–136.
8. Eggleston, P. A., Newill, C. A., Ansari, A. A., et al. (1989) Task-related variation in airborne concentrations of laboratory animal allergens: Studies with Rat n 1. *J. Allergy Clin. Immunol.* **84,** 347–352.

18

Assay of Air Sample Eluates

Anne Renström and Susan Gordon

Abstract

After air sampling and elution, the air sample eluate contains an unknown amount of allergens together with other materials. The proteins of interest can be quantified using immunoassays, which are sensitive, economical, and can be used for high throughput. However, the amount of antigen or allergen in an air sample may be very low and consequently the assays must be very sensitive and specific. Immunoassays use antibodies both to capture and visualize the chosen antigen. High specificity and sensitivity can best be achieved by the use of purified, characterized, and specific antibodies.

It is possible to choose between a wide variety of assay setups and reagents. The method described here has been developed for the measurement of airborne rodent allergens. It is a noncompetitive, two-site (sandwich) EIA that utilizes polyclonal antibodies. The detection system uses biotin and streptavidin for increased sensitivity and horseradish peroxidase as the substrate with 3,3′,5,5′-tetramethylbenzidine (TMB) for rapid color development and high sensitivity.

Key Words: Air sampling; aeroallergen; immunoassay; sandwich ELISA; streptavidin; horseradish peroxidase.

1. Introduction

After air sampling and elution, the air sample eluate contains an unknown amount of allergens together with other materials collected in the dust sample. The allergenic proteins or proteins of interest can be quantified using immunoassays. Immunoassays are sensitive and economic methods of analysis, and many samples can be analyzed by one person in a day (a consolation after time and labor-consuming aeroallergen sampling!).

The amount of antigen or allergen in an air sample may be very low – when measuring airborne pet allergens in public environments, levels may be in the pg/m^3 range. The assays used to quantify aeroallergens must therefore be very sensitive and specific. This can best be achieved by the use of purified,

From: *Methods in Molecular Medicine: Allergy Methods and Protocols*
Edited by: M. G. Jones and P. Lympany © Humana Press Inc., Totowa, NJ

characterized, and specific antibodies. Antibody preparation is described elsewhere in this book. Immunoassays use antibodies both to capture the chosen antigen and, when labeled, to visualize the antigen. It is possible to choose between a wide variety of assay setups and reagents. The assays may use monoclonal antibodies (MAbs) or polyclonal antibodies to capture and detect the antigen (see **Note 1**). The assay design may be competitive or noncompetitive, and the immunological (antigen–antibody binding) reaction may occur in the liquid or solid phase. If high sensitivity is necessary, a sandwich enzyme immunoassay (EIA) setup is often preferred, because such assays are usually 10 to 1000-fold more sensitive than inhibition EIAs using the same reagents (1). In addition, there are several methods of detection that may be employed; the detection antibody may be labeled with a choice of several enzymes, fluorescent or chemiluminescent compounds, or radioisotopes (which are more seldom used today for shelf-life, health, legal, and waste-handling reasons). The choice of assay setup and antibodies in particular may greatly influence the allergen levels found in the air samples and may account for differences in reported value of orders of magnitude (2,3).

The following method has been developed for the measurement of airborne rodent allergens. It is a noncompetitive, two-site (sandwich) EIA that utilizes polyclonal antibodies. The detection system uses the strong binding between the vitamin biotin and bacterial streptavidin molecule for increased sensitivity (see **Note 2**). The streptavidin molecule is bound to one or more enzymes that cause a color reaction on addition of a relevant substrate and that is proportional to the amount of bound antigen. In the described assay, horseradish peroxidase is used with the substrate TMB for rapid color development and high sensitivity. For even further sensitivity, the assay may be easily adapted to commercially available signal amplification systems (see **Note 3**).

The main steps of a sandwich enzyme immunoassay (EIA) utilizing biotin and streptavidin, are shown in **Fig. 1**.

2. Materials
2.1. Biotinylation of Purified Polyclonal Antibody

There are several varieties of biotin reagents and biotinylation protocols. The method described below has been used successfully in our antibody preparations. Use MilliQ or deionized, double-distilled water and good laboratory practice. Standard laboratory equipment such as pipetors, pipet tips, test tubes, and beakers, pH meter, scales, and magnetic stirrers are assumed to be available.

2.1.1. Equipment

1. Dialysis membrane (e.g., Spectrapore 6.4-mm diameter membrane with a cutoff of 12–14 kDa).

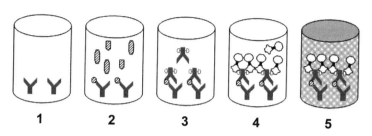

Fig. 1. Schematic sandwich assay setup. (**1**) Coat a microtiter plate with specific capture antibody; wash. (**2**) Add standard dilutions or test solution, incubate; wash. (**3**) Add excess of biotinylated detection antibody, incubate; wash. (**4**) Add streptavidin–enzyme conjugate, incubate; wash. (**5**) Add enzyme substrate, incubate. Read color reaction in plate reader.

2. Dialysis membrane seal.
3. Preweighed 1–3 mL test tube (preferably nonprotein-binding, such as Nunc Minisorp).

2.1.2. Buffers and Reagents

1. Carbonate buffer: 0.1 M $NaHCO_3$, pH 8.4. Dissolve 8.4 g of $NaHCO_3$ in about 900 mL of water in a 1-L container using a magnetic stirrer. Adjust the pH to 8.4 using 1 M NaOH and add water up to 1 L.
2. *N,N*-dimethylformamide (DMF, C_3H_7NO, e.g., Sigma-Aldrich).
3. Biotin reagent: aminohexanoyl-biotin *N*-hydroxysuccinimide (AH-BNHS, e.g., Zymed). Store desiccated at –20°C.
4. Phosphate-buffered saline (PBS), 10-fold concentrated (1.5 M). Dissolve 81.23 g of NaCl, 5.1 g of KH_2PO_4, 20.06 g of $Na_2HPO_4·2H_2O$ (or 40.3 g of $Na_2HPO_4·12H_2O$) in about 900 mL of water in a 1-L container using a magnetic stirrer. Adjust the pH to 7.4 if necessary and add water up to 1 L. Store at room temperature. For use in assays, dilute 1 part of the PBS 10-fold concentrate with 9 parts water (PBS, 0.15 M).
5. Biotinylated antibody storage buffer: 1 part 0.15 M PBS containing 0.15% v/v Kathon CG (Rohm & Haas) and 1 part glycerol. Store at +4°C. A 0.15% v/v solution of Kathon CG is used as a preservative, instead of sodium azide, to obviate the need to handle hazardous powders. Kathon is, however, an irritant and allergenic and should be handled using gloves.

2.2. Sandwich EIA

2.2.1. Equipment

1. High-protein-binding 96-well microtiter plates (e.g., Nunc Maxisorp plates).
2. Pipetors, single and multichannel.
3. Low-protein-binding test tubes (e.g., Nunc Minisorp).
4. Precut plate sealing tape (e.g., Nunc, Invitrogen, cat no. 236366).
5. Microplate washer (e.g., AquaMax DW4, Columbus, ELx50, Biotrak II, *see* **Note 4**).

2.2.2. Buffers and Reagents

MilliQ or deionized, double-distilled water is used for all buffers.

1. Coating buffer: 0.15 M PBS, 0.15% v/v Kathon CG. For 1 L, dilute 100 mL of PBS 10-fold concentrate (*see* **Section 2.1.**, **2.4.**) in 900 mL of water and add 1.5 mL of Kathon CG. Store at +4°C.
2. Wash buffer (20-fold concentrate): Dissolve 1.79 g of $NaH_2PO_4 \cdot 1H_2O$, 15.48 g of $Na_2HPO_4 \cdot 2H_2O$, 350.6 g of NaCl, and 40 mL of Tween 20 in 1.5 L of water in a 2-L container using a magnetic stirrer. Add water up to 2 L and store at room temperature. Prior to use, dilute 50 mL of wash buffer (20-fold concentrate) in 950 mL of water.
3. Dilution buffer: 0.15 M PBS, 0.1% v/v Tween, 1% w/v bovine serum albumin (BSA, heat fractionated, e.g., Sigma-Aldrich), 0.15% v/v Kathon CG. Dissolve 100 mL of PBS (10-fold concentrate), 1.5 mL of Kathon CG, 1 mL of Tween 20, 10 g of BSA in 850 mL of water in a 1-L container using a magnetic stirrer. Add water up to 1 L and store at +4°C for up to 2 d.
4. Coating antibody solution: Dilute the chosen polyclonal antibody in coating buffer (*see* **Section 2.2.**, **2.1.**) to between 2 and 10 µg/mL (*see* **Note 5**).
5. Standards and controls: A standard curve range should be determined from serial dilutions in, for instance, twofold steps in dilution buffer of the relevant standard preparation (*see* **Note 6**). Controls should be prepared, calibrated, diluted (*see* **Note 7**), divided into aliquots, and stored at −70°C.
6. Biotinylated detection antibody: Dilute the detection antibody solution, e.g., 1:1000 in dilution buffer.
7. Streptavidin–horseradish peroxidase conjugate: This is commercially available from many sources, e.g., Serotec, Mabtech AB, etc. Dilute, e.g., 1:1000 in dilution buffer or as recommended by the manufacturer. Other enzyme conjugates may be utilized, such as streptavidin–alkaline phosphatase (*see* **Note 8**).
8. Substrate solution: TMB, soluble form; readymade is available as, e.g., K-blue from Neogen.
9. Stop reagent: 1M H_2SO_4.

2.3. Analysis, Evaluation of Results

1. Microplate reader, set wavelength to 450 nm (or wavelength recommended for the substrate used). Several brands are available on the market, e.g., Spectramax (Molecular Devices), Multiskan (Labsystems).
2. Software program for analysis, compatible with plate reader, e.g., Softmax Pro (Molecular Devices). The program should have log–log and preferably four-parameter curve fit options, and for quality control purposes, coefficient of variation % (CV%) calculation and back-calculation of standard dilution values from the curve.

3. Method

3.1. Biotinylation of Polyclonal Antibody

1. Wet about 8 cm of dialysis membrane in MilliQ water. Tie a knot in one end or seal with dialysis membrane clip.

2. Pipet 0.5 mg of antibody preparation into the wet membrane tube and seal with clip, e.g., 0.5 mL of a 1 mg/mL antibody preparation.

3. Immerse tubing in 1 L 0.1 M NaHCO$_3$, pH 8.4, and dialyze with magnetic stirring at 4°C overnight.

4. Dissolve 1 mg of AH-BNHS in 100 μL of DMF by vortexing. Handle the DMF with gloves in a cabinet and dispose of the plasticware according to local regulations or as recommended by the supplier.

5. Remove the clip from one end of the dialysis membrane that contains the antibody and insert the dialysis tube into a preweighed test tube, so that contents spill into the tube. To ensure that the dialysis membrane is emptied of all the antibody solution, centrifuge the tube containing the membrane (with its opening fastened 1 cm above the bottom of the tube) for 5 min at 1000 rpm. Remove the dialysis membrane and weigh the tube. Note the weight (= volume) of the antibody solution.

6. Add approximately 5 μL of the AH-BNHS solution (the weight ratio of succinimide ester to antibody should be 1:10) and mix end over end for 1 h at room temperature.

7. Transfer the mixture to fresh dialysis tube (8 cm) and dialyze overnight at 4°C in 2 L of 0.15 M PBS to remove the unbound biotin and change the antibody solution buffer.

8. Centrifuge the membrane contents into a preweighed test tube as in step 5 and note the weight.

9. Add storage buffer up to 2 mL (*see* **Note 9**).

3.2. Sandwich EIA

1. Coat a microtiter plate with the coating antibody solution diluted to, e.g., 4 μg/mL in 0.15 M PBS, 0.15% v/v Kathon, 100 μL/well at +4°C overnight. For each incubation, cover the plate wells with a precut sealing tape plate cover. This prevents evaporation and contamination between wells.

2. Wash the microtiter plate three times with 300 μL of wash buffer per well (*see* **Note 4**).

3. Add 100 μL per well of the diluted standard curve series in duplicate (diluted in, for instance, twofold steps: e.g., 3.2, 1.6, 0.8, 0.4, 0.2, 0.1, 0.05 ng/mL), blank wells (i.e., only dilution buffer), positive (high and low) and negative controls, and samples diluted at least twofold, all in dilution buffer. Incubate for 2 h at room temperature.

4. Wash the microtiter plate as in step 2.

5. Dilute the biotinylated detection antibody to 1:1000 in dilution buffer. Add 100 μL/well and incubate for 1 h at room temperature.

6. Wash the microtiter plate as in step 2.

7. Dilute the streptavidin–horseradish peroxidase to 1:1000 in dilution buffer. Add 100 μL/well and incubate for 1 h at room temperature.

8. Wash the microtiter plate as in step 2.

9. Add TMB, 100 μL/well, and incubate at room temperature for 10–15 min. Stop the color reaction with 100 μL/well 1 M H$_2$SO$_4$ (the color will turn from blue to yellow). Other enzyme/substrate combinations or other detection systems may be used (*see* **Note 8**).

10. Read the absorbance (optical density, OD) of each well of the microtiter plate at 450 nm (or other appropriate wavelength, if TMB is not used). Use a four-parameter (or log–log) curve fit to plot the standard curve.

3.3. Analysis, Evaluation of Results, Quality Control

1. Criteria for the assay should be set up and used routinely for acceptance of EIA runs and sample values. The following criteria are used for our sandwich EIAs. The working range of the standard curve is determined as between a standard point reproducibly resulting in an OD >0.05 above the OD for background wells (with no standard, only dilution buffer added) to 75% of the maximum OD of the detection system. The standard points within the working range should give a four-parameter curve fit >0.99. The CV% of duplicate wells should not exceed 10%. The standard concentration values back-calculated from the curve equation should be close to the known values. The 'background' OD of the wells in which dilution buffer was added without antigen should be low, i.e., <0.2 OD. The control sample values should not deviate from the theoretical values more than 15% or from within a predetermined range. If all criteria are met, the run is accepted (*see* **Note 10**).
2. To determine the allergen concentration of the air sample eluate, the sample values are interpolated from the standard curve and corrected for sample dilution. Sample values with a CV of 10% or more between the duplicates are not acceptable and samples should be reassayed. If several dilutions of the sample have been used (recommended, e.g., 1:2, 1:4, 1:8), CV% between values within working range corrected for dilution should not differ >20%. Samples with high CV% are reassayed. Samples with OD values above working range are diluted further and reassayed. The amount collected on the filter per m^3 air is calculated as described in the previous chapter.
3. Check for contamination during filter handling or between wells during the assay run: negative filter controls, i.e., unexposed filters eluted simultaneously as the exposed filters, should be included on each plate, as well as randomly placed blank wells, neither of which should get a value within the standard curve range (*see* **Note 11**).
4. Further quality control measures for the assay are to determine inter- and intra-assay CV%, and variation resulting from both elution and assay steps by sampling in duplicate using parallel pumps placed about 30 cm apart (*see* **Note 12**).

4. Notes

1. MAbs are unique antibodies that ideally bind to one specific protein epitope. They have an advantage for standardization as they can be grown in long-term tissue culture and hence are available indefinitely. Commercial MAb assays are available for the measurement of major allergens from a number or sources including cat, cockroach, and mites. Polyclonal antibodies raised in rabbits are finite but have the advantage of capturing a wider spectrum of allergens from the same source, which might be present simultaneously in airborne dust.

2. The detection antibody is conjugated with biotin, a small molecule, which reduces the risk of loss of biological activity of the antibody. Streptavidin has four subunits, each with the capacity to bind one biotin molecule with strong hydrogen and van der Waals interactions. The streptavidin, being large, may in turn be labeled with several enzyme molecules *(4)*.

3. Commercially available signal amplification kits utilize enzyme cascade or cycle systems or conjugate with multiple enzymes that may enhance assay sensitivity up to 100-fold. Examples are AMPLIQ and AMPAK (DakoCytomation), the ELAST system (PerkinElmer), and polyHRP-streptavidin (RDI). When utilizing such systems, it is important to have very specific and clean reagents as well as laboratory equipment, as not only the analyte signal, but also background and contamination signals may be amplified. When using amplification systems, the standard curve range is set at lower concentrations, and detection antibody and conjugate dilutions usually need to be modified.

4. A microtiter plate washer is not strictly necessary, but very helpful. Ensure proper function with even washing of wells before use. Between-incubation washing without an automatic plate washer can be performed using a multichannel pipet, preferably automatic, for increased reproducibility and decreased ergonomic strain. Tap out contents of plate and add 300 µL wash buffer to each well. Repeat three times (or more, if assay background is high).

5. The geometric capacity of microtiter plates to bind protein has been calculated to be about 4 µg/mL or 400 ng in a well when incubated with 100 µL of solution *(5,6)*.

6. Standard preparation of the extract to which the antibodies are specific; if the antibodies are affinity purified using for instance dialyzed mouse urine, the preferred standard preparation is dialyzed mouse urine. Concentrations of allergen in the standard extract should be calibrated against international standards, where available, such as the NIBSC standards from WHO. Linscott's Directory may be of aid when searching for antigen preparations.

7. Controls containing the antigen in known amounts should be prepared, calibrated, and diluted to suitable concentrations for easy dilution to use in the assay. Include, for instance, a high and low concentration control in every plate, e.g., at 25 and 75% of standard curve range. Controls diluted in PBS containing stabilizing protein, such as 1% BSA, aliquoted in air-tight, low-protein-binding tubes kept at −70°C are usually stable for several years; allergen extracts with higher enzyme content, e.g., from plant sources, may be less stable.

8. Depending on the source of the samples, high background levels may occur, and other enzyme conjugates may be more suitable. An alternative is using streptavidin conjugated with the enzyme alkaline phosphatase and developed using a suitable substrate, such as *para*-nitro-phenyl phosphate tablets. Several other variants are possible, for instance using chemiluminescence or fluorescence for detection.

9. To minimize loss, e.g., if a tube becomes contaminated, aliquot the antibodies in 0.5-mL aliquots. Label the tubes with content and date; the biotinylated antibody solution is quite stable and functional for up to 3 yr when stored at +4°C. The

success of the biotinylation procedure can be checked by running the 'old' and 'new' biotinylated reagents in the assay in parallel. At 6-mo intervals or when contamination of an aliquot is suspected or when a new tube or antibody batch is needed, the performance of standard curve and controls in the assay should be checked by using the biotinylated reagent in parallel with another aliquot or batch.

10. The standard curve should utilize the major part of the OD range of the used enzyme/substrate, considering the capacity of the plate reader. The working range for a reproducible assay using the described assay system and equipment could be, for instance, 0.05–3 OD after reduction of the OD for the background wells (<0.2 OD), the standard points giving roughly a doubling in OD for every doubling in concentration. If other enzymes and substrates are used or if a four-parameter curve fit is not available, the quality criteria must be modified.

11. To successfully set up an assay as described in **Section 3.3.**, the reagents, concentrations, incubation times, numbers of washes between incubations, and so on must all be optimized. Test different combinations of reagent dilutions serially for determination of the standard curve range. Some combinations will increase sensitivity, others will mostly increase background. Optimize signal-to-noise ratio. For further reading on immunoassay performance and kinetics *see*, e.g., Tijssen's Practice and Theory of Enzyme Immunoassays *(7)*. *Check assay specificity*: when setting up the assay and choosing between antibody preparations, it is very important to include nonrelevant allergen extracts in several dilutions from other species or allergens related to the intended allergen or allergens that may be present in the environment to be tested. A suitable starting concentration of such samples may be 1000-fold higher than the highest standard point. Also include filters sampled in other environments, unlikely to contain the allergen in question. However, note that several allergens appear to be ubiquitous (cat and dog, for instance).

12. The study of sampling variation and exposure assessment is a science in itself, warmly recommended further reading is Boleij et al. *(8)*.

References

1. Grier, T. J. (2001) Laboratory methods for allergen extract analysis and quality control. *Clin. Rev. Allergy Immunol.* **21**, 111–140.
2. Hollander, A., Gordon, S., Renström, A., et al. (1999) Comparison of methods to assess airborne rat and mouse allergen levels. I. Analysis of air samples. *Allergy* **54**, 142–149.
3. Renström, A., Gordon, S., Hollander, A., et al. (1999) Comparison of methods to assess airborne rat or mouse allergen levels. II. Factors influencing antigen detection. *Allergy* **54**, 150–157.
4. Vilja, P. (1994) Non-competitive avidin-biotin immunoassay in antibody and antigen detection. Thesis. *Acta Universitatis Tamperensis ser A* pp.398.
5. Cantarero, L. A., Butler, J. E., and Osborne, J. W. (1980) The adsorptive characteristics of proteins for polystyrene and their significance in solid-phase immunoassays. *Anal. Biochem.* **105**, 375–382.

6. Esser, P. (1988) Principles in adsorption to polystyrene. *Nunc. Bull.* **6,** 1–5.
7. Tijssen, P. (1985) Practice and Theory of Enzyme Immunoassays, in *Laboratory Techniques in Biochemistry and Molecular Biology,* Elsevier Science, Amsterdam **15**.
8. Boleij, J., Buringh, E., Heederik, D., and Kromhout, H. (1995) Occupational hygiene of chemical and biological agents, Elsevier, Amsterdam, The Netherlands.

19

The Halogen Assay – A New Technique for Measuring Airborne Allergen

Euan Tovey, Sandra De Lucca, Leanne Poulos and Tim O'Meara

Abstract

The Halogen assay is a new technique for measuring airborne allergen. The assay is unique in that it is capable of analyzing allergens and particles together, combining the advantages of morphological approaches and immunoassay. The Halogen assay allows direct observation of the particles that carry the allergen as well as being capable of identifying all the allergen sources an individual is exposed and sensitized to. The assay is sensitive because the extracted allergen is bound to the membrane at a high local concentration within the minute area around each particle and so is easily detected by immunostaining. It is therefore easy to detect few pollen grains.

The Halogen method supersedes other methods commonly used to identify allergens as it is capable of identifying airborne particles that are allergen sources.

Key Words: Allergen; halogen; immunoassay; asthma; mite; cat.

1. Introduction

The term Halogen assay refers to a type of solid phase immunoassay where a visible *halo* of immunostained allergen is formed around the individual particles that are the source of that allergen *(1)*. To perform this, particles containing allergen such as pollen grains, fungal spores, mite feces, and cat dander are collected and permanently immobilized in contact with a protein-binding membrane. When the particles are wetted, the allergens are extracted from the particles and they bind to the membrane. The bound allergens are then immunostained by passing the reactants through the porous membrane, and the staining appears as halos around the particles (*see* **Fig. 1**).

A long-standing technical goal in aerobiology has been to identify the airborne particles that are allergen sources. The Halogen assay can be used to

From: *Methods in Molecular Medicine: Allergy Methods and Protocols*
Edited by: M. G. Jones and P. Lympany © Humana Press Inc., Totowa, NJ

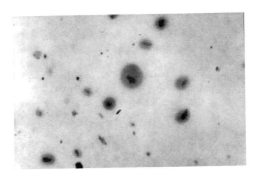

Fig. 1. A small area of the dust collected during active, domestic dust disturbance using a nasal sampler. This has been Halogen immunostained using a monoclonal antibody specific for cat allergen Fel d 1. Particles carrying allergen can be identified by the halo of immunostain around them. These particles differ in size and shape and also in the quantity of allergen per particle. Under these sampling circumstances and in this house, many of the inhaled particles carry cat allergen.

do this. A brief discussion of techniques previously used to detect the allergens associated with particles is provided (*see* **Note 1**).

The main methods commonly used to identify allergens and measure exposure have limitations. Whereas pollen grains and fungal spores can generally be identified based on their morphology, counting them does not provide a reliable measure of exposure to their allergens, as the allergens are also carried by small amorphous particles that cannot be identified (*2*). It is also not known how much different allergens are carried by pollen grains or fungal spores at different times. Exposure to the allergens of domestic pets and mites, which are carried by amorphous particles, is generally determined by extracting the allergens from the particles and then measuring them by methods such as ELISA. This approach gives no information about the particles carrying the allergen. Also, the quantities of allergen involved in personal exposure are close to detection limits of most ELISA systems and this limits the types of exposure measurements that can be made.

The Halogen assay combines the advantages of morphological approaches and immunoassays to provide a simple way to analyze allergens and particles together. For example, the use of an allergen-specific antibody allows the direct observation of the particles that carry a specific allergen as well as quantifying that allergen. Alternatively, immunostaining the air samples collected in a subject's environment with their own serum IgE allows the observation of all the allergen sources the subject is both exposed to and allergic to. No other technique can do this.

Halogen assays are also exquisitely sensitive. This sensitivity is achieved because the extracted allergen is bound to the membrane at a high local concentration within the minute area around each particle and so is easily detected by immunostaining. This means it is as easy to detect one pollen grain, as it is to detect thousands.

Finally, the assays have the potential to measure the quantity of allergen associated with each particle using calculations based on the integrated intensity of each halo measured using computer-based image analysis techniques. These quantities of allergen can then be related to other information about each particle (size, identity, etc.) and can be summed to provide the total amount of allergen in the sample. The technologies for performing these measurements are available in prototype form.

1.1. Three Variants of the Halogen Assay

Halogen immunostaining systems share the common principle of maintaining the collected particles in permanent contact with a matrix capable of nonspecifically binding proteins and other macromolecules. The matrix-bound proteins are then immunostained, allowing the particles that function as the allergen source to be identified. In practice, a protein-binding membrane is used as the matrix, though other options such as protein-binding gels are possible.

Three variants of this, which differ in the way particles are collected and fixed in contact with the protein-binding membrane, are shown in steps 1 and 2 of **Fig. 2**. These are:

1. Collection of particles onto a dry adhesive tape, which is later laminated to a dry protein-binding membrane.
2. Collection of particles onto the dry protein-binding membrane, which is later laminated with a dry adhesive tape.
3. Collection of particles onto a wet protein-binding membrane that has been precoated with an adhesive agarose gel. After collection, this is recoated with more gel to retain the particles.

Variants 1 and 3 are suitable for use with impaction-based collection systems and variant 2 is used with filter-type air samplers (*see* **Section 1.4.**). Binding of allergen to the membrane occurs immediately in the 'wet' system (variant 3) and only after the wetting the dry adhesive/membrane sandwich in variants 1 and 2. The remaining steps 3–5 of the assay process (**Fig. 2**) are common to all variants and are analogous to those used in protein blotting. The components required for performing variants 1–3 are described below.

1.2. Performance Requirements of Adhesive Tapes

There are two major functions of the adhesive tape in Halogen assays. First, it can form the surface on which samples are collected, as in variant 1. Second, if the samples have initially been collected onto the protein-binding membrane, as in variant 2, the tape is subsequently used to maintain the position of the particles on the membrane throughout the assay.

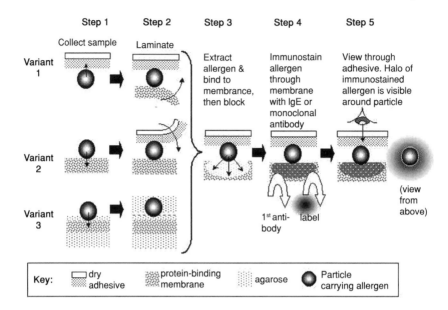

Fig. 2. A simplified schematic view of the five main steps involved in performing three variants of Halogen immunostaining. Interpretation of the symbols is contained in the key.

Of the extensive range of adhesive tapes available, in our experience no commercially available tapes have the required properties combining collection efficiency, optical clarity, noninterference with immunostaining as well as adhesiveness in the aqueous and solvent environments. This led to contracting the development and manufacture of a suitable tape (Inhalix, Woolcock Institute of Medical Research, NSW, Australia).

Low particle bounce is a critical property determining the collection efficiency of adhesive tapes when used for impaction collection. This performance requirement of adhesives could not be predicted from other published characteristics of adhesives. Particles in an impaction sampler may be traveling at well over 1 m/s (a million μm/s) when they hit the tape and they must be captured in the microseconds of contact time before they bounce off. Fibers, which do not make a large contact area with the adhesive surface compared to their contact area with the airstream (generating drag), and large particles, which have a high kinetic energy to surface contact area ratio, tend to be collected least efficiently, whereas small particles are less likely to be impacted. *See (3)* for discussion.

Adhesive tapes need to have excellent optical properties, as particles and staining are observed microscopically through them, not on them. When we compared the collection efficiency of four commercial adhesive tapes against the standard Vaseline-based coating in a Burkard trap, we found that although these tapes had a lower collection efficiency than did Vaseline for particles >10-µm diameter, we also found that the counts of smaller particles were apparently more than twice as high with the tapes than with Vaseline. This was probably because of greater visibility of the small particles on the tape *(4)*. As mentioned earlier, we subsequently developed more efficient adhesive tapes that collect 88% of *Lolium perenne* pollen at 10 L/min, which are better than the commercial adhesives used in this comparison.

The other properties required of tapes (aqueous adhesiveness, clarity, non-interference in assays) were all determined by experimental evaluation. The only property that was directly predictable from manufacturers' data was toxicity, as tapes used in nasal samplers must contain no hazardous solvents.

Adhesive tapes have been directly used for collection in a variety of impaction-type air samplers including nasal samplers *(5–7)*, Burkard spore traps *(4,8)*, and cascade impactors *(9)*. They could presumably be used in swinging arm impingers, although we have not tested these.

When the tape is used for nonimpaction sampling, such as with 'adhesive lifts' (*see* **Section 1.4.3.**) and 'sprinkle blots' *(10)* (and *see* **Section 1.4.4.**) and when used to laminate onto samples already collected onto a porous membrane, performance requirements do not need to include particle collection efficiency.

1.3. Performance Requirements of Protein-Binding Membranes

Many membranes that nonspecifically bind proteins (e.g., nylon, nitrocellulose [NC], mixed cellulose ester [MCE], and polyvinylidene difluoride [PVDF]) with different characteristics are available. Each of these differs in opacity, consistency of microscopic appearance, and protein-binding capacity, which contribute to differences in halo shape, sharpness, intensity, and signal to noise ratios. Good results can be obtained with NC, MCE, and PVDF membranes. In general, membranes with smaller pores, e.g., 0.2–0.45 µm produce more distinct and smaller halos than those with larger pores and in general PVDF and MCE membranes produce halos with a sharper appearance than NC membranes. In addition, some allergens seem to be better detected on PVDF, perhaps because interactions between the allergen and the membrane allow a better presentation of epitopes for binding by particular monoclonal antibodies. MCE membranes are easier to handle than PVDF membranes. The general subject of membrane choice has been widely discussed in the literature on protein blotting, for example see Kirschfink and Terness *(11)* who concluded with a similar preference for PVDF membranes. Our most recent experience has tended toward the use of MCE.

Sampling Systems		Halogen Assay Variant Used
impaction -time based	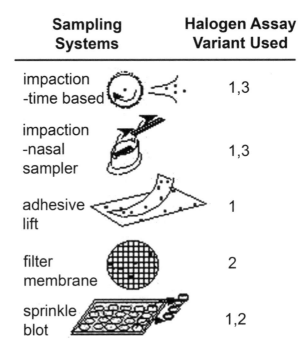	1,3
impaction -nasal sampler		1,3
adhesive lift		1
filter membrane		2
sprinkle blot		1,2

Fig. 3. Four different common methods of sampling allergens, to which one or more of the three variants of Halogen immunostaining systems can be applied, are shown schematically. These include impaction-based systems such as Hirst type spore traps and nasal samplers, collecting particles with an adhesive tape from soft or hard surfaces, and collection by filtering air through porous membranes. In addition, a large area of the laminate can be prepared which contains a known allergen source. This can be divided up for testing or validating assays in multiple assays.

1.4. Sampling of Allergens for Halogen Assay

As shown in **Figs. 2** and **3**, most of the common methods of air and surface sampling of allergens can be modified to allow analysis with Halogen assays. These include impaction systems (Burkard, nasal samplers) and air filtration systems using membranes, plus other applications such as the lifting of particles from collection surfaces as well as sprinkling particles directly onto the adhesive or the membranes. *See* **Note 2** for comments about sampling capacity of membranes and films.

As far as we are aware, Halogen systems can be used to detect all allergens carried by their natural carrier particles. We have measured cat Fel d 1 *(5)*, mite Der p 1 *(12,13)* (as well as Der p 2 and Der f 1, unpublished), Cockroach Bla g1 *(6)*, dog (unpublished), rat *(7)*, the grass pollens *L. perenne* and *C. dactylon*

(8,10,14). We have also detected more than eight species of fungi with IgE *(31)*. Fungi, however, present a challenge, as often only a low-percentage of spores appear to express allergens.

1.4.1. Nasal Air Sampling

The Halogen assay was originally developed for use with nasal air sampling and they are well suited to each other. The technical details of this sampler's performance are available in abstracts of *(15)* and *(16)*. Briefly, nasal air samplers are small impaction collectors that fit just inside the nostril and collect inhaled particles onto a removable adhesive tape (*see* Halogen methods 1 and 3) of approximate dimensions 12 × 3 mm/sampler. The samplers collect most particles of aerodynamic diameter >10 μm and 50% the particles >5-μm diameter. The samplers have negligible air resistance on normal breathing and provide a simple, inexpensive, and silent sampling platform that enables the dose of allergen exposure inhaled by a subject to be determined. The samplers are available from Inhalix, Australia (*see* **Note 3**).

1.4.2. Sampling by Air Filtration with Pumps

For conventional personal air filter sampling, we use portable, low-volume (2 L/min) air pumps, e.g., Airchek 52 (SKC, Eighty Four, PA) attached to IOM sampling heads (Institute of Occupational Medicine, Edinburgh, manufactured by SKC, Blandford, UK). Many other filter holder and air pump assemblies could be used. Again, different types of PVDF, MCE, and NC membranes can be used, provided they will allow sufficient airflow rates and offer the desired performance in immunostaining. We have commonly used 0.45-μm PVDF *(13)* and 1-μm pore size PVDF *(6)*. With more powerful vacuum pumps, airflow rates of up to 10 L/min can be achieved through 25-mm diameter membranes of 1-μm pore size.

1.4.3. Sampling by 'Adhesive Lifts'

Particles carrying allergens may be directly sampled from hard and soft surfaces with adhesive tape. We have measured the level of surface allergen on hard surfaces, such as vinyl floors (Sercombe, unpublished) and on soft surfaces, such as clothing and bedding fabrics. Depending on the circumstances, single or multiple presses can be made from the surface or the adhesive can be wrapped around a small cylinder and rolled across a large surface to sample a large area. In our observation, a single lift will pick up more than 85% of particles from a hard surface. An important consideration is that the tape does not become so saturated with dust that it cannot be later successfully laminated with the protein-binding membrane.

1.4.4. Sprinkle-Blot Assays for Screening

A homogeneous source of an allergen of known identity and purity, such as commercially available pollen grains or fungal spores from culture, may be directly sprinkled, or in other ways distributed, onto either the adhesive tape or the membrane. This is then laminated with the membrane or adhesive tape, respectively, and small disks cut which will fit ELISA wells. These can be used, for example, to screen monoclonal antibodies for functional activity *(10,14)* or to determine other aspects of assay development and optimization.

2. Materials
2.1. Collection and Lamination of Samples for Variants 1 and 2 of Halogen Assay

1. The recommended adhesive tape is supplied by Inhalix, Australia (*see* **Note 3**).
2. For a generally useful PVDF membrane, use 0.45-µm pore polyscreen (NEN Research Products, Boston, MA) or 1-µm pore Millipore BVXA (Millipore Corporation, Bedford, MA). For a generally useful NC membrane use 0.22-µm Nitrobind pure NC (Micron Separations Inc., Westborough, MA) and MCE protein-binding membranes (0.8-µm pore size; Millipore Corp., Bridgewater, MA).

2.2. Collection and Lamination of Samples for Variant 3 of Halogen Assay

1. Agarose ballast: 2% agarose type VI-A (Sigma-Aldrich) in 20% D-sorbitol (Sigma, St Louis) in PBS. PBS is prepared as 8.0 g/L NaCl, 0.2 g/L KCl, 1.44 g/L dibasic sodium phosphate Na_2HPO_4, 0.24 g/L monobasic potassium phosphate (K_2HPO_4). Dissolve in 800 mL MilliQ water, adjust to pH 7.2 with HCl or KOH, adjust volume to 1 L. The above agarose ballast solution is made by adding components together in a conical flask, stirring briefly to mix, and then heating in a microwave until the solution is at boiling point and the agarose has dissolved. Take care the solution does not boil over. Allow to cool to ~50°C for handling.
2. Adhesive coating: 1% agarose type VI-A (Sigma-Aldrich) in 20% D-sorbitol (Sigma), 2% sodium carboxy methyl cellulose (MW 90,000 Da, Sigma-Aldrich) in PBS.
3. Protein-binding membranes as in materials 2.1.2 can be used. New PVDF membranes require prior wetting in 80% ethanol or methanol for approx. 1 min before being transferred to PBS or water. After this, they should not be allowed to dry out.

2.3. Extraction, Blocking, and Immunostaining

1. Different extraction buffers which can be used include:
   a. *Phosphate-buffered saline, pH 7.4 (PBS)* (*see* **Section 2.2.1.**).
   b. *Borate buffer:* Dissolve 12.366 g boric acid in 900 mL MilliQ water. Adjust to pH 8.2 with NaOH and add MilliQ water to a final volume of 1 L.
   c. *Coca's solution:* In 0.5 L MilliQ water dissolve 0.14 g $NaHCO_3$, 0.41 g NaCl, and 0.23 g phenol. Adjust to pH 7.2.
2. Blocking buffer: 5% (w/v) skim milk powder in PBS (*see* **Section 2.2.1.**).

3. Washing buffer: Add 0.5 mL Tween 20 to 1 L PBS.
4. Incubation buffer for first and second antibodies: 2% (w/v) skim milk powder in washing buffer.
5. Immunostaining reagent: 1-step BCIP/NBT (5-bromo-4-chloro-5-indolyl phosphate/ nitroblue tetrazolium, Pierce; approximate staining time: 10–30 min). Use neat.
6. Immunostaining reagent: Fast Red TR/naphthol AS-MX (insoluble alkaline phosphatase substrate with 1 mM levamisole, Sigma Chemical Co.); approximate staining time: 30 min–1 h.

2.4. Visualizing Halogen Staining

Either binocular transmission microscope, equipped with 10× eyepieces and 10 and 20× objectives or a 35-mm slide scanner attached to a suitable computer. The slide scanner is useful as an economical way to obtain a digital image of the immunostaining, but is not useful for observation of particles.

2.5. Miscellaneous Materials

1. Precision pipets devices (0–20, 0–200, 0–1000 μL).
2. 24-Well plates (Sarstedt Inc., Newton, NC).
3. Scalpel blades, fine point tweezers, gloves.
4. Pipet attached to a vacuum line and liquid waste trap for removing liquid during washing steps.

3. Methods

3.1. Sample Collection onto Dry Adhesive Tape (Variant 1)

Samples are collected directly onto the adhesive tape as described in **Sections 1.4.1.**, **1.4.3.**, and **1.4.4**. Gloves, either powder free or washed free of powder, should be worn at all times and neither the adhesive nor the corresponding area of the membrane surface involved in particle and allergen presentation should be touched at any time.

The adhesive is removed from the collection device and laminated with the protein-binding membrane by gently 'rolling' the adhesive tape, adhesive side down, on top of the protein-binding membrane that has been placed on a clean, hard, smooth surface. The bond between the membrane and the tape is augmented by briefly massaging the back of the adhesive tape with a smooth item, such as a spatula, or a small hard rubber roller used for mounting photos. Take care during handling not to minutely crush areas of the membrane. In our experience, such laminated membranes can generally be stored for prolonged period prior to continuing the assay. The next step is **Section 3.4**.

3.2. Sample Collection onto Dry Protein-Binding Membranes (Variant 2)

Particles are directly collected by suction of the air containing the particles onto a protein-binding membrane as described in **Section 1.4.2**. *See* comments in **Sections 1.4.2.** and **2.1.** about airflow rates through membranes and the types of membranes that can be used.

After sample collection, the membranes are laminated with an adhesive tape to form a permanent sandwich containing the particles, using similar manual techniques described in **Section 3.1.** for laminating the adhesive carrying the particles with a membrane. The next step is **Section 3.4**.

1. Laminate the adhesive with the protein-binding membrane. Trim to size.
2. Place each laminated adhesive/membrane sandwich from a nasal sampler in the well of a labeled 24-well plate, with the membrane side facing upwards.
3. For PVDF only, not NC or MCE, wet in an 80% methanol solution for 60 s until evenly opaque. Do not oversoak or the laminate may separate.
4. For PVDF only, not NC or MCE, remove the methanol solution and rinse 3× with PBS over 5 min. Do not allow the membranes to become dry at any stage.
5. Add 500 μL of elution buffer to all membranes and elute allergens for 1–12 h at room temperature with gentle agitation. Incubation time depends on the allergen, but longer times give a stronger signal.
6. Block with 5% skim milk powder solution for 1 h, then rinse in PBS/Tween (0.05%) for 5 min.

3.3. Sample Collection onto a Wet, Protein-Binding Membrane Precoated with an Aqueous Adhesive Gel (Variant 3)

The preparation and handling of the wet adhesive membranes is technically rather tedious and demanding, although the method can give excellent results. It is included here as it can be used as an alternative to the dry adhesive film, described elsewhere, if these are not available.

NC *(12)*, MCE, or PVDF *(13)* membranes can be used. All these types of membranes should be kept moist once the adhesive gel has been applied and this imposes limits on impaction sampling conditions. The method is suitable for nasal sampling where the flow of humid air during exhalation minimizes drying out. It is only suitable for cascade impaction systems for short sampling times and there is the risk the high-velocity airstream in the final stages of the impaction collector will damage the agarose adhesive layer.

The first step is to coat the back of the membrane with a ~0.5-mm layer of the agarose, in PBS containing sorbitol as a humectant, to function as a water ballast. The calculated volume of agarose is pipeted onto a prewarmed surface in the collecting apparatus (held at about 45°C) and then the damp membrane is laid on top to this. A very thin (20–30 μm) layer of agarose is then applied to the top of the protein-binding membrane. This consists of agarose containing sorbitol plus 2% sodium carboxy methyl cellulose. This is applied using an ultrasonic nebulizer of the type used to deliver asthma medications at home. The jet of nebulized liquid agarose is directed onto the top surface of the membrane, where it gels. Successive, brief passages allow an even layer of 20–30 μm thickness to be deposited. The thickness is checked with a microscope and some experimentation is required to determine the exact conditions (we use 3–4 passages each of ~2–3 s with the surface to be coated held about 1 cm from the nebulizer's output orifice). After their construction, the adhesive-coated membranes are maintained in humid atmosphere prior to use.

Following sample collection, the membranes are stored in a sealed, humid container at 4°C for 1–24 h to allow the allergens to elute from the particles and to diffuse through the thin agarose layer and bind to the underlying protein-binding membrane. *See* **Section 3.4.1.** for comments on extraction times.

After this incubation, the membranes are again coated using the nebulizer to apply another thin (~50 μm) layer of 0.5% agarose to hold the particles in place during the rigors of immunostaining. It is important during the application of the second agarose coat that the layer is applied slowly so that no liquid agarose is allowed to accumulate. Any agarose flow on the surface at this time can redistribute the particles from the location where allergens have been bound.

The following is carried out to prepare the wet adhesive membrane for both sampling and immunostaining:

1. Wet membrane in 80% methanol solution for 60s until evenly opaque. Remove and rinse 3x with PBS (for PVDF only, not NC or MCE).
2. Coat back of wet PVDF or NC membrane with ~0.5-mm layer of agarose/humectant by pipeting out appropriate volume of agarose onto the base of collection device held at ~45°C and then placing the membrane gently on top of the thin layer of agarose. This needs to be done quickly as the agarose forms a gel in <1 min.
3. Construct the collection surface on the membrane by exposing it to an aerosol of agarose/humectant/adhesive until a thin coat is deposited. Exact conditions are established by prior experience—*see* **Section 3.3**. Store in humid location.
4. Collect sample (in nasal samplers).
5. Allow time for allergens to be extracted from particles (1–24 h).
6. Recoat particles on the collection surface with a layer of agarose using aerosol generator.
7. Block membranes with 5% skim milk powder solution for 1 h and then rinse in PBS/Tween 20 (0.05%) buffer.

3.4. Immunostaining Systems

The general scheme for immunostaining follows that used in protein blotting, *see (11,17,18)*. The scheme is outlined in **Fig. 2** and some variants for probing are shown in **Fig. 4**.

3.4.1. Elution of Allergens from Particles and then Blocking

In variant 3 (**Fig. 2**), which uses a wet collection surface, the elution of allergens from particles begins as soon as they are collected. In systems with dry

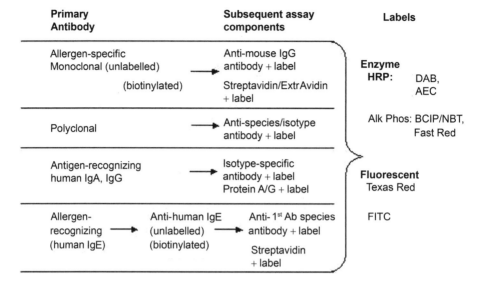

Fig. 4. An overview of some different combinations of primary antibodies and labeling systems that can be used for probing in Halogen assays.

collection surfaces (variants 1 and 2), extraction occurs only after lamination has been performed and the sandwich has been wetted. This event can be delayed until a convenient time.

The initial procedure for wetting the membrane/adhesive laminate depends on whether NC/MCE or PVDF membranes are used (*see* **Section 3.2.**).

Various extraction buffers can be used, *see* **Section 2.3.1**. These should not contain any detergents or proteins which can either block the membrane or interfere with the adhesive/membrane sandwich.

Extraction times vary from 1 to 24 h. Whereas for sources such as pollen this extraction mainly occurs in less than an hour, with mite, cat, and dog allergens, elution substantially occurs in the first hour, although longer incubations up to 12 h generally produce more intense halos. For fungi the extraction is slower and more variable and is best performed for up to 24 h. For membranes carrying fungi, storing the unlaminated membrane at 100% RH and 25°C for 24 h can lead to hyphal growth and enhanced allergen expression. This is followed by lamination, and this variation of the protocol shows improved immunostaining of both fungal conidia and hyphae *(31)*.

After extraction, the protein-binding membrane is blocked to prevent binding of antibodies to vacant protein-binding sites on the membrane. This is generally performed with 5% skim milk powder in PBS for an hour, although many blocking agents would be potentially suitable. The final choice may require experimentation. Based on the experience in the literature of blotting proteins from SDS gels, the choice of blocking agent can effect the subsequent detection of some allergens. In our experience with Halogen assays, the blocking agent may have a small effect on halo intensity.

The use of a sample for Halogen assay and for other types of assay is discussed (*see* **Note 4**).

3.4.2. Antibody Probing with a Monoclonal Antibody

Allergens are detected using a primary antibody of known specificity for that allergen. In our experience, monoclonal antibodies are preferred. Monospecific polyclonal antibodies have also been used *(8)*, but there is the risk that the animals they are raised in will have natural antibodies against a range of common environmental antigens which will also be detected by the serum. This requires either that these unwanted antibodies are adsorbed out or affinity purification of specific antibodies is performed. Techniques for this can be found in specialist text books of immunological methods. Small amounts of specific purified antibodies can also be prepared directly from protein blots *(20)*.

In Halogen assays, as the allergens are extracted from their native sources (unlike allergens blotted from SDS gels), the allergens are in their native conformation and should be detectable with monoclonal antibodies directed against conformational epitopes. However, there can be subtle differences in the shape of the allergen's epitopes following binding to different solid phases. Antibodies that were selected in an ELISA may not be optimal for Halogen applications and vice versa. In general, antibodies should be screened for performance in the application they will be used in.

Primary antibodies are generally used at a concentration of 1–2 μg/mL for incubation periods ranging from 1 h up to overnight. These times depend on the concentration and avidity of the antibody and the need to maximize the signal and minimize background and are best optimized by experiment. Incubation buffer is 2% skim milk in PBS–Tween.

After incubation with primary antibody the laminated membrane is washed three times for a total of 30 min, with rocking, to remove any unbound residual primary antibody. The bound primary antibody is detected with a secondary antibody, for example with antimouse antibody conjugated to alkaline phosphatase (Sigma) followed by washing and detection with BCIP/NBT (Pierce) substrate. Alternatively biotinylated primary antibody can be used and detected with ExtrAvidin or streptavidin–enzyme (peroxidase or alkaline phosphatase). In our experience the former system has lower backgrounds. Further comments on washing and incubation times are given (*see* **Note 5**).

1. Incubate with allergen-specific monoclonal antibody (generally at 1:500) in 2% skim milk in PBS/0.05% Tween 20 for 1 h at room temperature on the plate shaker.

A container is chosen to provide the minimum but sufficient area for the membrane to remain flat; for small items 24-well cell culture plates are convenient. The volume used should be the minimum needed to adequately cover the laminated membrane, for example 400 μL/well in a 24-well plate, and care should be taken that the adhesive side of the laminated membrane is kept facing down.

2. Wash 3 × 10 min in PBS/Tween.
3. Add 1:500 antimouse alkaline phosphatase conjugate. Incubate for 1 h at room temperature with agitation on the plate shaker.
4. Wash 3 × 10 min in PBS/Tween.
5. Develop membranes with BCIP/NBT substrate. The reaction is stopped after membranes have been stained light-medium purple (approximately 10–30 min) by rinsing 3× in deionized water.
6. Stained samples can be stored in deionized water at 4°C for up to 3 d before analysis.

3.4.3. Antibody Probing with IgE

IgE from allergic subjects can be used to specifically detect what are, by definition, allergens on the membrane. Usually the primary incubation is performed with RAST class 3 or 4 serum, overnight, at 4°C. However, depending on the antibody titer of the serum and the allergen involved, the serum can sometimes be diluted up to fivefold with no loss of halo quality or number and a reduction of background staining. In one study we found a direct correlation between the numbers of halos detected and the titer of the sera, with serum dilutions going down to 128-fold for a 35% reduction in the numbers of halos. After incubation with serum and then washing, the bound IgE is detected using suitable second antibody, such as biotinylated antihuman IgE (for example KPL, Gaithersburg, MA), at a dilution of 1 in 500. This is followed by incubation with streptavidin–alkaline phosphatase conjugate (1 in 1000) and BCIP/NBT development.

1. Add neat human sera from allergic patient (preferably RAST class 3 or 4) to the laminated membrane. Dilutions of serum may later be used after confirming their activity by trial. *See* **Note 1** in **Section 3.4.2.** on advice about containers and volumes to use.
2. Incubate overnight on an orbital shaker at room temperature.
3. Wash 3 × 10 min in PBS/Tween.
4. Incubate with biotin-labeled goat antihuman biotin IgE diluted 1:500 in 5% skim milk, PBS–Tween for 1.5–2 h at room temperature.
5. Wash 3 × 10 min in PBS/Tween.
6. Incubate with ExtrAvidin alkaline phosphatase conjugate diluted 1:1000 in 2% skim milk, PBS–Tween for 1.5–2 h at room temperature.
7. Wash 3 × 10 min in PBS/Tween.
8. Develop membranes with either BCIP/NBT for 10–30 min or Fast Red TR/naphthol AS-MX for 30–60 min at room temperature.
9. Stop the staining reactions by rinsing in distilled water.

10. Stained samples can be stored in deionized water at 4°C for up to 3 d before analysis.

3.5. Enzyme and Fluorescent Immunostaining Systems

Halogen staining uses similar immunostaining techniques that have been used for protein blotting. When the enzyme label horse radish peroxidase is used, the insoluble, colored enzyme substrates are used, for example, a precipitating TMB (3,3′,5,5′-tetramethyl benzidine; Pierce) and when the enzyme label alkaline phosphatase is used the substrates used are BCIP/NBT or Fast Red.

In general, the intensity of background color is developed to a darker level in Halogen than in protein-blotting assays. For example, BCIP/NBT is allowed to develop until the membrane background is stained to a medium blue to the eye, although when viewed through the microscope using illumination directed from the underside, this background appears quite light. Epi-illumination can also be used if available, which allows the particles to be more closely observed.

We have found enzyme-labeling systems to be more sensitive than fluorescent labels such as Texas Red and FITC and would be easier to quantify. We have recently published a highly sensitive method using dual immunofluorescence and confocal microscopy *(32)*.

Immunogold staining was found not to be sensitive, presumably because of the hindrance of migration of the gold–second antibody complexes by the membrane. Chemiluminescence has not been evaluated, as it would require a sophisticated system of signal capture.

PVDF membranes can be cleared by briefly incubating in ethylene glycol/ glycerol solution (9:1) *(21)*. This is useful particularly when heavy staining has been used to maximize sensitivity. NC membranes can be cleared when dry using microscope immersion oil (e.g., Olympus nd 1.516).

Further comments about multiprobe labeling can be found (*see* **Note 6**).

3.6. Staining of all Proteins or Particles

For some applications it maybe of additional interest to be able to stain all the proteins or other types of macromolecules extracted from particles and bound to the membrane. For example, it is surprising to see the amounts of protein extracted from fungal spores even though there may be little immuno-staining of allergens. Proteins can be biotinylated directly on the membrane (prior to blocking) using kits such as NHS-Biotin Total Protein Detection kit (BioRad) and then probed with a streptavidin–enzyme system. It should also be possible to do this with India ink on NC after Tween blocking or with other protein-staining systems prior to blocking, although we have not tested this. Additionally it may be of interest to stain all the translucent dust particles to aid their counting. This can be done with 0.25% Safranin O in 10% ethanol (DeLucca, unpublished).

3.7. Interpretation of Halogen Assays

The simplest way to interpret Halogen assays is to directly visualize the membranes using a conventional laboratory compound light microscope. If a video camera is attached, this has the advantage that images can be preserved, captured, and communicated.

An image can provide a more dramatic interpretation than the quantity of allergen expressed as weight. Any patient shown a picture can fully grasp the story "you did not think you were exposed to cat allergen, but you can see in the staining of this air sample from your house, that many of the airborne particles carry cat allergen".

The next level of interpretation is to count the number of particles carrying allergen. This provides a useful proxy for quantity that is dependent on the distribution of allergen content/particle being similar between samples. This is likely to be the case when large numbers of particles are collected under similar circumstances, but is less likely when the total number of particles is small or some samples contain a disproportionate number of large particles carrying more allergen. These impose limitations on the interpretation of counts of numbers of particles with halos.

The most accurate interpretation of quantity is provided by image analysis of stained membranes to determine the integrated optical density of each halo and then interpret this into absolute quantities of allergens. This is performed by reference to a set of standards of known allergen concentration which have been microdotted onto the membrane and immunoprobed simultaneously. Prototype hardware and software for performing this is available in our laboratory, but overall, the results were inconsistent and the method is technically demanding.

The use of an image analysis-based system provides additional information about the size and shape of particles carrying allergen and about the quantity of allergen per particle. Experience with 'thunderstorm asthma' shows that inhaling many small particles has quite different clinical outcomes than inhaling a few large particles even if the total amount of allergen is similar *(22)*. The important distinction of particle size, which determines the site of deposition of the particles in the respiratory system, would be missed by an assay that relied on allergen quantification only.

The original aim of the project that led to our development of the nasal air sampler and Halogen assay was to provide an integrated system complete with automated pollen and fungal identification. Although considerable progress has been made *(23–25)* including a stand-alone CD-ROM Database (Inhalix, Sydney) of allergenic pollen grains and fungal spores *(26)*, such a fully integrated system remains a future project.

4. Notes

1. Halogen immunostaining differs from other published methods of immunostaining particles and their allergens. It differs from precipitation systems (27) that involve specific antibodies of a predetermined specificity to immobilize only the specified antigens around the particle; from press-blotting systems (28,29) where the association of particle and allergens is not permanently maintained and immunostaining cannot be associated on a one-to-one basis with individual particulate sources; from fixation techniques where the allergen is either fixed inside the particle (22) and from fixation techniques where allergens are fixed to nonprotein-binding membranes (30,31).

2. The sampling capacity is limited by the particle loading of the adhesive or the membrane surface used for sample collection. It would probably be unwise for the samples to exceed 5% of the total surface area, as further loading may reduce sampling efficiency, interfere with subsequent lamination and/or with the resolution of halos. With adhesive tapes, we are not aware that they directly lose their adhesiveness from exposure to air alone. Time *per se* is not an issue and we have intermittently sampled onto tapes in Burkard samplers and onto membranes (using a timer on the pump) for sampling periods of over a week.

3. Inhalix, was a spin-off from the Institute of Respiratory Medicine, now called the Woolcock Institute of Medical Research. Although Inhalix was wound up in 2002, most materials are still available for research purposes by contacting Dr Euan Tovey, Rm 461, Blackburn Building, DO6, University of Sydney, NSW 2006, Australia or fax: 61-2-9351 7451.

4. More than one type of assay can be performed on samples collected both in methods 1 and 2. Assuming there is sufficient density of sample on a tape or membrane to enable smaller sections to be representative, the adhesive tapes can be cut into sections and allergen extracted off a section by immersion in buffer that is then subject to liquid phase immunoassay. The remaining section can be analyzed by Halogen assay. Conversely, if samples are collected on PVDF membranes, prior to lamination of the membrane, allergens can be eluted from part of the membrane in an elution buffer such as 1% BSA, PBS with no Tween. PVDF does not 'wet' under these conditions, whereas NC would bind the allergens. In this way, samples collected on filters or membranes can be divided and one section can be analyzed by Halogen assay and the remaining section analyzed in parallel by amplified ELISA.

5. Because all reactants both enter and leave through only one side of the protein-binding membrane in Methods 1 and 2 (the other side being sealed with the adhesive), reagent incubation and washing times are longer in comparison with those used for protein-blotting methods. Larger pore membranes and gentle shaking of reactions aid the more rapid diffusion of reagents.

6. We have attempted to develop multiprobe immunolabeling systems with only partial success. It is feasible to probe two different antigen sources with two different antibodies on the same blot. This is performed by using an unlabeled primary antibody followed by an antimouse antibody labeled with for example alkaline phosphatase, then followed with a biotin-labeled primary antibody of different specificity and

with HRP–streptavidin. This produces a blot with different colored halos for each allergen. However, the colabeling of the same allergen with two differently labeled primary antibodies (for example, an allergen-specific monoclonal and human IgE) so far has been less satisfactory using either different fluorescent probes (e.g., FITC and Texas Red) or a fluorescent probe and an insoluble substrate. It would seem the presence of one antibody system interferes with the expression of the other's signal either by quenching or by steric hindrance. Four recent papers *(32–35)* describe methods for dual staining of fungi with human IgE and a monoclonal. These techniques are operational but require on-going development. We would be very pleased to receive correspondence on techniques suitable for dual staining of the same allergen.

References

1. Tovey, E. (1995) *Patent US* 08/7934887, *Detection of Molecules Associated with Airborne Particles.* University of Sydney, Assignee.
2. Spieksma, F. T. M., Kramps, J. A., Plomp, A., and Koerten, K. (1991) Grass-pollen allergen carried by the smaller micronic aerosol fraction. *Grana* **30,** 98–101.
3. Hinds, W. (1982) *Aerosol Technology.* Wiley, New York.
4. Razmovski, V., O'Meara, T., Hjelmroos, M., et al. (1998) Adhesive tapes as capture surfaces in Burkard sampling. *Grana* **37,** 305–310.
5. O'Meara, T., DeLucca, S., Sporik, R., et al. (1998) Detection of inhaled cat allergen. *Lancet* **351,** 1488–1489.
6. De Lucca, S., Taylor, D., O'Meara, T., et al. (1999) Measurement and characterisation of cockroach allergens detected during normal domestic activity. *J. Allergy Clin. Immunol.* **104,** 672–680.
7. Renstrom, A., Karlsson, A. S., Manninen, A., and Tovey, E. (1999) Measuring inhaled occupational allergens: a comparison between nasal sampling and conventional air sampling on filters using pumps. *Eur. Respir. J.* **14(30),** 538s.
8. Razmovski, V., O'Meara, T., and Tovey, E. (2000) A new method for simultaneous immuno-detection and morphologic identification of individual sources of pollen allergens. *J. Allergy Clin. Immunol.* **105,** 725–731.
9. Tovey, E., De Lucca, S. D., Pavlicek, P., et al. (2000) The morphology of particles carrying mite, dog, cockroach and cat aeroallergens affects their efficiency of collection by nasal samplers and cascade impactors. *J. Allergy Clin. Immunol.* **105,** S228, Abstract 676.
10. Lovborg, U., Baker, P., Taylor, D. J. M., et al. (1999) Subtribe-specific monoclonal antibodies to *Lolium perenne. Clin. Exp. Allergy* **29,** 973–981.
11. Kirschfink, M. and Terness, P. (1998) Immunoblotting. In *Molecular Diagnosis of Infectious Disease* (Reischl, U. ed.), Humana, Totowa, NJ, pp. 361–371.
12. Poulos, L., O'Meara, T., Sporik, R., and Tovey, E. (1999) Detection of inhaled Der p 1. *Clin. Exp. Allergy* **29,** 1232–1238.
13. De Lucca, S., Sporik, R., O'Meara, T., and Tovey, E. (1999) Mite Allergen (Der p 1) is not only carried on mite faeces *J. Allergy Clin. Immunol.* **103,** 174–175.
14. Lovborg, U., Baker, P., and Tovey, E. (1998) A species-specific monoclonal antibody to *Cynodon dactylon. Int. Arch. Allergy Immunol.* **117,** 220–223.

15. Sercombe, J. K., Pavlicek, K., Xavier, M. L., et al. (1998) (Abstract 337) Assessment of nasal and pocket air samplers. *J. Allergy Clin. Immunol.* **101,** S80.
16. Graham, J., Pavlicek, J., Sercombe, M., and Xavier, M., et al. (2000) The nasal sampler. A device for sampling inhaled aeroallergens. *Ann. Allergy, Asthma and Immunol.* **84,** 599–604.
17. Bjerrum, O. and Heegard, H. (ed.) (1988) *Handbook of Immunoblotting of Proteins,* CRC, Baco Raton, FL.
18. Garfin, D. and Bers, G. (1989) Basic aspects of protein blotting. In *Protein Blotting: Methodology, Research and Diagnostic Applications* (Baldo, B. and Tovey, E. R. ed.), Karger, Basel.
19. Black, S. (1998) Diagnostic application of a multi-channel immunoblot apparatus. In *Molecular Diagnosis in Infectious Disease* (Reischel, U. ed.), Humana, Totowa, NJ, pp. 373–396.
20. Tovey, E., Johnson, M., Roche, A., et al. (1989) Cloning and sequencing of a cDNA expressing a recombinant House Dust Mite protein that binds human IgE and corresponds to an important low molecular weight allergen. *J. Exp. Med.* **170,** 1457–1462.
21. Tarlton, J. and Knight, P. J. (1996) Clarification of immunoblots on polyvinylidene difluoride (PVDF) membranes for transmission densitometry. *J. Immunol. Methods* **191,** 65–69.
22. Knox, R. B. (1993) Grass pollen, thunderstorms and asthma. *Clin. Exp. Allergy* **23,** 354–359.
23. Benyon, F., Jones, A., and Tovey, ERT. (1998) Spores of airborne, allergenic fungi are differentiated and identified by image analysis. *J. Allergy Clin. Immunol.* **101,** S132, Abs 550.
24. Jones, A., Hjelmroos-Koski, M., and Tovey, E. (1999) Image analysis can be used to identify airborne allergenic pollen. *J. Allergy Clin. Immunol.* **103,** S188, Abs 721.
25. Benyon, F., Jones, A., Tovey, E., and Stone, G. (1999) Differentiation of allergenic fungal spores by image analysis, with application to aerobiological counts. *Aerobiologia* **15,** 211–223.
26. Hjelmroos, M., Benyon, F., Culliver, S., et al. (1999) *Airborne Allergens. Interactive Identification of Allergenic Pollen and Fungal Spores,* CD-ROM, Inhalix Institute of Respiratory Medicine, Sydney.
27. Tovey, E. R., Chapman, M. D., and Platts-Mills, T. A. E. (1981) The distribution of house dust mite allergen in the houses of patients with asthma. *Am. Rev. Respir. Dis.* **124,** 630–635.
28. Schumacher, M. J., Griffith, D., and O'Rourke, M. K. (1988) Recognition of pollen and other particulate aeroantigens by immunoblot microscopy. *J. Allergy Clin. Immunol.* **82,** 608–616.
29. Suphioglu, C., Singh, M. B., Taylor, B. B., et al. (1992) Mechanism of grass pollen-induced asthma. *Lancet* **339,** 569–572.
30. Acevedo, F., Vesterberg, O., and Bayard, C. (1998) Visualization and quantification of birch-pollen allergens directly on air-sampling filters. *Allergy* **53,** 594–601.

31. Holmquist, L. and Vesterberg, O. (1999) Luminescence immunoassay of pollen allergens on air sampling polytetrafluoroethylene filters. *J. Biochem. Biophys. Methods* **41**, 49–60.

32. Green, B. J., Sercombe, J. K., and Tovey, E. R. (2005) Fungal fragments and undocumented conidia function as new aeroallergen sources. *J. Allergy Clin. Immunol.* **115**, 1043–1048.

33. Green, B. J., Millecchia, L. L., Blachere, F. M., Tovey, E. R., Beezhold, D. H., and Schmechel, D. (2006) Dual fluorescent halogen immunoassay for bioaerosols using confocal microscopy. *Anal. Biochem.* **354**, 151–153.

34. Green, B. J., Schmechel, D., Sercombe, J. K., and Tovey, E. R. (2005) Enumeration and detection of aerosolized *Aspergillus fumigatus* and *Penicillium chrysogenum* conidia and hyphae using a novel double immunostaining technique. *J. Immunol. Methods* **307**, 127–134.

35. Green. B. J., Schmechel, D., and Tovey, E. R. (2005) Detection of aerosolized *Alternaria alternata* conidia, hyphae, and fragments by using a novel double-immunostaining technique. *Clin. Diagn. Lab. Immunol.* **12**, 1114–1116.

20

Measurement of Specific IgG Anti-Fel d 1 Antibodies

Meinir G. Jones

Abstract

There is currently considerable interest in the role of specific IgG antibodies in allergy. Several studies suggest that specific IgG antibodies may play a protective role in allergy. Successful immunotherapy is associated with increases in allergen-specific IgG antibodies which correlate with clinical outcome. Other studies have identified an inverse relationship between exposure to cat and sensitization, which was associated with high titer specific IgG and IgG_4. This immune response was described as a modified Th2 response, because both IgE and IgG_4 require Th2 cytokine IL-4 for their production. A modified Th2 response was described with laboratory animal allergy, where there was almost a twofold reduction in the risk of developing work-related chest symptoms.

In this chapter, we review the major factors to be considered in the development of an ELISA for the determination of specific IgG and IgG_4 antibodies.

Key Words: IgG antibodies; IgG_4 antibodies; IgE; modified Th2 response; blocking antibodies.

1. Introduction

There has been considerable interest in the role of IgG in allergy: recent evidence suggests it may play a protective role. An inverse relationship between exposure to cats and sensitization was described which was associated with high titer specific IgG and IgG_4 *(1)*. This immune response is described as a modified Th2 response, because both IgE and IgG_4 require Th2 cytokine IL-4 for their production. The modified Th2 response is suggestive of clinical tolerance as the shift from specific IgE antibodies to IgG_4 resulted in a decrease in both sensitization and asthma *(2)*.

We have recently established a modified Th2 response in laboratory animal workers. Within our cohort and cross-sectional studies on laboratory animal allergy we observed increasing risks of sensitization and work-related symptoms

From: *Methods in Molecular Medicine: Allergy Methods and Protocols*
Edited by: M. G. Jones and P. Lympany © Humana Press Inc., Totowa, NJ

with increasing exposures to rats, except at highest exposure level where risks of both outcomes were lower *(3,4)*. We established a significantly increased ratio of IgG_4:IgE in those workers most heavily exposed. There was an almost twofold reduction of symptoms in those who produced both specific IgG_4 and IgE as compared to those producing specific IgE only. The attenuation of sensitization and symptoms at high exposures and the increased ratio of IgG_4:IgE in laboratory animal workers is suggestive of a natural form of immunotherapy.

Ratios of IgE to IgG_4 have been found to change during specific immunotherapy *(5)*. Specific serum levels of both IgE and IgG_4 increase during the early phase of therapy, but the increase in specific IgG_4 is more pronounced and the ratio of specific IgG_4:IgE is increased 10- to 100-fold, suggesting a protective role for IgG_4 *(5)*. IL-10 is a potent suppressor of both total and allergen-specific IgE, whereas it simultaneously increases IgG_4 production *(6)*.

Successful immunotherapy is associated with increases in allergen-specific IgG_1 and IgG_4 antibody concentrations that correlate with the clinical outcome *(7–10)*. It is not known whether allergen-specific IgG or IgG_4 antibodies associated with the modified Th2 response exhibit functional activity. It is possible that IgG antibodies may play a protective role by blocking leukocyte histamine release, inhibiting signal transduction and mediator release through the high-affinity IgE receptors (FcεR1) and IgG (FcγRIIB) receptors *(11–14)* and blocking allergen-induced IgE-dependent histamine release by basophils *(15)*. IgG antibodies may exert their effect by competitive inhibition of allergen–IgE complexes, which prevents complexes binding to the low-affinity IgE receptor, CD23, and subsequent antigen presentation. Others have suggested that not only quantitative changes occur with the IgG antibody but also the spectrum of the specificity of the IgG is altered *(16)*. One grass pollen immunotherapy study demonstrated a blunting of seasonal increases in serum allergen-specific IgG and IgG_4. Further examination showed the postimmunotherapy serum to exhibit inhibitory activity, which coeluted with IgG_4 and blocked IgE-facilitated binding of allergen–IgE complexes to B cells. Increases in IgG and the IgG blocking activity correlated with the patients' overall assessment of improvement *(9)*.

2. Materials

2.1. ELISA

1. ELISA plate (Thermo Electron Corporation, Basingstoke, UK).
2. 1X phosphate-buffered solution (PBS).
3. Allergen at 1 µg/mL Fel d 1 in PBS (Indoor Biotechnology, Cardiff, UK).
4. Positive control: a pool of serum samples known to have IgG anti-Fel d 1 antibodies.
5. Negative control: a pool of serum samples known to be negative for IgG anti-Fel d 1 antibodies.
6. Test serum samples for the measurement of IgG anti-Fel d 1 antibodies.

7. Coating buffer: 50 mM carbonate bicarbonate buffer pH 9.6.
8. Blocking buffer: PBS, 1% bovine serum albumin (BSA). Make up fresh on day of assay.
9. Reagent buffer: PBS, 1% BSA, and 0.05% Tween 20. Make up fresh on day of assay.
10. Wash buffer: PBS, 0.05% Tween 20. Add sodium azide 0.05% for storage.
11. Biotinylated anti-IgG antibody (Becton Dickinson, Cowley, UK) diluted 1:1000 in reagent buffer; 10 mL is sufficient for 96-well ELISA plate.
12. ExtrAvidin peroxidase (Sigma, Poole, UK) diluted 1:1000 in reagent buffer.
13. Phosphate citrate buffer pH 5.0: 2.48 g Na_2HPO_4 to 50 mL water –buffer A. 1.92 g citric acid to 50 mL water – buffer B. Add 50 mL of buffers A and B to 100 mL deionized water and bring pH to 5.0. Store at 4°C.
14. Stock substrate: Dissolve 100 mg 3,3′,5,5′-tetramethyl-benzidine (TMB) in 10 mL dimethyl sulfoxide. Store in 200-µL aliquots at −20°C.
15. Substrate solution: Add 100 µL TMB stock solution to 10 mL phosphate citrate pH 5.0 and add 3 µL H_2O_2 (w/w) immediately before use. The substrate solution must be made prior to addition to wells; 10 mL substrate solution is sufficient for one 96-well ELISA plate.
16. Stop solution: 1.9 M sulfuric acid. Store at room temperature. Note: Always add acid to water in fume cupboard.

2.2. Inhibition Assay

In addition to the reagents for the ELISA, a higher concentration of Fel d 1 at 10 µg/mL is required for preincubation with serum.

3. Methods

The method described for the measurement of IgG antibodies specific for Fel d 1 has been optimized. A checkerboard was set up with varying concentrations of allergen, biotinylated antibody, and strepAvidin peroxidase (*see* **Note 1**). The optimum concentrations were used for the ELISA. The time and temperature of the incubation periods were also optimized.

We believe it is essential to subtract the binding of IgG antibodies to the blocking agent BSA. Some sera have much higher binding to BSA than other sera; however, it is essential to subtract the background binding for each individual.

We have measured specific IgG antibodies to a panel of allergens. The protocol given for the measurement of IgG-specific antibodies to Fel d 1 can be optimized for each allergen using the checkerboard approach. IgG_4-specific antibodies can also be measured using the same protocol but substituting the biotinylated anti-IgG antibody with biotinylated anti-IgG_4 antibody. The IgG_4 ELISA will need to be optimized as above.

3.1. Protocol for IgG-Specific Antibodies to Fel d 1

1. Coat each well in the upper half of the ELISA plate with 100 µL of 1 µg/mL Fel d 1.
2. Coat each well in the lower half of the ELISA plate with 100 µL of 1% BSA.

3. Store in a polystyrene box with a damp tissue overnight at 4°C.
4. Wash plates 3× with wash buffer. Plates can be washed by hand using a squeezy bottle or using a dedicated ELISA washer (*see* **Note 2**). The hand method is suitable for a small number of plates. At the end of the third wash, bang the plate on a tissue to get most of the remaining buffer out of the wells.
5. Add 200 μL of blocking buffer to each well in the whole plate. Incubate in a damp box for 2 h at 4°C.
6. Wash plates 4× with wash buffer.
7. Gently mix serum samples on vortex. Add 100 μL of reagent buffer to wells A1–2 and E1–2. Add 10 μL of positive control and 90 μL reagent buffer to wells A3–4 and E3–4. Add 10 μL negative control and 90 μL reagent buffer to wells A5–6 and E5–6. Add 10 μL of test serum to wells in duplicate to both the upper allergen-coated plate and also the BSA-coated plate. Incubate for 2 h at 4°C.
8. Wash plates 5× with wash buffer.
9. Add 100 μL of biotinylated antihuman IgG (diluted 1:1000 in reagent buffer) to each well and incubate for 1 h at 4°C.
10. Wash plates 6× with wash buffer.
11. Add 100 μL of ExtrAvidin peroxidase (diluted 1:1000 in reagent buffer) to each well and incubate for 30 min at 4°C.
12. Wash plates 7× with wash buffer.
13. Add 100 μL of freshly made substrate solution to each well. Leave for 10 min at room temperature.
14. Add 50 μL of stop solution to each well.
15. Wipe the bottom of ELISA plate with a tissue and ensure there are no air bubbles in any of the wells. Read ELISA plate at 450-nm absorbance.
16. Calculate the average of duplicates.
17. Subtract the background BSA OD measurement from the allergen OD measurement for each sample. The results are arbitrary values based on OD values.

3.2. Protocol for Determining Specificity of ELISA by Inhibition Assay

1. Coat each well in the upper half of the ELISA plate with 100 μL of 1 μg/mL Fel.
2. Coat each well in the lower half of the ELISA plate with 100 μL of 1% BSA.
3. Store in a polystyrene box with a damp tissue overnight at 4°C.
4. Incubate serum with varying quantities of allergen to set up an inhibition curve. In our Fel d 1 assay, we incubated equal volume of serum sample with Fel d 1 solution at 1.0, 0.5, 0.1, and 0 μg/mL final concentration in the well. The serum and allergen were left on a roller at 4°C overnight.
5. Wash plates 3× with wash buffer.
6. Add 200 μL of blocking buffer to each well in the whole plate. Incubate in a damp box for 2 h at 4°C.
7. Wash plates 4× with wash buffer.
8. Add 10 μL of the preincubated serum and allergen to the wells and incubate for 2 h at 4°C.

Table 1
Inhibition of IgG Anti-Fel d 1 Antibodies Binding
with the Solid-Phase Fel d 1 with Inhibitor Fel d 1 Allergen

Inhibitor µg/mL	OD Fel d 1	OD HSA	OD Fel d 1 − HSA	Inhibition (%)
0	0.947	0.430	0.517	0
0.1	0.761	0.388	0.373	27.8
0.5	0.740	0.369	0.371	28.3
1.0	0.521	0.445	0.076	85.3

Table 2
Inhibition of IgG Anti-Fel d 1 Antibodies with
the Solid-Phase Fel d 1 with Inhibitor Fel d 1 Allergen

Inhibitor µg/mL	OD Fel d 1	OD HSA	OD Fel d 1 − HSA	Inhibition (%)
0	1.073	0.425	0.648	0
0.1	0.980	0.453	0.527	18.6
0.5	0.849	0.424	0.425	34.4
1.0	0.722	0.789	0	100.0

We were able to get 85 and 100% inhibition by preincubating two different sera with 1 µg/mL Fel d 1. Less than 1 µg/mL of inhibitor Fel d 1 did not significantly inhibit the binding of specific IgG anti-Fel d 1 antibodies to the solid phase. This demonstrated that the binding to Fel d 1 in the assay was specific to Fel d 1 and was not as a result of nonspecific or low-affinity antibody binding.

9. Continue with ELISA as for above protocol from step 8 onwards.
10. The degree of allergen inhibition is taken as ([uninhibited − inhibited]/inhibited) × 100. An example of our inhibition curve for Fel d 1 is shown in **Tables 1** and **2** for two different sera.

3.3. Analysis of ELISA Data

We did not have the appropriate reagents to set up a standard curve for our Fel d 1 assay; we therefore reported our results as arbitrary values based on the optical density. We had to ensure that samples run in different assays were compatible, so we ran a pool of serum with low, medium, and high levels of IgG antibody on each plate in every assay run. We ran these samples in 10 different assays to establish the coefficient of variance. Our assays would only be accepted if the coefficient of variance of the quality control samples was less than 20%.

4. Notes

1. Optimization of assay.
   Every step within the ELISA needs to be optimized *(17)*. In particular the following were considered when setting up the IgG assay:
   a. Concentration of allergen on solid phase: The capacity of microtiter plates to bind proteins is limited. At high concentration of protein, there is a tendency for protein molecules to bind to each other, resulting in dissociation of bound protein during the assay. In practice, 1–10 µg/mL is the desired concentration to use for coating the solid-phase ELISA plate. A steep reference curve is desirable as a small change in concentration will give a large color change. In practice, we would aim for a 2–3 log range in our dilution curves.
   b. Choice of coating buffer: The choice of coating buffer should be determined by testing the binding of allergen with pH 9.6 carbonate/bicarbonate buffer, a pH 7.4 PBS and a pH 5.0 acetate/citrate buffer. The charge of a protein depends on the buffer it is dissolved in. Therefore the charge of the coating buffer plays an important role in the ability of the allergen to bind to the ELISA plate.
   c. Incubation time for coating plate: A time of 1 h is usually sufficient. However, it is often desirable to coat the ELISA plate overnight, to allow time to perform the assay the following day. Again it is prudent to optimize the incubation time. It is possible to coat and block ELISA plates and keep frozen until ready for use. Again it is essential to check that this works for your particular assay.
   d. Blocking plates: Several blocking reagents can be used ranging from human serum albumin, BSA, casein, and gelatin. Again when setting up your assay it is worthwhile comparing the various blocking agents. Typically the blocking agents are used at a concentration of 1–2%.
   e. Volume of reagents: Typically we use 100 µL of reagents per well, apart from the blocking stage where we typically use 200 µL. If the sensitivity of the assay needs to be increased we use 200 µL reagent per well. Anything over 200 µL per well has the potential for crossover of reagent between wells.
   f. Choice of buffer: The concentration and molarity of buffers is generally between 0.05 and 0.1 M. Antibody–antigen reactions normally take place between pH 6.0 and 9.0. Normally the buffers used in the assay will contain blocking buffer. It is essential that the buffers are made fresh on the day because addition of serum albumin can lead to bacterial contamination which will result in erroneous ELISA results.
   g. Incubation times: For the reaction to be complete, 1 h is usually sufficient. The incubation times can be shortened by placing the ELISA plate on a shaker – the times can typically be cut by half. Again the incubation times will need to be optimized for each assay.
   h. The dilution of the sample will depend on the concentration; low concentration will require high sample volume, whereas high concentration will need to be diluted. At high serum concentrations there is a tendency to get nonspecific binding and the binding of low-affinity antibodies. The serum sample needs to be optimized by setting up a dilution curve.

i. Detecting antibodies: As with other steps in the ELISA these will need to be optimized. It is essential to ensure that the detecting reagent binds only to the sample and not to the other reagents in the ELISA.

j. We normally use a wash bottle to wash our ELISA plate which is perfectly adequate. This is a very simple, effective, cheap method of washing ELISA plates. It is essential for the user to be very thorough in the washing steps, ensuring all wells are washed and that the buffer is flicked out of the plate. Some prefer to use an automated plate washer which is useful if running several plates in one assay. The downside of an automated plate washer is the expense; however, it is useful if you intend running ELISAs on a regular basis and it overcomes user error in the washing process. Others use a bucket of buffer and simply immerse the plate in the bucket of buffer which is a perfectly adequate system of washing.

References

1. Platts-Mills, T., Vaughan, J., Squillace, S., Woodfolk, J., and Sporik, R. (2001) Sensitisation, asthma, and a modified Th2 response in children exposed to cat allergen: a population-based cross-sectional study. *Lancet* **357,** 752–756.
2. Hesselmar, B., Aberg, B., Eriksson, B., Bjorksten, B., and Aberg, N. (2003) High-dose exposure to cat is associated with clinical tolerance—a modified Th2 immune response? *Clin. Exp. Allergy* **33,** 1681–1685.
3. Akdis, C. A. and Blaser, K. (1999) IL-10-induced anergy in peripheral T cell and reactivation by microenvironmental cytokines: two key steps in specific immunotherapy. *FASEB J.* **13,** 603–609.
4. Akdis, C. A., Blesken, T., Akdis, M., Wuthrich, B., and Blaser, K. (1998) Role of interleukin 10 in specific immunotherapy. *J. Clin. Investig.* **102,** 98–106.
5. Cullinan, P., Cook, A., Gordon, S., et al. (1999) Allergen exposure, atopy and smoking as determinants of allergy to rats in a cohort of laboratory employees. *Eur. Respir. J.* **13,** 1139–1143.
6. Jeal, H., Draper, A., Harris, J., Taylor, A. N., Cullinan, P., and Jones, M. (2006) Modified Th2 responses at high-dose exposures to allergen: using an occupational model. *Am. J. Respir. Crit. Care Med.* Jul 1;174(1):21–25. *Epub.* 2006 Apr 7.
7. Gehlhar, K., Schlaak, M., Becker, W., and Bufe, A. (1999) Monitoring allergen immunotherapy of pollen-allergic patients: the ratio of allergen-specific IgG4 to IgG1 correlates with clinical outcome. *Clin. Exp. Allergy* **29,** 497–506.
8. Jutel, M., Akdis, M., Budak, F., et al. (2003) IL-10 and TGF-beta cooperate in the regulatory T cell response to mucosal allergens in normal immunity and specific immunotherapy. *Eur. J. Immunol.* **33,** 1205–1214.
9. Nouri-Aria, K. T., Wachholz, P. A., Francis, J. N., et al. (2004) Grass pollen immunotherapy induces mucosal and peripheral IL-10 responses and blocking IgG activity. *J. Immunol.* **172,** 3252–3259.
10. Djurup, R. and Osterballe, O. (1984) IgG subclass antibody response in grass pollen-allergic patients undergoing specific immunotherapy. Prognostic value of serum IgG subclass antibody levels early in immunotherapy. *Allergy* **39,** 433–441.

11. Golden, D. B., Meyers, D. A., Kagey-Sobotka, A., Valentine, M. D., and Lichtenstein, L. M. (1982) Clinical relevance of the venom-specific immunoglobulin G antibody level during immunotherapy. *J. Allergy Clin. Immunol.* **69,** 489–493.
12. Daeron, M., Malbec, O., Latour, S., Arock, M., and Fridman, W. H. (1995) Regulation of high affinity IgE receptor-mediated mast cell activation by murine low-affinity IgG receptors. *J. Clin. Investig.* **95,** 577–585.
13. Daeron, M. (1997) Negative regulation of mast cell activation by receptors for IgG. *Int. Arch. Allergy Immunol.* **113,** 138–141.
14. Zhu, D., Kepley, C. L., Zhang, M., Zhang, K., and Saxon, A. (2002) A novel human immunoglobulin Fc gamma Fc epsilon bifunctional fusion protein inhibits Fc epsilon R1-mediated degranulation. *Nat. Med.* **8,** 518–521.
15. Ball, T., Sperr, W. R., Valent, P., et al. (1999) Induction of antibody responses to new B cell epitopes indicates vaccination character of allergen immunotherapy. *Eur. J. Immunol.* **29,** 2026–2036.
16. Wachholz, P. A. and Durham, S. R. (2003) Induction of 'blocking' IgG antibodies during immunotherapy. *Clin. Exp. Allergy* **33,** 1171–1174.
17. Kemeny, D. M. (1991) A Practical Guide to ELISA. Pergamon Press plc, Headington Hill Hall, Oxford OX3 0BW, England.

21

The Facilitated Antigen Binding (FAB) Assay – A Protocol to Measure Allergen-Specific Inhibitory Antibody Activity

James N. Francis

Abstract

Specific allergen immunotherapy is an effective treatment for IgE-mediated allergic disease and involves T- and B-cell mediated events. IgE receptors on the surface of antigen-presenting cells facilitate the presentation of allergens in the presence of specific IgE antibody resulting in T-cell activation. Interference with these IgE-dependent mechanisms by 'blocking' IgG antibodies may downregulate T-cell responses and manifest as a reduction in allergic responses in vivo.

The vigor of proliferative responses by T-cell clones is representative of the binding of allergen–IgE complexes to B cells. Therefore, a simplified assay can be employed that measures the binding of allergen–IgE complexes to B cells instead of a more complex assay involving proliferative assays using antigen-specific T-cell clones. Allergen–IgE complexes can be easily detected by flow cytometry and this simplified technique is called the IgE-facilitated allergen binding (IgE-FAB) assay which is described in this chapter.

Key Words: T cell; B cell; immunotherapy; flow cytometry; IgG.

1. Introduction

Specific allergen immunotherapy is an effective treatment for IgE-mediated allergic disease (1). The mechanisms that are associated with successful immunotherapy involve both T- and B-cell mediated events (2). Cellular changes include immune deviation favoring T helper 1 responses (3) and the induction of regulatory cells producing interleukin (IL)-10 (4). Treatment is also associated with the induction of allergen-specific serum IgG4 antibodies (5–7). IgG4 antibodies are thought to have blocking activities as they compete with IgE for allergen binding to mast cells, basophils, and other IgE receptor-expressing cells (8).

Receptors for IgE expressed on the surface of antigen-presenting cells have been shown to facilitate the presentation of allergens in the presence of specific

From: *Methods in Molecular Medicine: Allergy Methods and Protocols*
Edited by: M. G. Jones and P. Lympany © Humana Press Inc., Totowa, NJ

IgE antibody resulting in effective T-cell activation at low concentrations of allergen *(9)*. Interference with these IgE-dependent mechanisms by 'blocking' IgG antibodies may downregulate T-cell responses and manifest as a reduction in allergic responses in vivo.

Previous studies by van Neerven and colleagues *(10,11)* have shown that serum obtained from subjects receiving birch immunotherapy was able to inhibit IgE-facilitated presentation of allergen by B cells to an allergen-specific T-cell clone. Another study has also demonstrated that serum obtained from a double-blind placebo-controlled trial of grass pollen immunotherapy can inhibit IgE-facilitated allergen presentation to a grass-specific T-lymphocyte clone *(12)*. This report demonstrates that the vigor of proliferative responses by T-cell clones is representative of the binding of allergen–IgE complexes to B cells. Therefore, a simplified assay can be employed that measures the binding of allergen–IgE complexes to B cells instead of a more complex assay involving proliferative assays using antigen-specific T-cell clones. Allergen–IgE complexes can be easily detected by flow cytometry and this simplified technique is called the IgE-facilitated allergen binding (IgE-FAB) assay.

Briefly, the IgE-FAB assay involves incubation of serum, known to contain high levels of allergen-specific IgE, with low concentrations of allergen extract in the presence or absence of 'test serum' with potential inhibitory activity. The resulting allergen–IgE complexes are subsequently incubated with an EBV-transformed human B-cell line. These cells express high levels of the low-affinity IgE receptor (CD23, FcεRII) which binds allergen–IgE complexes. Detection of allergen–IgE complexes on the surface of B cell can be achieved using either a biotinylated allergen or a fluorescent antibody against IgE and analyzed using flow cytometry (**Fig. 1**). In the presence of inhibitory serum, number of allergen–IgE complexes bound to B cells is decreased.

2. Materials

2.1. Assay Buffers

2.1.1. FAP Buffer (pH 7.2)

8.10 g NaCl, 0.16 g NaH_2PO_4, 0.98 g Na_2HPO_4, 1.0 g BSA (0.1%) (all from Sigma or any qualified commercial company). Dissolve in 1 L of distilled H_2O, adjust pH to 7.2. Store for up to 2 wk at 4°C.

2.1.2. EBV Growth Medium

RPMI 1640 supplemented with 1% (v/v) L-glutamine (Invitrogen, Paisley, UK), 10% heat-inactivated FCS (PAA laboratories, Yeovil, UK), and 1% (v/v) penicillin/streptomycin mixture (Invitrogen). Store at 4°C for up to 4 wk.

1. Mix indicator serum (specific IgE>100 kU/mL), test serum and allergen

1 hour @ 37°C

2. Add B cells to antibody/allergen complexes

1 hour @ 4°C

3. Wash B cells and stain with anti-IgE-FITC

45 mins @ 4°C

4. Analyse by flow cytometry

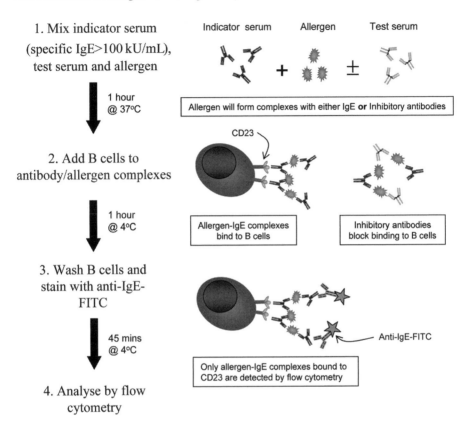

Indicator serum   Allergen   Test serum

Allergen will form complexes with either IgE **or** Inhibitory antibodies

CD23

Allergen-IgE complexes bind to B cells

Inhibitory antibodies block binding to B cells

Anti-IgE-FITC

Only allergen-IgE complexes bound to CD23 are detected by flow cytometry

Fig. 1.

2.2. Serum and Allergen Requirements

1. Indicator serum should be obtained from an atopic (allergic) donor with high allergen-specific IgE levels (as measured by CAP-RAST). Serum with levels of >100 kU/L are generally found to be suitable indicator serum as the level of binding to EBV-transformed B cell is proportional to the amount of IgE contained within the serum. If serum with >100 kU/mL is not available then it is worthwhile testing serum with 50–100 kU/mL. Generally, serum with less than 50 kU/mL does not bind in the assay. Serum (plasma) from allergic donors can also be purchased from Plasmalabs, Washington.

2. Inhibitory serum to be tested in the assay can be obtained from subjects undergoing a specific treatment or with signs of clinical remission/tolerance. Serum can be collected using standard blood tubes with clotting agent.

3. Allergen can be purchased from a number of commercial companies or isolated by standard laboratory methods. Freeze-dried allergen should be dissolved in sterile RPMI at 1–5 mg/mL, aliquotted, and stored at −20°C.

3. Methods

3.1. Cultivation of EBV-Transformed B Cells

Detailed description of the generation of EBV-transformed B cells is beyond the remit of this protocol. Briefly, supernatant from a EBV-producing cell line (e.g., B-958) is cultured with peripheral blood mononuclear cells (PBMC) from an atopic donor (allergic to the allergen of interest). Transformed B cells are enriched for high CD23 expression by the use of magnetic bead separation and stored in liquid nitrogen.

1. EBV-transformed B cells are rapidly thawed at 37°C and washed twice in 50 mL of RPMI.
2. The cell line is maintained in vented-cap, canted-neck cell culture flasks from Falcon/VWR (Poole, UK) at 37°C, 5% CO_2, and 95% relative humidity (RH).
3. Cells should be subcultured two to three times a week to maintain cell density of $0.5-1.5 \times 10^6$ cells/mL.
4. Cell viability should be maintained above 95%.
5. Cells can be used in the assay a minimum of 10–14 d after the start of the culture period and up to a maximal of 60 d.
6. CD23 expression on B-cell lines should be routinely checked by flow cytometry, e.g., using CD23-FITC (DakoCytomation). Numbers of B cells expressing CD23 should be very high (>98%) and levels of expression should lie within 10^2 and 10^3 MCF.

3.2. Analytical Procedure

3.2.1. Serum Preparation

Serum stored at −80°C should be left for 24 h at −20°C, then thawed in a water bath at 37°C for 10 min. Serum containing precipitants may be filtered before use in the assay.

3.2.2. Allergen Dilutions

Allergen should be freshly prepared in RPMI to a working dilution 10 × greater than the required final concentration, e.g., if a final allergen concentration of 1 µg/mL is required the substock solution should be prepared at 10 µg/mL.

3.2.3. Complexing Allergen with Serum Antibodies

1. 20 µL of serum, the inhibitory activity of which is to be tested, is added to a tube (BD Falcon 5-mL polystyrene round-bottom tube). Control tubes should contain 20 µL of RPMI.
2. Add 20 µL of 'high-IgE' indicator serum.
3. Add 5 µL of the allergen dilution.
4. Place a cap on the tube to minimize evaporation.
5. Incubate serum/allergen for 1 h at 37°C.

3.2.4. Preparation of EBV-B Cells

1. Transfer cells from culture flask into a 50-mL centrifuge tube.
2. Wash cells by centrifugation at $490g$ at 4°C for 7 min.
3. Repeat wash step with 50 mL cold RPMI (centrifuge at $490g$ at 4°C for 7 min).
4. Resuspend cells in 10 mL of RPMI.
5. Count cells by trypan blue exclusion (1:1 dilution: 20 µL cell suspension in 20 µL trypan blue) using a hemocytometer. Duplicate sampling for cell counts is recommended.
6. Centrifuge the cells and resuspend to 2×10^7 cells/mL in FAP buffer.
7. Store cells on ice and mix thoroughly prior to use.

3.2.5. Incubation of EBV-B Cells with Precomplexed Allergen

Add 5 µL of EBV-B cell solution (100,000 cells per test) to allergen–serum complexes. Mix gently and incubate for 1 h on ice.

3.2.6. Staining of Allergen–IgE Complexes Bound to B Cells (see **Note 1**)

1. Wash B cells from the previous step twice with 1 mL of FAP buffer (centrifuge at $490g$ at 4°C for 7 min).
2. Dilute anti-IgE-FITC antibody 1:50 (e.g., 20 µL in 980 µL of FAP buffer).
3. Add 20 µL of diluted anti-IgE-FITC antibody to each tube.
4. Incubate for 45 min on ice, in the dark.
5. Wash cells 1 mL per tube and resuspend in 200 µL of ice-cold FAP buffer.
6. Analyze surface staining immediately on flow cytometer.

3.2.7. Acquisition Using the Flow Cytometer

1. Open forward scatter vs side scatter dot-plot and identify EBV cell population as the main population.
2. Gate around the population in FSC/SSC and adjust the FL-1 gain so that cells appear between 10^0 and 10^1 on a histogram plot.
3. Ensure that a positive signal is detected using the indicator serum-positive control (*see* below).
4. Acquire 5000 gated cells per sample.
5. The following controls should be included in each experiment:
   a. Cells only (i.e., no FITC stain; however, cells should be incubated with human serum as this can increase fluorescence).
   b. Cells + isotype control for IgE-FITC.
   c. Cells + IgE-FITC.
   d. Indicator serum/allergen + IgE-FITC (serum-positive control).
   e. Internal negative control (for inhibition).
   f. Internal positive control (for inhibition).

3.2.8. Running Multiple Samples

The above protocol uses standard 5-mL Falcon 'FACS' tubes in the assay. For multiple samples, a 96-well U-bottomed plate (Nunc) may be used. In this case, a centrifuge equipped with microplate carriers is required and wash steps should be carried out using a multichannel pipet. In addition, wash volumes should be reduced to 250 μL (or so that the maximal volume of the well is not exceeded). For FACS analysis, contents of the wells should be mixed well and transferred to microtubes (Bioquote, UK). Microtubes can be place in a standard FACS tube and used as normal.

3.2.9. Optimization of the Assay

It is essential to optimize the FAP assay for your allergen of choice. The following experiments should be completed before using the assay on large numbers of test samples:

1. Identification of a suitable indicator serum (containing high allergen-specific IgE levels, *see* **Section 2.2.**). Potential serum to be used as indicator serum should be first tested for binding with a limited dose–response of allergen (e.g., 0.01, 1, and 100 μg/mL) without inclusion of inhibitory serum.
2. Any serum showing binding of >30% (at any allergen concentration) should be further tested using a more comprehensive dose–response curve (e.g., half logarithmic doses from 1 pg/mL to 100 μg/mL). Typical optimal binding occurs at 0.1–5 μg/mL. It is desirable to achieve binding of >50% although binding in the range of 70–80% is optimal. Indicator serum binding of approx. 30% can be used in the assay although increased variability is observed.
3. Once a suitable indicator serum is identified, the time course of allergen–IgE complex binding to B cells should be optimized (*see* **Section 3.2.5.**). Binding time between 2 and 120 min can be tested (e.g., 2, 10, 30, 60, and 120 min).
4. If indicator serum is of limited availability, dilutions (in RPMI) of serum can be tested for binding in the assay. Also, pooled serum can be used in place of serum from a single donor.
5. If serum with potential inhibitory activity is available, this should be tested in the assay before running large numbers of test samples. The assay should be run using a dose range of allergen concentrations in the presence or absence of potential inhibitory serum. As inhibition of FAP occurs at low allergen concentrations, an allergen concentration should be chosen that generates binding of >50% (or less, *see* above) but also allows the maximal inhibition of binding by test sera.

4. Notes

1. Allergen–IgE complexes can also be detected using biotinylated allergen. In such a case optimal binding/inhibition should first be established using the biotinylated allergen. Detection of complexes (4.6) is achieved using streptavidin-PE (BD biosciences).

Acknowledgment

The author would like to thank Drs Peter Wurtzen, Petra Wachholz, and Mohamed Shamji for their contributions to this protocol.

References

1. Bousquet, J., Lockey, R., Malling, H. J., et al. (1998) Allergen immunotherapy: therapeutic vaccines for allergic diseases. World Health Organization. American academy of Allergy, Asthma and Immunology. *Ann. Allergy Asthma Immunol.* **81,** 401–405.
2. Till, S. J., Francis, J. N., Nouri-Aria, K., and Durham, S. R. (2004) Mechanisms of immunotherapy. *J. Allergy Clin. Immunol.* **113,** 1025–1034.
3. Wachholz, P. A., Nouri-Aria, K. T., Wilson, D. R., et al. (2002) Grass pollen immunotherapy for hayfever is associated with increases in local nasal but not peripheral Th1:Th2 cytokine ratios. *Immunology* **105,** 56–62.
4. Francis, J. N., Till, S. J., and Durham, S. R. (2003) Induction of IL-10+CD4+CD25+ T cells by grass pollen immunotherapy. *J. Allergy Clin. Immunol.* **111,** 255–261.
5. Gehlhar, K., Schlaak, M., Becker, W., and Bufe, A. (1999) Monitoring allergen immunotherapy of pollen-allergic patients: the ratio of allergen-specific IgG4 to IgG1 correlates with clinical outcome. *Clin. Exp. Allergy* **29,** 497–506.
6. Jutel, M., Akdis, M., Budak, F., et al. (2003) IL-10 and TGF-beta cooperate in the regulatory T cell response to mucosal allergens in normal immunity and specific immunotherapy. *Eur. J. Immunol.* **33,** 1205–1214.
7. Nouri-Aria, K. T., Wachholz, P. A., Francis, J. N., et al. (2004) Grass pollen immunotherapy induces mucosal and peripheral IL-10 responses and blocking IgG activity. *J. Immunol.* **172,** 3252–3259.
8. Garcia, B. E., Sanz, M. L., Gato, J. J., Fernandez, J., and Oehling, A. (1993) IgG4 blocking effect on the release of antigen-specific histamine. *J. Investig. Allergol. Clin. Immunol.* **3,** 26–33.
9. van der Heijden, F. L., van Neerven, R. J., and Kapsenberg, M. L. (1995) Relationship between facilitated allergen presentation and the presence of allergen-specific IgE in serum of atopic patients. *Clin. Exp. Immunol.* **99,** 289–293.
10. van Neerven, R. J., Wikborg, T., Lund, G., et al. (1999) Blocking antibodies induced by specific allergy vaccination prevent the activation of CD4+ T cells by inhibiting serum-IgE-facilitated allergen presentation. *J. Immunol.* **163,** 2944–2952.
11. van Neerven, R. J., Arvidsson, M., Ipsen, H., et al. (2004) A double-blind, placebo-controlled birch allergy vaccination study: inhibition of CD23-mediated serum-immunoglobulin E-facilitated allergen presentation. *Clin. Exp. Allergy* **34,** 420–428.
12. Wachholz, P. A., Soni, N. K., Till, S. J., and Durham, S. R. (2003) Inhibition of allergen-IgE binding to B cells by IgG antibodies after grass pollen immunotherapy. *J. Allergy Clin. Immunol.* **112,** 915–922.

22

Microscopic Identification and Purity Determination of Pollen Grains

Magdalena Rahl

Abstract

Identification of pollen is like entering a world of great variation in size, shape, and structure. To obtain a correct result, a good microscope, basic information on pollen grain morphology and a reference sample of the plant to be identified are needed.

Purity determination of pollen can be performed by particle count or by volumetric analysis. In our experience, particle counting is the better and most reproducible method and is not greatly influenced by interindividual variation. In this chapter, we have described the detailed procedure to obtain satisfactory results for identification and determination of pollen purity.

Key Words: Pollen.

1. Introduction

Identification of pollen is like entering a world of great variation in size, shape, and structure. To obtain a correct result, a good microscope, basic information on pollen grain morphology and a reference sample of the plant to be identified are needed.

Purity determination of pollen can be performed by particle count or by volumetric analysis. In our experience, particle counting is the better and most reproducible method and is not greatly influenced by interindividual variation.

Below we have described the detailed procedure to obtain satisfactory results for identification and determination of pollen purity.

2. Materials

2.1. Equipment

1. Phase contrast microscope or light microscope with at least the following magnifications: 100, 200, 400, and 1000.

From: *Methods in Molecular Medicine: Allergy Methods and Protocols*
Edited by: M. G. Jones and P. Lympany © Humana Press Inc., Totowa, NJ

2. Glass microscope slides and cover slips.
3. Spatula.
4. 15-mL centrifuge tubes.
5. Multiblock heater.
6. Centrifuge.

2.2. Chemicals and Solutions

1. 95% ethanol.
2. Acetic acid anhydride.
3. Concentrated sulfuric acid.
4. Lactophenol: Add 10 mL distilled water to 10 g phenol crystals and heat. Add 10 g lactic acid and 20 g pure glycerol.
5. Colberla's stain: 1:3:3 glycerol:95% ethanol:distilled water. Add 0.2% Basic Fuchsin until color changes to red.

3. Methods

3.1. Identification of Pollen Grains

To understand what to observe when identifying pollen grains, it is necessary to have a brief introduction regarding pollen morphology. Pollen grains can vary in size from 5 to 200 μm, although 20–50 μm is the most common. The size of the different pollen grains is related to the chromosome numbers. The size variation in living grains is because of the changes in the osmotic balance of the protoplast. Furrow membranes, for example, well with increased internal volume and furthermore the entire outline changes from angular to distend with an increase in the internal turgid pressure.

If grains are prepared through acetolysis, they will be more constant in size. This is the reason for performing acetolysis in the method described below.

The wall: Each pollen grain is sealed in a double-layered wall. The outer pollen wall is called the exine and the inner wall is called the intine.

Intine: The intine surrounds the living protoplasm. It consists partly of cellulose, pectic substances, callose, and other polysaccharides.

Exine: The exine is a waxy or resinous, chemically resistant layer, which serves to minimize damage and prevent drying of the pollen grain. The substances forming the exine are called sporopollenins. Many anemophilus (wind-pollinating) plants have walls modified to enhance spreading, whereas entomophilus (insect-pollinated) types have surface rods, spines, and other sculptural features which serve to improve spreading. The exine provides important features for microscopic identification such as size, shape, number, and arrangement of apertures, structure, and ornamentation.

Apertures: The apertures of pollen grains are the primary basis for identification. True apertures are found in most pollen types and are either furrows or pores in the exine (**Fig. 1**).

Gymnosperms	Inaperturate	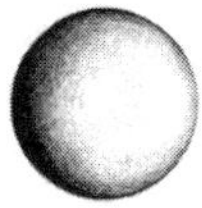
	Winged with an obscure furrow	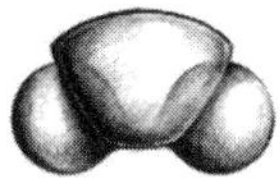
Monocotyledons	Inaperturate	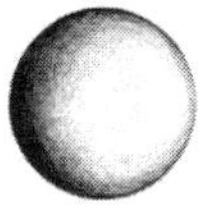
	Monocolpate	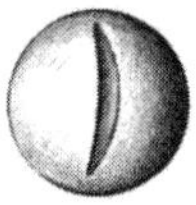
	Monoporate	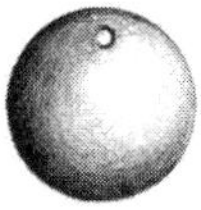
Dicotyledons	Inaperturate	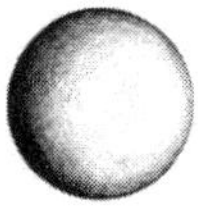
	Periporate	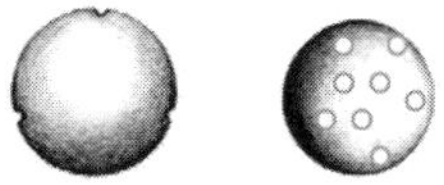
	Colpate	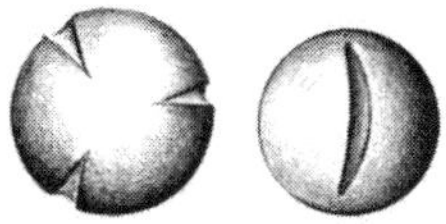
	Colporate	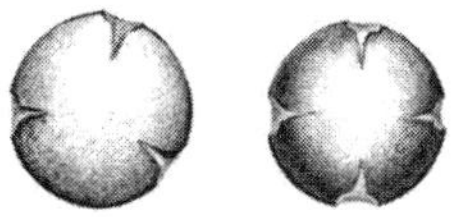

Fig. 1. Different types of apertures found in pollen grains.

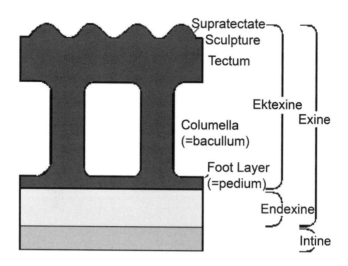

Fig. 2. Structural features of the exine.

Furrows are boat-shaped apertures which are more than twice as long as broad, whereas pores are circular to elliptical apertures. The furrow or pore membrane may be smooth and featureless, has a granular surface, or bears a perculum (an exinous covering over a pore). Pollen grains with pores are called porate, whereas pollen grains with furrows are called colpate. Pollen grains with both furrows and pores are called colporate.

3.1.1. Structural Features of the Exine

Structural differences refer to various shapes and arrangements of the columellae (**Fig. 2**). The columellae may be simple or branched elongated rods or low granules. Their arrangement may be scattered and irregular, continuous and regular, or they may form a reticulate, striate, or regular pattern. If the columellae are fused distally to form a more or less continuous tectum, the condition is tectate. If there are numerous openings in the tectum, it is perforate tectate. Intectate forms lack an extensive or continuous tectum (**Fig. 3**). The characteristics of the sculptural elements are described in **Table 1** (for further details *see* **Refs. [1,2]**). Detailed study of the pollen exine structure requires phase contrast microscopy with polarizing accessories.

3.2. Acetolyzation of Pollen Grains

1. Mix the acetolyzation solution as follows in a fume cupboard: take 9 parts pure acetic acid anhydride and add 1 part concentrated sulfuric acid dropwise. For calculation purposes, note that approximately 10 mL acetolyzation solution is required per sample.

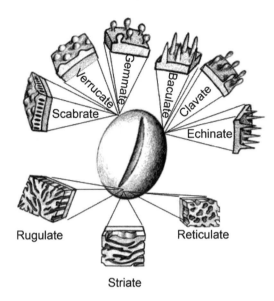

Fig. 3. Sculptural elements and patterns of the pollen exine.

2. Place some pollen in the bottom of a centrifuge tube.
3. Add approx. 10 mL acetolyzation solution to each tube.
4. Heat the tubes in a multiblock heater at 85°C for 10 min, which is when the samples begin to "cook." Turn off heater.
5. Centrifuge the samples for 3–4 min.
6. Pour out the acetolyzation solution into a suitable receptacle in a fume cupboard and discard according to local health and safety guidelines.
7. Add 5 mL of a mixture of water/95% ethanol (3:1).
8. Wash the sediment by careful shaking of the tube.
9. Centrifuge for 3–4 min.
10. Pour off the supernatant.
11. Add 2 mL glycerine:water mixture (1:1).
12. Shake as in 8.
13. Leave the mixture for a minimum of 15 min before placing pollen sample on a slide to be identified.

3.3. Purity Determination of Pollen

1. Take a random sample from the pollen container and place in a small aluminum tube. Label the tube with article name and batch number.
2. Shake the tube carefully. Take a small amount with a spatula and place on a slide.
3. Add a few drops of 95% ethanol and spread the material on the slide with the spatula.
4. Leave the ethanol to evaporate.

Table 1
The Characteristics of Sculptural Elements

Sculptural element	Characteristics
Scabrate	Small sculptural elements <1 μm in any dimension
Verrucate	Elements as broad as or broader than length >1 μm wide
Gemmate	Diameter of elements equal to or greater than height, constricted base ≥1 μm wide
Baculate	Elements post or rod-like, longer than width ≥1 μm long
Clavate	Elements longer than width, with a constricted base or club shaped ≥1 μm long
Echinate	Elements in form of pointed spines, sometimes called spinulate if between 1 and 3 μm in length
Rugulate	Horizontally elongated elements in an irregular pattern
Striate	Horizontally elongated elements in a more or less parallel pattern
Reticulate	Horizontally elongate elements forming a net-like patter of holes and walls

5. Count the number of pollen grains and the number of plant parts in each field. Note the number for purity determination.
6. Count about 500 pollen grains in randomly chosen fields all over the slide. The fields counted should not contain pollen grains in several layers.
   Calculate the purity of the sample:
   (No. pollen grains/[No. pollen grains + plant parts]) $\times 100 = x\%$

3.4. Determination of Foreign Particles

1. Study the pollen grains under light microscope. (Use magnification 20×10 or 40×10 depending on the size of the pollen grains).
2. Shake the pollen sample carefully, then take a sample using a spatula.
3. Place the sample on a slide.
4. Add a few drops of lactophenol and disperse the pollen. Put on a cover slip.
5. Examine the whole slide carefully. Start in the upper left corner and systematically cover the whole slide, ending in the lower right corner.
6. Count the number of pollen grains, A = foreign pollen grains and B = spores in different fields of the slide.
7. Count at least 2000 pollen grains of actual species.
8. Calculate the number of foreign particles (A/B) as follows:
   (Foreign particles [A/B]/Total number of particles) $\times 100 = x\%$
   Total number of particles is the actual pollen grains + foreign particles ($A + B$)
   Calculate actual values for each type of foreign particle.
9. Calculate the total number of foreign particles: $A\% + B\%$ = total number of foreign particles in %.

4. Notes

Identification of pollen grains:

The most important thing is to acetolyse the pollen grains. Through this you get rid of almost everything inside the pollen and it is then easier to look at the exine characteristics.

It is useful to build up one's own reference system, as it is convenient to compare a new sample against a reference.

It can sometimes be difficult to distinguish details of closely related species under light microscopy, and so a scanning electron microscope may be required to obtain the best result.

Purity determination of pollen grains:

Pollen grain toward plant parts:

Some pollen species have pollen grains that seem to dry out quickly. If this is the case, then add more ethanol to allow the pollen to swell.

Occasionally, some grains can appear darker than others because of the oxidation of the grain.

Pollen grain toward foreign particles:

Foreign pollen grains can be hard to distinguish in lactophenol or Colberla's stain if they are closely related to the actual pollen species. In this case, it is important to look at acetolysed slide where it can be easier to see such differences.

Lactophenol is good for spore identification, as they will appear brown in solution.

Rarely do we find unrelated plant material such as soil particles, insect parts, or other material related to the utensils used in production.

References

1. Kapp, R. O. (1969) *How to Know Pollen and Spores*, W. C. Brown Co. Publ., Dubuque, IA.
2. Wodehouse, R.-P. (1965) *Pollen Grains*, Hafner, New York.
3. Stanley, R. G. and Linskens, H. F. (1974) *Pollen Biology, Biochemistry, Management*, Springer, New York.

23

Biopanning for the Characterization of Allergen Mimotopes

Isabella Pali-Schöll and Erika Jensen-Jarolim

Abstract

Proper understanding of the pathogenesis of type I allergy relies on the identification of allergen epitopes. The phage display technique is a relatively new one to define peptide structures that mimic natural epitopes, including conformational B-cell epitopes. Peptides displayed on the phage recognized by an antiallergen antibody mimic the physicochemical properties of the amino acids and are, therefore, called mimotopes. The main advantage of the biopanning technique described in this chapter is that the structure of the antigen/allergen may be completely unknown; the only material needed is an antibody binding to it. The mimotopes generated by this technique display the features of the antigen/allergen but do not crosslink the mast cell-bound IgE-antibodies. Thus mimotopes could be used as a safe alternative to the commonly applied allergen extracts in immunotherapy of allergic patients and direct the immune response toward the desired allergen epitopes. In the selection procedure called biopanning, phages with the mimotopes best recognized by the selecting antibody are amplified. The titers of phages specifically binding to the selection antibody are checked. In this chapter we describe two alternative methods for colony screening: the immunoblot and ELISA.

Key Words: Biopanning; mimotope; epitope; phage.

1. Introduction

Molecular biology and biochemical techniques have considerably advanced the knowledge of allergens. Until now, descriptions of allergens were based on recombinant DNA technology, chromatography, spectrometry of proteolytic fragments, crystallization, X-ray investigations, and, lately, computational modeling (1). These methods supported the characterization of isoforms and the determination of the primary, secondary, and tertiary structures of these proteins. For further understanding of the pathogenesis of type I allergy, allergen epitopes

From: *Methods in Molecular Medicine: Allergy Methods and Protocols*
Edited by: M. G. Jones and P. Lympany © Humana Press Inc., Totowa, NJ

should be known. Attempts to identify B-cell epitopes of allergens on a molecular basis have been unsuccessful because these epitopes are generally conformational and discontinuous in nature. The phage display technique is a relatively new technique to define peptide structures that mimic natural epitopes, including conformational B-cell epitopes *(1–12)*. Peptides displayed on the phage recognized by an antiallergen antibody do not necessarily reassemble the natural allergen epitopes; they mimic the physicochemical properties of the amino acids and are therefore called mimotopes. There are several advantages of the biopanning technique: (i) the structure of the antigen/allergen may be completely unknown, the only material needed is an antibody binding to it; (ii) the epitopes which this antibody binds to can be either of linear (continuous) or conformational (discontinuous) nature; (iii) the generated mimotopes presented in a monovalent way display the features of the antigen/allergen, but do not crosslink the mast cell-bound IgE-antibodies, thus avoiding side reactions. Mimotopes could therefore be used as a safe alternative to the commonly applied allergen extracts in immunotherapy of allergic patients and direct the immune response toward the desired allergen epitopes. This epitope-specific immunotherapy would further prevent the induction of anaphylactogenic antibodies, which are an additional undesired side-effect of the currently applied hyposensitization therapy. We have successfully performed epitope characterization of respiratory and alimentary allergens *(6,8,13)* and of cancer antigens *(1,14–16)*, as well as immunization studies in mouse models *(1,7,17)* in our group.

1.1. Random Phage Display Peptide Libraries

Phage peptide libraries consist of filamentous phages displaying random peptides of defined length on their surface, which can be cloned either into surface protein pVIII (resulting in a high-density display with 1000–2700 copies/phage) or into protein pIII (giving only about 3 copies/phage, but being easily accessible on the phage tip pole) *(7,12)*. Alternatively, phagemid libraries can be used for longer peptides, which only contain the genetic information for the assembling of the phage, but are not able to replicate or expulse from bacteria. Therefore, helper phages are needed for phagemid libraries. The procedures described here are for random peptide phagemid libraries, using *Escherichia coli* XL-1 as host and M13 as helper phage *(9,18)*. Libraries contain about 10^8 different random peptides from 6 to15 amino acids, depending on the size of the cloned insert. Some examples including references are given in **Table 1**. In these random peptide phage display libraries, the peptides can be displayed either in linear form or in circular manner, when two flanking cysteins form a disulfide bond and, thereby, a loop *(18)*.

Table 1
Libraries of Random Peptides

Amino acid insert	Diversity	Ref.
Libraries of random linear peptides		
6 mer	2×10^8	*(2)*
6 mer	2×10^7	*(24)*
9 mer	1×10^9	*(9)*
9 mer	Unknown	*(25)*
10 mer	4×10^8	*(26)*
15 mer	Unknown	*(2)*
Libraries of random peptides constrained by flanking cysteins		
7 mer	4×10^9	*(27)*
9 mer	1×10^9	*(18)*
10 mer	1×10^9	*(25)*

In the selection procedure called biopanning, phages bind via their displayed peptides to a specific (selection) antibody and can be isolated and amplified. Several rounds of biopanning (three to four usually) are done, starting with the original library. The phage eluents from the preceding round are used for a new selection. This procedure renders an amplification of the phages with the mimotopes best recognized by the selecting antibody. First, the outcome of biopanning is controlled by determination of the total phage titer. An increase in the phage titer from one to the subsequent round is usually an indication for successful biopanning. Second, the increase of the titers of phages specifically binding to the selection antibody has to be checked by immunodotting or ELISA. The selection antibody and an isotype control antibody are dotted and incubated with the amplified original library and phage eluents from the different biopanning rounds. The extent of binding to the selection antibody will ideally increase from round 1 to the last. To identify certain positive single phage clones, a colony screening assay is performed. In this chapter, we describe two alternative methods for colony screening, first the immunoblot according to Scott et al. *(2)* and second the detection via ELISA *(19,20)*. Individual clones of interest are amplified and can be further analyzed by DNA sequencing.

2. Material

2.1. Biopanning

1. Microtiter plates (Maxisorp, NUNC, Roskilde, Denmark).
2. Bicarbonate buffer: 0.1 M bicarbonate, pH 9.6.

Biopanning

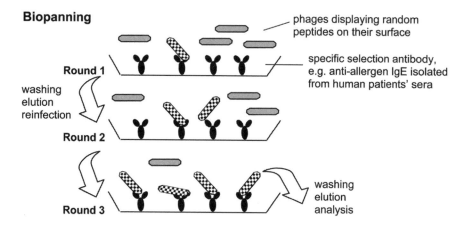

Fig. 1. Principle of the biopanning procedure for selection of specific ligands for an antibody. A solid phase is coated with the selection antibody. After each round of biopanning, specifically bound phages (squared pattern) are eluted and amplified, whereas nonbinding phages (gray) are washed away. Usually three to four rounds of biopanning are necessary for an enrichment of specifically binding phage clones. Using an antiallergen antibody for coating, the selected phages will display peptides on their surface, which mimic the natural allergen epitope (mimotope) *(28)*, reprint kindly permitted by Allergo Journal.

3. Phosphate-buffered saline (PBS): 137 mM NaCl, 3 mM KCl, 6.5 mM Na_2HPO_4, 1.7 mM KH_2PO_4.
4. Blocking buffer: PBS, containing 3% (w/v) BSA.
5. PBS/casein buffer: PBS, containing 0.15% (w/v) casein, dissolved in 56°C water bath. This buffer may be kept for several weeks at 4°C when autoclaved.
6. PBS-T: PBS, containing 0.1% (v/v) Tween 20.
7. Elution buffer: 0.1 M HCl, adjusted to pH 2.2 with solid glycine.
8. Neutralization buffer: 2 M Tris.
9. Use aerosol-resistant tips when pipeting phage preparations to avoid cross-contamination via the pipet.
10. Because of the danger of infections the phage-contaminated waste may potentially pose, it must be disposed of according to local safety regulations, e.g., decontaminated in hypochlorite.
11. Perform experiments with phages under half-sterile conditions (best in a laminar flow). Clear bench from contaminating phages by using UV light for 30 min.

2.2. Amplification of Phages

1. SB medium: 30 g/L peptone from casein, 20 g/L yeast extract, 10 g/L MOPS (3-(*N* morpholino) propane sulfonic acid), add deionized H_2O and shake until the solutes have dissolved. Adjust the pH to 7.0 and the volume of the solution to 1 l with deionized H_2O. Sterilize by autoclaving for 20 min.

2. Antibiotics stocks:
   Carbenicillin (100 mg/mL H_2O)
   Kanamycin (25 mg/mL H_2O)
   Tetracycline (10 mg/mL 70% (v/v) ethanol).

3. Bacterial strain *E. coli* XL-1 Blue.

4. LB-agar plates:
   a. First prepare liquid media (LB medium): 10 g/L bacto trypton, 5 g/L yeast extract, 5 g/L NaCl, add deionized H_2O and shake until the solutes have dissolved. Adjust the pH to 7.0 with 5 M NaOH before adding 15 g/L bacto-agar. Sterilize by autoclaving for 20 min on liquid cycle. When the medium is removed from the autoclave, swirl it gently to distribute the melted agar throughout the solution (*see* **Note 1**). Allow the medium to cool to 50°C. To avoid producing air bubbles, mix the medium by swirling.
   b. Medium can then be poured directly from the flask into sterile Petri dishes; allow about 30–35 mL of medium per 90-mm plate. When the medium has hardened completely, invert the plates to prevent contamination by condensation water, and store them at 4°C until needed. The plates should be removed from storage 1–2 h before usage (*see* **Note 2**).

5. Helper phage M13 (10^{12} plaque forming units (pfu)/mL PBS) (VSCM13 from Stratagene or M13 K07 from Pharmacia).

6. PEG/NaCl: 160 g/L polyethylene glycol 8000, 40 g/L NaCl.

7. PBS/casein buffer (*see* above).

8. A bent glass rod is used for plating bacteria on LB-agar plates. Decontaminate rod using a Bunsen burner, let it shortly cool down, and only then use for plating another sample.

9. In all culturing steps seal bottles/tubes with foil or cap tight enough to prevent contamination, but also guaranteeing sufficient aeration of the bacterial culture during incubation.

2.3. Determination of Total Phage Titer

1. SB medium.

2. Antibiotics stocks:
   Carbenicillin (100 mg/mL H_2O)
   Tetracycline (10 mg/mL 70% (v/v) ethanol).

3. LB/carb plates: First prepare LB media containing 10 g/L bacto-agar as described above. When the medium has cooled down to 50°C, add 1 mL/L carbenicillin stock solution (100 mg/mL H_2O) and swirl gently to distribute the antibiotic throughout the solution. Medium can then be poured into plates as described above.

2.4. Monitoring of Specific Phage Titer: Immunodot Assay

1. Nitrocellulose with appropriate pore size (4 μm). Membranes with printed raster of 0.5 cm^2 are recommended for precise dotting (Millipore Corp., Bedford, MA, USA).

2. Dot buffers:
   a. Tris-buffered saline (TBS) washing buffer: 2 M Tris, 1 M HCl, 2 M NaCl, pH 7.0.
   b. TBS/casein buffer for blocking and antibody dilution: TBS, containing 0.15% (w/v) casein, dissolved in 56°C water bath. This buffer may be kept for several weeks at 4°C when autoclaved.
   c. Developing stock solution: Prepare 4-chloro-1-naphthol (carcinogenic, wear gloves!) 3 mg/mL methanol (light sensitive, wrap with foil). Can be kept at 4°C for 3–4 weeks.

3. Dotting 50-µg syringe with 1-µL drop dispenser (Hamilton, Bonaduz, Switzerland).
4. Plastic reservoirs, eight-well (Labsystems, Finland).
5. Antibody HRP/anti-M13 conjugate (Pharmacia).

2.5. Colony Screening Assay (Two Alternative Methods)

The colony screening can be performed either by the immunoblot method (**Section 2.5.1.**) or by the ELISA method (**Section 2.5.2.**).

2.5.1. Immunoblot Method

2.5.1.1. RANDOM SELECTION OF PHAGE COLONIES AND TRANSFER ON FILTER MEMBRANES

1. LB/carb plates: Prepare the same number as single clones will be tested by selecting and control antibodies, respectively.
2. Wooden tooth sticks sterilized at 180°C for 3 h or sterile pipet tips.
3. Nitrocellulose filters (use square diameter of 82 mm for 100-mm plates) (Schleicher & Schuell BA 85).
4. Filter paper (Whatman).
5. Induction reagents: 5 mM isopropyl-β-D-thiogalactopyranoside (IPTG) in sterile H$_2$O.
6. Chloroform atmosphere (work in fume hood): Place several small flat bottom glass dishes containing chloroform in larger glass Petri dish (square diameter 20 cm and above), cover with glass lid.

2.5.1.2. COLONY SCREENING IMMUNOBLOT

1. Basic buffer for colony screening immunoblot: 50 mM Tris, 150 mM NaCl, 5 mM MgCl$_2$, pH 8.0.
2. Blocking buffer: basic buffer, containing 3% (w/v) BSA.
3. Lysozyme buffer: basic buffer containing, 400 µg lysozyme/mL and 20 U DNAse/mL.
4. PBS/casein blot buffer: PBS, containing 0.15% (w/v) casein.
5. PBS-T washing buffer: PBS, containing 0.1% (v/v) Tween 20.

2.5.2. ELISA Method

2.5.2.1. RANDOM SELECTION OF PHAGE COLONIES AND TRANSFER ONTO MICROTITER PLATES

1. SB medium.
2. Microtiter plates (Maxisorp, NUNC).

2.5.2.2. COLONY SCREENING ELISA

1. Selection antibody.
2. Coating buffer: 50 mM NaHCO$_3$, pH 9.6.
3. Microtiter plates.
4. Blocking buffer: PBS-T, containing 1% BSA.
5. Antibody HRP/anti-M13 conjugate.
6. ABTS solution: 10 mg 2,2'-azino-bis(3-ethylbenzothiazoline-6-sulfonic acid) substrate (ABTS; Sigma) in 10 mL citrate buffer (100 mM NaH$_2$PO$_4$·H$_2$O, 6 mM citric acid, pH 4.0) and 10 µL H$_2$O$_2$.

3. Methods

3.1. Biopanning

1. Coat four wells of a microtiter plate with 50 µL antibody solution each (20–50 µg/mL) in bicarbonate buffer.
2. Incubate overnight at 4°C.
3. Remove the coating solution and wash twice with water by filling wells with 150-µL volumes from a multidispenser microliter pipet and emptying again.
4. Block the wells by completely filling with blocking buffer (200 µL each) and incubate at 37°C in a humidified container for 1 h.
5. Remove the blocking solution and add 50 µL of the phage library (about 10^{11} pfu/well) in PBS/casein buffer. For determination of the library's phage titer, *see* **Section 3.3**.
6. Incubate in a humidified container at 37°C for 2 h.
7. Remove the phages by pipeting thoroughly and wash the plate once with water.
8. Wash with PBS-T by completely filling the wells and resuspending. Wait 5 min, then remove PBS-T. In the first round, wash in this fashion 3×, in the second round 5×, and in subsequent rounds 10×.
9. Wash once more with ddH$_2$O and empty wells.
10. For eluting the phages, add 50 µL of elution buffer to each well and incubate at room temperature for 10 min.
11. Pipet the elution buffer several times up and down to collect all eluted phages (do not aspirate into filter of pipet tip, phages will be lost!). Remove and transfer phages to microliter tubes. Immediately, neutralize solution by adding 3 µL neutralizing buffer per 50 µL of elution buffer used. Ideally use eluents freshly for further biopanning or store overnight at 4°C.

3.2. Amplification of Phages

1. Inoculate 10 mL SB medium containing 10 µg/mL tetracycline with a colony picked from a fresh plate of *E. coli* XL-1 Blue cells and grow by shaking overnight at 37°C (= overnight culture).
2. Infect 10 mL SB medium containing 10 µg/mL tetracycline with 100 µL of the overnight culture. Incubate at 37°C until an OD at 600 nm of 0.7 is reached.
3. Incubate the eluted phages (200 µL) with 2 mL of prepared *E. coli* XL-1 Blue cells (OD$_{600nm}$ = 0.7) for 15 min at room temperature. Before doing so, remove aliquots of eluted phages for determination of the titers in this round of biopanning (*see* **Section 3.3.**).

4. Add 10 mL of 37°C prewarmed SB medium containing 20 µg/mL carbenicillin and 10 µg/mL tetracycline.
5. Shake tube at 300 rpm for 1 h at 37°C.
6. Transfer to 100 mL of SB medium containing 50 µg/mL carbenicillin and 10 µg/mL tetracycline and shake at 300 rpm for 2 h at 37°C.
7. Add 1 mL of helper phage M13 (10^{12} pfu/mL) and shake at 300 rpm for 2 h at 37°C.
8. Add 70 µg/mL kanamycin and incubate at 300 rpm overnight at 37°C.
9. Centrifuge at 4000g for 20 min at 4°C.
10. Transfer the phage supernatant to a clean bottle and add 35 mL of PEG/NaCl to 100 mL phage supernatant, mix gently.
11. Precipitate the phage on ice for 30 min.
12. Centrifuge at 10,000g for 20 min at 4°C and remove supernatants.
13. Resuspend the phage pellet in 2 mL PBS/casein, centrifuge for 5 min at 13,000 rpm (Eppendorf microcentrifuge), and store the supernatant at 4°C (*see* **Note 3**).
14. For subsequent rounds of biopanning reapply 50 µL of eluted phage suspension from point 13 above in PBS/casein to antibody-coated ELISA plate wells and repeat as described above in **Section 3.1.**, point 5.

3.3. Determination of Total Phage Titer

1. Prepare fresh *E. coli* XL-1 Blue cells with an $OD_{600nm} = 0.7$ as above (**Section 3.2.**, points 1 and 2).
2. Prepare dilutions (10^{-3}, 10^{-6}, and 10^{-8}) of the PBS/0.15% (w/v) casein resuspended phages from **Section 3.2.**, point 13, eluted in different rounds of biopanning in 1 mL SB medium. Alternatively, use original library.
3. Use 5 µL of each dilution to infect 50 µl of fresh *E. coli* XL-1 Blue cells ($OD_{600nm} = 0.7$).
4. Incubate at room temperature for 15 min.
5. Directly apply samples onto LB/carb plates with a microliter pipet and plate infected cells evenly on the agar plate using a glass rod. Incubate overnight at 37°C (plates in regular position).
6. Count colonies and calculate pfu/mL, taking the dilutions into account.
7. Alternatively, prepare different dilutions of phages in 1 mL SB medium and measure concentration in a glass cuvet in the photometer at 269 and 320 nm, distracting empty SB medium as background. Calculate particles per mL (p/mL) according to

$$\text{p/mL} = \frac{(ABS_{269nm} - ABS_{320nm}) \times \text{dilution} \times 6 \times 10^{16}}{3488}$$

3.4. Monitoring of Specific Phage Titer: Immunodot Assay

Procedure essentially described elsewhere in this volume, with slight modification:

1. Dilute selection antibody which was used for biopanning and, for control purposes, nonrelevant isotype control antibody to 1 mg/mL PBS for dotting.

2. Prepare 1 µL dots in triplicates per sample or dilution.
3. Air-dry membrane at least 2 h at RT before starting the immunoblot or store ready-to-use dot strips dry at 4°C for several weeks.
4. Number and cut strips from membrane. Perform all of the following steps on a rocking table.
5. Saturate with blocking buffer for 30 min at RT.
6. Dilute phage from original library or phage eluents from round 1, 2, 3, and so on to a final concentration of 10^7 pfu/mL (total phage titer) in PBS/casein and incubate dot strip overnight at RT. For negative control, incubate with buffer only.
7. Rinse well with sufficient volume of washing buffer, 3×10 min, changing the buffer each time.
8. Dilute detection antibody (HRP/anti-M13 conjugate) 1:2000 in dilution buffer and incubate for 2 h at RT.
9. Wash with washing buffer 3×10 min.
10. Freshly prepare the immunodot-developing buffer: 2 mL developing stock solution, add 10 mL TBS and 5 µL H_2O_2. Put immediately 1 mL per blot strip and develop color reaction for approximately 30 min in the dark under constant agitation. Stop the reaction by washing with ddH_2O and allow strips to air-dry.

3.5. Colony Screening Assay

3.5.1. Immunoblot Method

3.5.1.1. RANDOM SELECTION OF PHAGE COLONIES AND TRANSFER ON FILTER MEMBRANES

1. Use plates from the last panning round (or another round of interest) which were used for determination of phage titers. Select single bacterial clones randomly and streak approximately 50 single clones on an LB/carb plate, using in each case a new sterilized tooth stick or sterile pipet tip. Prepare two identical plates. Number the clones on the back of the two identical plates to guarantee later identification.
2. Grow colonies on both plates overnight at 37°C.
3. Seal copy colony plate with parafilm and store reversed at 4°C. Use the other plate for the following procedure.
4. Chill plate at 4°C for 30–60 min.
5. Wet nitrocellulose filters 30 min prior to use by placing them in Petri dishes with IPTG solution and then place them on filter paper to air-dry (determine the number of filters according to planned, following immunoassay) (*see* **Note 4**).
6. Apply IPTG-treated nitrocellulose filter on the colony plate, wait 1 min, then remove the filter, and place it on a new LB/carb plate overnight at 30°C (several copies can be done, *see* **Note 5**). Store original colony plate at 4°C for later identification of clones.
7. Chill all the plates at 4°C for 30–60 min.
8. The following procedures can be done on a normal bench.

9. Chill shock: Carefully remove the nitrocellulose filters from the agar using a forceps and put them (colony side up) for 10 min onto aluminum foil separating them from dry ice (*see* **Note 6**).
10. Transfer filters into a chloroform atmosphere for 30 min.
11. The filters may now be used for the immunoblot (*see* **Section 3.5.1.2.**) or stored separated by in-between paper in a plastic Petri dish at −20°C until usage.

3.5.1.2. COLONY SCREENING IMMUNOBLOT

1. Immerse each filter in 25 mL blocking buffer and put on a shaker for 30 min.
2. Remove the blocking buffer, add 25 mL of lysozyme buffer on each filter, and agitate for 1 h.
3. Remove the buffer, add PBS/casein (10 mL per Petri dish), and agitate for 1 h.
4. Incubate each filter with 10 mL of the antibody used for biopanning diluted in PBS/casein and one filter with a control antibody.
5. Wash each filter 3 × 10 min using 10 mL PBS-T.
6. Add second antibody binding to the selection antibody conjugated with HRP for 1 h, and thereafter develop each filter with developing solution.
7. Align positive clones on the colony screening filter with the clone number on plate and pick the corresponding clone from the copy plate for amplification and further analysis (*see* **Note 7**).

3.5.2. ELISA Method

3.5.2.1. RANDOM SELECTION OF PHAGE COLONIES AND TRANSFER
ONTO MICROTITER PLATES

Procedure is the same as in **Section 3.5.1.1.**, points 1–4, for selection of random colonies.

1. Place 270 μL SB medium per well onto microtiter plates.
2. Transfer single colonies from plates in **Section 3.5.1.1.**, point 4, by sterile pipet tips into the wells.
3. Incubate overnight at 37°C, sealed with parafilm, agitating at 160 rpm.
4. Centrifuge plates at 3000 rpm, 30 min, 4°C.
5. Use supernatants for detection of specificity in **Section 3.5.2.2**.

3.5.2.2. COLONY SCREENING ELISA

1. Coat fresh microtiter plates with selection antibody in coating buffer, 100 μL/well, overnight at 4°C (negative control: no coating and coating with irrelevant antibody, positive control: direct coating of phages).
2. Wash 5× with PBS-T, 200 μL/well.
3. Block plates with blocking buffer, 120 μL, 1 h at 37°C, and 1 h at 4°C.
4. Wash 5× with PBS-T, 200 μL/well.
5. Add supernatants with phages from ELISA plates I (**Section 3.5.2.1**, point 5), 80 μL/well in duplicates (on negative controls: SB medium or XL-1 supernatant without phages, on positive control: SB medium).

6. Incubate overnight at 4°C.
7. Collect supernatants with phages and store at −20°C for further usage. (*see* **Note 7**).
8. Wash plates 5× with PBS-T, 200 µL/well.
9. Apply antibody HRP/anti-M13 conjugate, diluted 1:1000 in PBS-T/0.1% BSA, 100 µL/well and incubate 1 h at 37°C and 1 h at 4°C.
10. Wash 5× with PBS-T, 200 µL/well.
11. Apply ABTS solution and measure optical density at 405–490 nm.

4. Notes

1. Be careful! The fluid may be superheated and may boil over when swirled, use protection gloves.
2. Fresh plates will "sweat" when incubated at 37°C. This allows bacterial colonies to spread across the surfaces of the plates and increases the risk of cross-contamination. To avoid this, the plates should be incubated 1–2 h at 37°C in an inverted position before they are used. Moreover, any condensation from the lids of the plates should be wiped off. The liquid can be removed by shaking the lid with a single, quick motion. To minimize the possibility of contamination, hold the open plate in an inverted position while removing the liquid from the lid.
3. Longer storage of phages in PBS/casein or in glycerol can be done at −20 or −70°C.
4. This assay is primarily a means for the identification of phages specifically selected by the antibody used for biopanning. However, filters with phage clones may also be tested with other antibodies suspected to crossreact with this epitope. This is a very direct method for proof of crossreactive epitopes (e.g., IgG vs IgE epitope of allergen).
5. On the same plate four or more filters can be applied, but each filter should be fixed on the plate for about 5 min before removal and then placed on a new LB/carb plate overnight at 30°C.
6. If dry ice is not available, ice for chilling can be treated with NaCl salt achieving a temperature of approximately −25°C.
7. Further procedures with single phage clones may for instance comprise DNA sequence analysis and alignment of the deduced amino acid sequence of the mimotopes with the natural antigen's or allergen's sequence (*6,16,21*), immunological cross-inhibition assays for determination of crossreactive allergen epitopes (*22*), or immunization experiments (*7,17,23*).

Acknowledgements

This work was supported by SFB F1808–08 and Hertha Firnberg stipend T293–B13 of the Austrian Science Fund (FWF).

References

1. Ganglberger, E., Grünberger, K., Sponer, B., et al. (2000) Allergen mimotopes for 3-dimensional epitope search and induction of antibodies inhibiting human IgE. *FASEB J.* **14**, 2177–2184.
2. Scott, J. K. and Smith, G. P. (1990) Searching for peptide ligands with an epitope library. *Science* **249**, 386–390.

3. Mittag, D., Batori, V., Neudecker, P., et al. (2006) A novel approach for investigation of specific and cross-reactive IgE epitopes on Bet v 1 and homologous food allergens in individual patients. *Mol. Immunol.* **43**, 268–278.

4. Moreau, V., Granier, C., Villard, S., Laune, D., and Molina, F. (2006) Discontinuous epitope prediction based on mimotope analysis. *Bioinformatics* **22**, 1088–1095.

5. Riemer, A. B., Hantusch, B., Sponer, B., et al. (2005) High-molecular-weight melanoma-associated antigen mimotope immunizations induce antibodies recognizing melanoma cells. *Cancer Immunol. Immunother.* **54**, 677–684.

6. Untersmayr, E., Szalai, K., Riemer, A. B., et al. (2006) Mimotopes identify conformational epitopes on parvalbumin, the major fish allergen. *Mol. Immunol.* **43**, 1454–1461.

7. Schöll, I., Wiedermann, U., Förster-Waldl, E., et al. (2002) Phage-displayed Bet mim 1, a mimotope of the major birch pollen allergen Bet v 1, induces B cell responses to the natural antigen using bystander T cell help. *Clin. Exp. Allergy* **32**, 1583–1588.

8. Hantusch, B., Krieger, S., Untersmayr, E., et al. (2004) Mapping of conformational IgE epitopes on Phl p 5a by using mimotopes from a phage display library. *J. Allergy Clin. Immunol.* **114**, 1294–1300.

9. Felici, F., Castagnoli, L., Musacchio, A., Jappelli, R., and Cesareni, G. (1991) Selection of antibody ligands from a large library of oligopeptides expressed on a multivalent exposition vector. *J. Mol. Biol.* **222**, 301–310.

10. Devlin, J. J., Panganiban, L. C., and Devlin, P. E. (1990) Random peptide libraries, a source of specific protein binding molecules. *Science* **249**, 404–406.

11. Cwirla, S. E., Peters, E. A., Barrett, R. W., and Dower, W. J. (1990) Peptides on phage, a vast library of peptides for identifying ligands. *Proc. Natl Acad. Sci. USA* **87**, 6378-6382.

12. Zwick, M. B., Shen, J., and Scott, J. K. (1998) Phage-displayed peptide libraries. *Curr. Opin. Biotechnol.* **9**, 427–436.

13. Szalai, K., Fuhrmann, J., Pavkov, T., et al. (2007) Mimotopes identify conformational B-cell epitopes on the two major house dust mite allergens Der p 1 and Der p 2. *Mol. Immunol.*, in press.

14. Förster-Waldl, E., Riemer, A. B., Dehof, A. K., et al. (2005) Isolation and structural analysis of peptide mimotopes for the disialoganglioside GD2, a neuroblastoma tumor antigen. *Mol. Immunol.* **42**, 319–325.

15. Riemer, A. B., Klinger, M., Wagner, S., et al. (2004) Generation of Peptide mimics of the epitope recognized by trastuzumab on the oncogenic protein Her-2/neu. *J. Immunol.* **173**, 394–401.

16. Riemer, A. B., Kraml, G., Scheiner, O., Zielinski, C. C., and Jensen-Jarolim, E. (2005) Matching of trastuzumab (Herceptin) epitope mimics onto the surface of Her-2/neu—a new method of epitope definition. *Mol. Immunol.* **42**, 1121–1124.

17. Ganglberger, E., Grünberger, K., Wiedermann, U., et al. (2001) IgE mimotopes of birch pollen allergen Bet v 1 induce blocking IgG in mice. *Int. Arch. Allergy Immunol.* **124**, 395–397.

18. Luzzago, A., Felici, F., Tramontano, A., Pessi, A., and Cortese, R. (1993) Mimicking of discontinuous epitopes by phage-displayed peptides, I. Epitope mapping of human H ferritin using a phage library of constrained peptides. *Gene* **128,** 51–57.
19. Fack, F., Deroo, S., Kreis, S., and Muller, C. P. (2000) Heteroduplex mobility assay (HMA) pre-screening, an improved strategy for the rapid identification of inserts selected from phage-displayed peptide libraries. *Mol. Divers.* **5,** 7–12.
20. Fack, F., Hugle-Dorr, B., Song, D., et al. (1997) Epitope mapping by phage display, random versus gene-fragment libraries. *J. Immunol. Methods* **206,** 43–52.
21. Leitner, A., Vogel, M., Radauer, C., et al. (1998) A mimotope defined by phage display inhibits IgE binding to the plant panallergen profilin. *Eur. J. Immunol.* **28,** 2921–2927.
22. Jensen-Jarolim, E., Wiedermann, U., Ganglberger, E., et al. (1999) Allergen mimotopes in food enhance type I allergic reactions in mice. *FASEB J.* **13,** 1586–1592.
23. Jensen-Jarolim, E., Leitner, A., Kalchhauser, H., et al. (1998) Peptide mimotopes displayed by phage inhibit antibody binding to Bet v 1, the major birch pollen allergen, and induce specific IgG response in mice. *FASEB J.* **12,** 1635–1642.
24. Stoute, J. A., Ballou, W. R., Kolodny, N., et al. (1995) Induction of humoral immune response against Plasmodium falciparum sporozoites by immunization with a synthetic peptide mimotope whose sequence was derived from screening a filamentous phage epitope library. *Infect Immun.* **63,** 934–939.
25. Mazzucchelli, L., Burritt, J. B., Jesaitis, A. J., et al. (1999) Cell-specific peptide binding by human neutrophils. *Blood* **93,** 1738–1748.
26. Christian, R. B., Zuckermann, R. N., Kerr, J. M., Wang, L., and Malcolm, B. A. (1992) Simplified methods for construction, assessment and rapid screening of peptide libraries in bacteriophage. *J. Mol. Biol.* **227,** 711–718.
27. Koivunen, E., Gay, D. A., and Ruoslahti, E. (1993) Selection of peptides binding to the alpha 5 beta 1 integrin from phage display library. *J. Biol. Chem.* **268,** 20,205 –20,210.
28. Schöll, I., Boltz-Nitulescu, G., and Jensen-Jarolim, E. (2003) Mimotopes and their impact on allergology. *Allergo J.* **12,** 382–387.

24

Identification of Mast Cells and Mast Cell Subpopulations

Mark Buckley and Andrew F. Walls

Abstract

Mast cells generate mediators of inflammation which are stored in granules and secreted on activation either by allergen crosslinking of membrane-bound IgE or through other stimuli. Most methods for mast cell identification rely on the histochemical detection of constituents of the secretory granules. Although staining for mast cells with histochemical stains can be rapid and relatively inexpensive, it is not always possible to distinguish reliably between mast cells and basophils in tissues. A further problem with the staining of mast cells with commonly used basic dyes is that the reagents employed to fix the tissues can influence the results, leading to confusion regarding the numbers of mast cells present in various tissues. Recognition that there is considerable heterogeneity between mast cell populations in the degree to which staining properties are lost with formalin fixation has led to mast cell subsets being defined on this basis.

The development and application of procedures for identifying mast cell proteases has led to important advances in our understanding of the role of mast cells and in the nature of heterogeneity in man. The techniques described here should allow the reliable detection of mast cells and mast cell subsets in a range of tissues and cell preparations. There will be a continuing need for validation, for consideration of potential sources of error, and for the development of new and more reliable techniques for mast cell identification.

Key Words: Mast cell; basophil; protease; chymase; Alcian blue.

1. Introduction

Mast cells were originally described by Ehrlich in 1879 as granular cells staining metachromatically with a basic dye (*1*). Thinking that the granules had been phagocytosed, he named them "mast zellen" (well-fed cells). It has since become clear that the granules contain mediators of inflammation which are generated within the mast cells and which are secreted following cell activation,

From: *Methods in Molecular Medicine: Allergy Methods and Protocols*
Edited by: M. G. Jones and P. Lympany © Humana Press Inc., Totowa, NJ

either induced by allergen crosslinking membrane-bound IgE or through a range of other stimuli. Certain mediators (including heparin and a trypsin-like enzyme named tryptase) are stored in the granules of all mast cells, and have been used as markers for mast cells in cell preparations and tissues, as have IgE and the membrane component c-*kit*. Other unique mast cell products such as chymase and mast cell carboxypeptidase are present only in a subset of these cells and have become markers for mast cell heterogeneity *(2,3)*.

For over a hundred years following their discovery, mast cells continued to be identified using basic dyes. The dyes most commonly used today are Alcian blue and toluidine blue. At neutral pH both these dyes bind to a variety of tissue components. However, under the highly acidic conditions at which they are employed for the identification of mast cells, only the highly sulfated proteoglycans remain positively charged and therefore capable of binding these basic dyes. Binding of toluidine blue to the repetitively charged side chains of heparin in the mast cell granule brings the colored ionic portions of the dye into close alignment, causing a shift in the wavelength of light absorbed. This color shift is termed metachromasia and is seen for toluidine blue but not for Alcian blue. Staining for mast cells with histochemical stains can be rapid, and the dyes are relatively inexpensive. However, these reagents do not provide means for distinguishing reliably between mast cells and basophils in tissues as the highly charged proteoglycans of basophils may also bind them.

A further problem with the staining of mast cells with basic dyes is that the reagents employed to fix the tissues can influence the results. Fixation in the most commonly used formaldehyde preparations can lead to the loss of mast cell staining with toluidine blue or Alcian blue. Until the late 1960s, the extent of this problem was not appreciated, leading to confusion regarding the numbers of mast cells present in various tissues.

Recognition that there is considerable heterogeneity between mast cell populations in the degree to which staining properties are lost within formalin fixation has led to mast cell subsets being defined on this basis. Mucosal tissues of humans and rodents readily lose their ability to stain with basic dyes following formaldehyde fixation (as can be seen when compared with findings from certain other fixatives such as Carnoy's fluid). The staining of mast cells in connective tissue on the other hand is relatively little affected by formaldehyde fixation. Staining properties of mast cells may be altered by disease; for example, selective increases in the proportions of the formaldehyde-resistant mast cells have been noted in bronchoalveolar lavage fluid from patients with certain fibrotic lung conditions *(4)*.

The ability of mast cells in formaldehyde-fixed tissues to be stained may be restored by prolonging the staining period to several days or by treating tissue sections with trypsin *(4,5)*. This suggests that formaldehyde may induce crosslinking of the protein shell around the proteoglycan and thus restrict dye binding. In this case, the proteinaceous content of the mast cell secretory granule as well as the proteoglycan may contribute to the dye-binding properties of mast cells. With toluidine and Alcian blue dyes, it is important for mast cell specificity that the staining is performed at very low pH values (e.g., pH 0.5). Even so, with prolonged staining periods, it may be difficult to distinguish mast cells from other cell types on the basis of staining alone. With a staining period greater than 6 h, metachromatic staining of eosinophils has been observed with toluidine blue and after 24 h, erythrocytes and some lymphocytes become intensely stained *(4)*. Careful standardization of fixation and staining procedures is crucial.

Toluidine and Alcian blue have come to be the most widely employed histological stains for mast cells in fixed tissues or cell preparations, and protocols for their use are provided here. Differences in performance between these two dyes have been reported but not consistently, perhaps because of variation between individual batches. A staining procedure developed by Kimura and colleagues *(6)* also involves staining with toluidine blue and a protocol for this is also provided.

There are numerous other procedures in which the detection of mast cells relies on principles similar to those involved with Alcian or toluidine blue. Other basic dyes include safranin O, astra blue, azure A and B, and thionine. Safranin, a red stain which resembles toluidine blue in chemical structure and which stains mast cells orange, has been used in a staining procedure either in sequence or together with Alcian blue (reviewed in **Ref.** *[7]*). Differential staining of mast cell granules with Alcian blue and safranin has been observed in human and rodent tissues, which may be related to the degree of sulfation of proteoglycans. Other approaches employed to detect mast cells have relied on the binding of proteoglycans of fluorescent dyes such as berberine sulfate or acridine orange or avidin conjugated to enzymes or fluorescent compounds.

Constituents of the mast cell secretory granule other than proteoglycans may offer advantages as markers for this cell type. Some success has been reported using an immunohistochemical procedure with an antibody specific to histamine *(8)*. However, the advent of well-characterized monoclonal antibodies specific for some of the mast cell proteases has led to immunohistochemical procedures with specific antibodies becoming the method of choice for the detection of mast cells in human tissues. The tryptic serine protease tryptase appears to be almost unique to mature mast cells and as such is an excellent maker for this cell type. Immunocytochemical procedures allow selective targeting of this major granule constituent, and employing secondary antibody and enzyme conjugate amplification procedures allows higher signal to noise ratios to be achieved than with conventional basic dye procedures *(9)*. Chymase, a chymotryptic serine

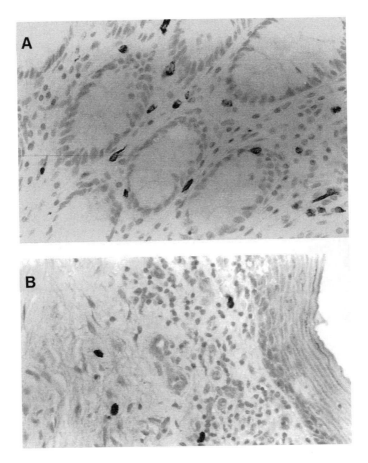

Fig. 1. Mast cells identified **(A)** around the crypts in human colonic tissue, using an immunohistochemical procedure specific for tryptase (AA1) and **(B)** in the dermis of skin using an antibody specific for chymase (CC1).

protease, is unique to a subpopulation of mast cells which predominates in normal connective tissue sites and as such has become an important marker for mast cell heterogeneity in human mast cell populations. The identification of mast cells with antibodies specific for tryptase or chymase is illustrated in **Fig. 1**. On the basis of double-labeling procedures in immunohistochemistry, mast cells can be categorized according to the presence of both tryptase and chymase (MC_{TC}) or of tryptase but not chymase (MC_T) *(2,10)*.

Selective depletion of the (MC_T) population has been noted in the gut of AIDS patients and a selective expansion in the affected tissues in a range of conditions involving inflammation or tissue remodeling including rhinitis, conjunctivitis, scleroderma, rheumatoid arthritis, and osteoarthritis (reviewed in **Ref. *[11]***). Available evidence suggests that certain other mast cell proteases including a carboxypeptidase and cathepsin G are localized preferentially in the MC_{TC} subset, and certain inflammatory cytokines may be selectively present in each of the major subsets defined, although this has not been investigated systematically with a range of tissues.

Sensitive immunocytochemical procedures for mast cell proteases have now largely supplanted earlier approaches involving the application of chromogenic substrates for histochemical detection of these enzymes. Immunocytochemistry probably offers a greater chance for standardization, and antigenicity may be better conserved than enzymatic activity during storage and processing of tissues. Nevertheless, the relative proportions of MC_T and MC_{TC} reported have varied between studies, even when results with nondispersed tissues have been compared. The use of different antibodies and different staining protocols has undoubtedly contributed to this, and there is a constant need for optimization and standardization. When double-labeling procedures are employed for tryptase and chymase, it is essential that there is effective detection of both these proteases. Variations in periods of incubation of primary antibodies on tissue sections can result in major differences in the proportions of MC_T and MC_{TC} subpopulations detected and even in the appearance of cells with chymase but not tryptase MC_c *(12)*.

The development and application of procedures for identifying mast cell proteases has led to important advances in our understanding of the role of mast cells and in the nature of heterogeneity in man. With nonhuman species, suitable antibodies which could allow similar approaches to be pursued are not generally available. Moreover, there are major interspecies differences in the types and distributions of proteases present in mast cells, and simple categorization of MC_T and MC_{TC} populations will in most cases be inappropriate. Thus, for example, multiple chymases (with quite different patterns of expression) have been characterized in several species of small mammal, but just one in man (reviewed in **Ref. *[11]***). It also seems likely that several subsets of human mast cell will be defined using immunohistochemical procedures with antibodies specific for proteases or other mast cell components.

An unresolved issue is the extent to which basophils may be detected as mast cells using the immunocytochemical techniques currently available. The early studies suggested that the quantities of tryptase or chymase present in basophils were too small to be detected. However, a report that substantial quantities of tryptase or chymase may be present in basophilic cells in peripheral blood from certain allergic subjects *(13)* calls for further evaluation of the potential for basophil staining. The advent of antibodies specific for unique constituents of the human basophil *(14)* should allow this point to be addressed.

Most methods for identification of mast cells rely on the detection of con-stituents of secretory granules. In most cases, mast cell degranulation may be partial rather than total, but there may be particular difficulties in detecting mast cells where a substantial degree of degranulation has occurred. The potential for "phantom mast cells" which fail to stain with basic dyes is well established *(15)* and it seems likely that even with the more sensitive techniques, numbers of mast cells may sometimes be underestimated. To date, the only marker selective for mast cells which is not granule-associated is c-*kit*. Immunochemistry with the c-*kit*-specific antibody YB5.B8 has been used for the identification of mast cells *(16)*, but it has proved unsuitable for paraffin-embedded tissues.

The techniques described here should allow the reliable detection of mast cells and mast cell subsets in a range of tissues and cell preparations. There will be a continuing need for validation, for consideration of potential sources of error, and for the development of new and more reliable techniques for mast cell identification.

2. Materials

2.1. Fixatives

1. Neutral buffered formalin: 100 mL 40% formaldehyde solution, 3.48 g NaH_2PO_4, 6.5 g Na_2HPO_4, 900 mL distilled water.
2. Carnoy's fixative: 60% ethanol, 30% chloroform, 10% acetic acid. The chloroform in this solution can corrode certain plastics, so it should be prepared and stored in glassware.

2.2. Histochemistry with Embedded Tissues

1. Histoclear II histological clearing agent (Raymond Lamb, Eastbourne). This is a less toxic alternative to xylene.
2. Alcian blue: 0.5% Alcian blue 8GX (certified stain CI 74240) in 0.5 M HCl (*see* **Note 1**).
3. Toluidine blue: 0.5% toluidine blue (certified stain CI 52040) in 0.5 M HCl. Add the stain to the acid gradually, with continual magnetic stirring. Filter each time before use.

2.3. Staining Wet Cell Preparations

Kimura stain *(6)*: Prepare stock solutions a–d which have a longer shelf life individually than the complete stain.

a. Dissolve 0.05 g toluidine blue in 22 mL 90% ethanol, add 1.8 g NaCl, and dilute to 100 mL with distilled water.
b. 0.03% light green stain SF yellowish (certified stain CI 42095) in distilled water.
c. Saturate 50% ethanol with saponin (Sigma, Poole, UK).
d. 0.07 M sodium phosphate, pH 6.4.

The complete stain can be made by mixing 11 mL (a), 0.8 mL (b), 0.5 mL (c), and 5 mL (d). This stain is stable for 3–4 wk at 4°C.

2.4. Peroxidase Method

1. Peroxidase blocking solution: 0.5% H_2O_2, 0.1% NaN_3 in methanol. Sodium azide is highly toxic, so PPE should be worn.
2. PBS-Albumin: 1% fraction V bovine serum albumin in phosphate-buffered saline.
3. Monoclonal antibody response to tryptase, AA1 *(9)* (Dako, Glostrup, Denmark, or AbD serotec, Oxford, or Lab Vision, Freemont, CA).
4. Monoclonal antibody to chymase, CC1 *(10)* (serotec or Lab Vision).
5. Negative control monoclonal antibody to *Aspergillus niger* glucose oxidase, X931 (Dako).
6. Wash buffer A: 0.4 M NaCl, 50 mM Tris, 0.05% Tween-20, pH 8.5.
7. Wash buffer B: 0.15 M NaCl, 50 mM Tris, 0.05% Tween-20, pH 8.5.
8. Wash buffer C: 50 mM Tris, 0.1% Tween-20, pH 8.5.
9. Biotinylated goat antiserum to mouse immunoglobulins and Extravidin®-peroxidase conjugate (EXTRA 2 kit, Sigma).
10. Acetate buffer: 0.1 M sodium acetate, pH 5.0.
11. AEC stock solution: 10 mg/mL 3-amino 9-ethylcarbazole in dimethylformamide. This stock can be stored in the dark for up to 1 wk at 4°C. Avoid polystyrene vessels because these are attacked by the solvent.
12. AEC substrate solution: 1 mL AEC stock, 19 mL acetate buffer, 3.3 µL 30% H_2O_2. Filter immediately before use.
13. Mayer's hemalum (BDH, Poole). Filter each time before use.

2.5. Alkaline Phosphatase Method

1. TBS-albumin: 1% fraction V bovine serum albumin in Tris-buffered saline.
2. Biotinylated goat antiserum to mouse immunoglobulins and Extravidin®-alkaline phosphatase conjugate (EXTRA 2A kit, Sigma).
3. Alkaline phosphatase buffer: 0.1 M glycine, 1 mM $MgCl_2$, 1 mM $ZnCl_2$, pH 10.4.
4. 50 mg/mL 5-bromo-4-chloro-3-indolyl phosphate (*p*-toluidine salt; BCIP) in dimethylformamide. Store at 4°C, avoiding polystyrene vessels.
5. 75 mg/mL *p*-nitrotetrazolium blue (NBT) in 70% dimethylformamide, can be stored at 4°C.
6. Alkaline phosphatase substrate solution: add 75 µL BCIP stock and 100 µL NBT stock to 20 mL alkaline phosphatase buffer containing 0.25 mg/mL levamisole to block most endogenous alkaline phosphatases.

2.6. Equipment

For immunohistochemistry, it is imperative that the sections do not dry out or else substantial nonspecific staining will occur. Therefore, incubations lasting more than 5 min should take place on a slide tray which holds the slides above a pool of tap water. A close fitting lid for the tray allows a humidified atmosphere to be maintained.

3. Methods

3.1. Fixation and Processing

1. Fix tissues as soon as possible after removal to preserve architecture.
2. If the tissue sample is large, cut the tissue into smaller pieces (1 cm^3 or less) to aid penetration of the fixative. Handle the tissue with care and cut with a scalpel to minimize crush artifacts.
3. Add a generous amount of neutral buffered formalin or Carnoy's fixative and leave to fix overnight at room temperature (*see* **Note 2**). Carnoy's fluid erodes plastics, so use glass vessels with this fixative.
4. Remove the fixative and dispose of according to local regulations. Carnoy's fluid can first be neutralized by the addition of $NaHCO_3$. Add PBS and mix gently on a spiral or rotary mixer at 4°C for 1–2 h to wash out the fixative.
5. At intervals of an hour or more, dehydrate the specimens through a series of graded alcohols (70, 90, 100, and 100%) with gentle mixing at 4°C.
6. Embed the tissues in paraffin wax and cut into 4 to 6-µm sections. For immunohisto-chemistry, sections can be wrapped and stored at 4°C for up to 2 wk before staining.

3.2. Histochemical Staining of Mast Cells

1. Remove the slides from the refrigerator and allow to come to room temperature before unwrapping them and warming them in an incubator at 37°C for a few minutes.
2. Remove the wax from the sections by immersion in Histoclear for 5 min, then transfer to another batch for a further 5 min.
3. Rehydrate the sections through a series of alcohols in the order: 100, 100, 90, and 70% ethanol, then transfer to distilled water, spending 5 min in each.
4. Place the sections in Alcian blue or toluidine blue solution between 30 and 150 min.
5. Dehydrate the sections very quickly in 70, 90, and 100%, and a brand new batch of absolute ethanol. It is crucial that dehydration is rapid; aim for 1 s in each of the alcohols.
6. Mount a coverslip using DPX mountant. DO NOT use aqueous mounting medium or staining will be lost. Alcian blue gives a pale blue staining of mast cells whereas toluidine blue produces an intense blue/purple color.

3.3. Staining of Wet Cell Preparations

Kimura stain (*6*) can be used to identify mast cells in dispersed cell preparations; staining is based on toluidine blue metachromasia. The stain also contains saponin which lyses red blood cells.

1. Incubate 90 µL cell suspension with 10 µL Kimura stain for 5 min at 37°C.
2. Examine the cells using a hemocytometer. Mast cells stain a bright cerise color.
3. If erythrocytes are too numerous, they will not all lyse and may interfere with staining. Therefore, before counting, dilute the cells further or lyse the red blood cells with hypotonic saline or 0.85% ammonium chloride solution.

3.4. Immunohistochemistry: Peroxidase Method

Note: sodium azide inhibits the peroxidase enzyme used in this method, so MUST NOT BE USED as a preservative for the buffers.

1. Remove the wax and rehydrate the sections as described in **Section 3.1.** (steps 1–3).
2. Inhibit endogenous peroxidase activity with the peroxidase blocking solution for 10 min.
3. Block nonspecific protein-binding sites with PBS-albumin for 10–30 min.
4. Discard the PBS-albumin and wipe around the sections with a piece of tissue. This minimizes the spread of liquid and therefore reduces the amount of antibody required to stain the section and the chances of the section drying out.
5. Apply 100 μL primary antibody diluted in PBS-albumin to the section and incubate for 90 min at room temperature. It is advisable to titrate the antibodies before use; we find that concentrations of monoclonal antibodies of around 1 μg/mL usually give good results. Remember to include a negative control antibody in the staining run.
6. Collect the slides in a rack and wash in a trough of running tap water for 5 min. Avoid a direct jet which may dislodge the sections. Next, wash the slides in wash buffers A, B, and C (5 min each).
7. Wipe around the sections and apply 100 μL of the biotinylated secondary antibody diluted 1/20 in PBS-albumin. Incubate the slides for an hour at room temperature.
8. Wash the slides as described in step 6.
9. Wipe around the sections and apply 100 μL Extravidin®-peroxidase diluted 1/20 in PBS-albumin. Incubate the slides for an hour at room temperature.
10. Wash the slides as described in step 6. Whilst the sections are being washed, prepare the AEC substrate solution.
11. Apply the AEC substrate solution for 3–4 min or until color develops. In practice this means starting to collect slides in a rack after 2 min; staining can continue with the slides in a vertical position.
12. Wash the sections in running tap water for 5 min, then rinse briefly in distilled water.
13. Counterstain in Mayer's hemalum for 2 min, then wash as described in step 12. DO NOT USE hematoxylin which must be blued in acid alcohol as this will remove the AEC.
14. When the sections have dried completely, mount a coverslip using aqueous mounting medium. DO NOT USE xylene-based medium such as DPX as this will solubilize the AEC stain. The AEC gives a reddish-brown staining pattern.

3.5. Immunohistochemistry: Alkaline Phosphatase Method

Phosphate ions inhibit the enzyme used in this staining protocol, so a TBS-albumin rather than a PBS-albumin solution is employed.

1. Perform steps 1 and 3–8 in **Section 3.4**. Step 2 is omitted because there is no need to block endogenous peroxidase, as a peroxidase substrate will not be used.
2. Wash the slides as described in **Section 3.4.**, step 6.

3. Wipe around the sections and apply 100 µL of a 1/20 solution of Extravidin®-alkaline phosphatase in TBS-albumin for 30 min.
4. Wash the slides as in step 2 above. Whilst the slides are being washed, prepare the alkaline phosphatase substrate solution. Levamisole is an inhibitor of many endogenous alkaline phosphatases, but not the intestinal form generally used for conjugation.
5. Apply the substrate solution for 10–15 min.
6. Wash the sections in running tap water for 5 min, then rinse briefly in distilled water.
7. Counterstain with Mayer's hemalum for 2 min, then wash the slides as in step 2.
8. Because the blue/black precipitate formed is insoluble in water or xylene, either aqueous or xylene-based media can be used to mount a coverslip.

3.6. Double-Labeling Immunohistochemistry

It is difficult to cut paraffin wax sections thin enough to get several sections through a single cell. Therefore, for colocalization of antigens in wax-embedded tissue, it is necessary to adopt a double-labeling procedure. Some workers combine fluorescent and chromogenic staining. However, we prefer to use different colored stains as this allows counterstaining and sections can be examined and photographed a long time after staining. If the two primary antibodies to be used come from different species, secondary antibodies conjugated to different enzymes can be used. However, where both primary antibodies are of mouse origin, it is necessary to have different labels conjugated directly to them. In the following section, we describe the detection of tryptase and chymase using mouse monoclonal antibodies. As chymase is the less abundant antigen *(17)*, the chymase antibody should be biotinylated because more than one biotin molecule can be conjugated to each immunoglobulin, thus providing an amplification step. The tryptase antibody can be directly labeled with horseradish peroxidase. To allow distinction between the different antibodies, contrasting chromogens should be used. In the example below, tryptase antibody binding causes reddish-brown staining whereas binding of chymase antibodies produces a blue/black color. Care must be exercised to get the correct balance of staining of the two target proteins; antibody concentrations should be titrated and incubation times selected carefully.

1. Dissolve the wax, rehydrate the tissue, and block peroxidase activity as described in **Section 3.4.**, steps 1–2.
2. Block nonspecific protein-binding sites with TBS-albumin for 10–30 min. Do not use PBS-albumin as the phosphate will interfere with the alkaline phosphatase enzyme used later.
3. Wipe around the sections and apply (a) 1/100 peroxidase-conjugated antitryptase antibody (*see* below), (b) 1 µg/mL biotinylated antichymase antibody, (c) 1 µg/mL negative control antibody, or (d) both antibody conjugates together. Perform dilutions in TBS-albumin and incubate for 3 h at room temperature.

4. Wash the sections as described in **Section 3.4.**, step 6.
5. Apply the filtered AEC substrate solution for 5 min.
6. Wash the sections as described in **Section 3.4.**, step 6.
7. Wipe around the sections and apply 1/20 Extravidin®-alkaline phosphatase in TBS-albumin for 1 h.
8. Wash the sections as described in **Section 3.4.**, step 6.
9. Apply the BCIP/NBT substrate solution for 10 min.
10. Wash the slides in running tap water for 5 min, rinse in distilled water, then counterstain in Mayer's hemalum for 2 min, and wash with tap water and distilled water again.
11. Because the AEC is soluble in alcohol, aqueous medium should be used to mount coverslips.

3.7. Cytocentrifuge Preparations

It is possible to store cell suspensions for staining at a later date by making cytocentrifuge preparations (Cytospins).

Establish the number of cells using a hemocytometer, then adjust to 1,000,000 per mL using a physiological strength buffer.

Assemble the cytocentrifuge according to the manufacturer's instructions, then load 100 µL of cell solution per slide, and centrifuge for 5 min at 500 rpm (28g).

Remove the slides, taking care not to smear the cells. Allow the cells to air dry, then fix in methanol or acetone for 1 min.

For histochemical staining, the cytospins can be stored at room temperature. For immunocytochemistry, wrap them tightly in aluminum foil and store at 4°C.

4. Notes

1. Alcian blue is very difficult to dissolve, so prepare it well in advance. Add the stain to the acid very slowly with continual magnetic stirring. Do not add any more stain until the last batch has dissolved completely, otherwise the dye will come out of solution permanently. Be prepared for this to take all day. Filter each time before use.
2. If antibodies against tryptase and chymase other than those described in this chapter are to be employed, then the antigen may be sensitive to fixation. Therefore it may be advisable to fix tissue samples in 85% ethanol for 1 wk at 4°C instead of formalin, then dehydrate them through 90% and absolute ethanols. However, care must be taken in handling these specimens before embedding, as 85% ethanol may be less efficacious than many other fixatives in eliminating biohazards. Fixation in ethanol alone will lead to some tissue shrinkage.

References

1. Ehrlich, P. (1879) Contributions to the theory and practice of histological staining. In *The Collected Papers of Paul Ehrlich* (Himmelweit, F. ed.), 1956, Pergamon, New York, pp. 65–68.
2. Irani, A.-M. A., Bradford, T. R., Kepley, C. L., Schechter, N. M., and Schwartz, L. B. (1989) Detection of MC_T and MC_{TC} types of human mast cells by

immunohistochemistry using new monoclonal anti-tryptase and anti-chymase antibodies. *J. Histochem. Cytochem.* **37**, 1509–1515.

3. Irani, A.-M. A., Bradford, T. R., and Schwartz, L. B. (1991) Human mast cell carboxypeptidase. Selective localization to MC_{TC} cells. *J. Immunol.* **147**, 247–253.

4. Walls, A. F., Roberts, J. A., Godfrey, R. C., Church, M. K., and Holgate, S. T. (1990) Histochemical heterogeneity of human mast cells: disease-related differences in mast cell subsets recovered by bronchoalveolar lavage. *Int. Arch. Allergy Appl. Immunol.* **92**, 233–241.

5. Wingren, U. and Enerback, L. (1983) Mucosal mast cells of the rat intestine: a re-evaluation of fixation and staining properties, with special reference to protein blocking and solubility of the granular glycosaminoglycan. *Histochemistry* **15**, 571–582.

6. Kimura, I., Moritani, Y., and Tanizaki, Y. (1973) Basophils in bronchial asthma with reference to reagin-type allergy. *Clin. Allergy* **3**, 195–202.

7. Heard, B. E. (1986) Histochemical aspects of the staining of mast cells with particular reference to heterogeneity and quantification. In *Asthma, Clinical Pharmacology and Therapeutic Progress* (Kay, A. B. ed.) Blackwell Scientific Publications, Oxford, pp. 286–294.

8. Johansson, O., Virtanen, M., Hilliges, M., and Yang, Q. (1994) Histamine immuno-histochemistry is superior to the conventional heparin-based routine staining methodology for investigations of human skin mast cells. *Histochem. J.* **26**, 424–430.

9. Walls, A. F., Jones, D. B., Williams, J. H., Church, M. K., and Holgate, S. T. (1990) Immunohistochemical identification of mast cells in formaldehyde-fixed tissue using monoclonal antibodies specific for tryptase. *J. Pathol.* **162**, 119–126.

10. Buckley, M. G., McEuen, A. R., and Walls, A. F. (1999) The detection of mast cell subpopulations in formalin-fixed human tissues using a new monoclonal antibody specific for chymase. *J. Pathol.* **189**, 138–143.

11. Walls, A. F. (2000) The roles of neutral proteases in asthma and rhinitis. In *Asthma and Rhinitis* (Busse, W. W. and Holgate, S. T. eds.), 2nd Ed., Blackwell, Boston, pp. 968–998.

12. Beil, W. J., Schulz, M., McEuen, A. R., Buckley, M. G., and Walls, A. F. (1997) Number, fixation properties, dye-binding and protease expression of duodenal mast cells: comparisons between healthy subjects and patients with gastritis or Crohn's disease. *Histochem. J.* **29**, 759–773.

13. Li, L., Reddel, S. W., Cherrian, M., et al. (1998) Identification of basophilic cells that express mast cell granule proteases in the peripheral blood of asthma, allergy and drug-reactive patients. *J. Immunol.* **161**, 5079–5086.

14. McEuen, A. R., Buckley, M. G., Compton, S. J., and Walls, A. F. (1999) Development and characterization of a monoclonal antibody specific for human basophils and the identification of a unique secretory product of basophil activation. *Lab. Investig.* **79**, 27–38.

15. Claman, H. N., Choi, K. L., Sujansky, W., and Vatter, A. E. (1986) Mast cell "disappearance" in chronic murine graft-vs-host disease (GVHD) – ultrastructural demonstration of "phantom mast cells". *J. Immunol.* **137**, 2009–2013.

16. Mayrhofer, G., Gadd, S. J., Spargo, L. D., and Ashman, L. K. (1987) Specificity of a mouse monoclonal antibody raised against acute myeloid leukaemia cells for mast cells in human mucosal and connective tissues. *Immunol. Cell Biol.* **65,** 241–250.

17. Schwartz, L. B., Irani, A.-M. A., Roller, K., Castells, M. C., and Schechter, N. M. (1987) Quantitation of histamine, tryptase and chymase in dispersed human T and TC mast cells. *J. Immunol.* **138,** 2611–2615.

25

Purification and Characterization of Mast Cell Tryptase and Chymase from Human Tissues

Alan R. McEuen and Andrew F. Walls

Abstract

Mast cells are key effector cells of the allergic response. When stimulated by specific allergen through the high-affinity IgE receptors or through other stimuli, these cells release a number of potent mediators of inflammation. Amongst these are the serine proteases tryptase and chymase. In humans, tryptase is the most abundant mediator stored in mast cells. Chymase is present in more moderate amounts in a subpopulation of mast cells (MC_{TC}). This subtype of mast cells predominates in connective tissue, whereas the other major subtype, the MC_T, predominates in mucosal tissue.

Both proteases have been shown to act on specific extracellular proteins and peptides, as well as to alter the behavior of various cell types. Inhibitors of tryptase have been found to be efficacious in animal and human models of asthma, and both proteases are currently being investigated as potential targets for therapeutic intervention. Such pharmacological, physiological, and biochemical studies require the availability of purified tryptase and chymase.

In this chapter, we shall describe procedures for the purification of tryptase and chymase from human tissues and provide protocols for monitoring purification and characterization of the final product. The preparation of recombinant proteases will not be covered, though some of the procedures described may be readily adapted for their purification from recombinant expression systems. The procedures described here have been developed for the purification of the human proteases and will require some modification if applied to purify mast cell proteases from the tissues of other species.

Key Words: Chymase; tryptase; mast cell.

1. Introduction

Mast cells are key effector cells of the allergic response. When stimulated by specific allergen through the high-affinity IgE receptors or through other stimuli, these cells release a number of potent mediators of inflammation.

From: *Methods in Molecular Medicine: Allergy Methods and Protocols*
Edited by: M. G. Jones and P. Lympany © Humana Press Inc., Totowa, NJ

Amongst these are the serine proteases tryptase (EC 3.4.21.59) and chymase (EC 3.4.21.39), which have trypsin-like and chymotrypsin-like substrate specificity, respectively *(1)*. In humans, tryptase is present in all mast cells in quantities of 15–30 pg/cell, which makes it the most abundant mediator stored in this cell type (cf. histamine content of 2–3 pg/cell). Chymase is present in a subpopulation of mast cells, designated MC_{TC}, in more moderate amounts of 5–10 pg/cell. This subtype of mast cells predominates in connective tissue, whereas the other major subtype, the MC_T, predominates in mucosal tissue. Initially it was thought this latter cell type lacked chymase, but more recent evidence indicates that these cells may also contain chymase, but in lesser amounts *(2,3)*.

Both proteases have been shown to act on specific extracellular proteins and peptides, as well as to alter the behavior of various cell types *(1,4)*. Inhibitors of tryptase have been found to be efficacious in animal and human models of asthma *(5,6)*, and both proteases are currently being investigated as potential targets for therapeutic intervention. Such pharmacological, physiological, and biochemical studies require the availability of purified tryptase and chymase. There is considerable heterogeneity in mast cell proteases, with several DNA sequences for distinct human tryptases (α, β, γ, δ, ε), and a growing number of polymorphic variants for both tryptase and chymase. Differences in glycosylation may underlie differences in size, charge, and substrate affinity of tryptase *(7)* and chymase *(8)* purified from human tissues. Recombinant forms of tryptase and chymase have offered a valuable means for the preparation of forms of these proteases with a defined sequence, though it may be difficult to relate these to the forms present in human tissues. In this chapter, we shall describe procedures for the purification of tryptase and chymase from human tissues, and provide protocols for monitoring purification and for characterizing the final product. The preparation of recombinant proteases will not be covered, though some of the procedures described may be readily adapted for their purification from recombinant expression systems. Mast cell proteases from humans appear to differ substantially from those in other mammalian species in the forms present, their distribution, and in the functions they perform. The procedures described here have been developed for the purification of human proteases and will require some modification if applied to purify mast cell proteases from the tissues of other species.

In most studies with native enzymes, human tryptase has been isolated from lung or skin and human chymase from skin or heart. In the case of tryptase, lung is the tissue of choice. It is a richer source of the enzyme and it can be readily homogenized in a blender, whereas skin is too tough for this process. Skin tryptase may be produced as a byproduct of chymase purification. We have purified or partially purified chymase from a number of tissues and found the richest sources to be skin, heart, and duodenum. Of these, duodenum is the easiest to process, but perhaps the most difficult to obtain, though undiseased tissue may be obtained as a byproduct of the Whipple's procedure or radical pancreactomy *(3)*. Skin may be readily obtained from amputated limbs, but is the most difficult to process. In the first report of chymase isolation *(9)*, the skin was manually minced with scissors. This was subsequently replaced by an improved procedure in which pieces of skin were compacted into cylinders, frozen, partially thawed, sliced into thin shavings with a razor, the shavings packed back into the cylinders, frozen again, and the process repeated twice more *(10)*. Our initial work with chymase involved passing the skin several times through a meat grinder *(11–13)*. We have since developed the method of freezing pieces of skin in liquid nitrogen and milling them to a fine powder in a blender *(8)*. This latter procedure makes extraction of skin as straightforward as that of lung.

Each group that works with tryptase and chymase has its own purification protocols. In developing our own methods, we have adopted from others those procedures that have worked well with us, as well as devising our own. Alternative protocols which have been reported, but not here, include immuno-affinity chromatography for the purification of tryptase *(14,15)*, hydrophobic interaction chromatography for the purification of tryptase *(16,17)*, and purification of chymase by affinity chromatography with soybean trypsin inhibitor agarose *(18)*.

Our protocol relies on a pre-extraction of tissue with low ionic strength buffer, extraction of the mast cell proteases with high ionic strength buffer *(9,19)*, and chromatographic separations based on heparin agarose affinity chromatography and gel filtration *(11,20)*. At low or physiological, ionic strength, most tissue proteins are readily soluble, whereas chymase and tryptase remain tightly associated with proteoglycans and are insoluble. Therefore, for both of these enzymes, the tissue is first extracted with low salt buffer (LSB) several times to remove soluble proteins, including plasma inhibitors of chymase, before proceeding to extraction with high salt buffer (HSB), which disrupts the protease–proteoglycan complexes.

The salt concentration of the extract must be reduced from 2.0 to 0.4 M before being applied to the column of heparin agarose. The simplest way to do this is by dialysis. However, there was concern that proteoglycans in the extract might interfere with the heparin chromatography. One option was to precipitate the proteoglycans with cetylpyridinium chloride. The large volumes of extract were then concentrated in a tangential flow ultrafiltration system (Pellicon, Millipore), diluted to the appropriate ionic strength, reconcentrated, and finally diafiltered with the starting buffer for heparin chromatography. However, we have found that the recovery of tryptase and chymase from these additional steps has not always been as good as one would like, and the Pellicon system has proved troublesome and time-consuming. Reverting to the simpler protocol has produced very good results for the purification of tryptase, but mixed results for chymase. Therefore, we give the simpler procedure for tryptase purification from lung, but both procedures for chymase and tryptase purification from skin.

The greatest single increase in purity is achieved by heparin agarose affinity chromatography. Both enzymes bind strongly to heparin and require relatively high concentrations of NaCl to be eluted. The initial reports in the literature used isocratic elution with 2 M salt solution, but we have improved resolution from other impurities by using a gradient elution *(11,20)*. Furthermore, the use of gradient elution revealed previously undetected heterogeneity in human chymase with one isoform eluting at 1.0–1.2 M NaCl (Peak B) and another at 1.8–2.0 M NaCl (Peak C) *(8)*. In our earlier work, the partially purified tryptase and chymase went straight onto the final purification step, which was gel permeation chromatography on Sephacryl S-200. However, impurities were still sometimes observed in these final preparations. The introduction of a second heparin chromatography step before S-200 chromatography yielded preparations of lung tryptase that were homogeneous by silver-stained SDS-polyacrylamide gel electrophoresis (PAGE) gels and fully active by active site titration *(21)*. We have improved on this by introducing benzamidine agarose affinity chromatography *(22)*. As this procedure involves binding of the tryptase to the affinity matrix by its active site, it has the advantage of selecting active tryptase over inactive or denatured tryptase.

For chymase, the principal impurity is tryptase. Indeed, it is not uncommon for the chymase-containing fractions from the heparin chromatography step to contain more tryptase than chymase. Although tryptase and chymase are well resolved by chromatography on S-200 (tryptase elutes first at 134 kDa, followed by chymase at 32 kDa), there is often a long "tail" after the tryptase peak, running into the chymase peak, which can only be detected by using a highly sensitive substrate. Any procedure that reduces the amount of tryptase in the applied sample will also reduce the magnitude of this tail. We have therefore introduced benzamidine agarose affinity chromatography to achieve this aim.

Both tryptase and chymase have particular stability problems that need to be taken into account during purification and subsequent storage. Tryptase requires either heparin or high salt (>1 M NaCl) to maintain the active tetrameric structure. Therefore, once tryptase is eluted from the heparin column it is kept in 2 M NaCl for all subsequent procedures. Whether the final product is stored in a HSB without heparin or in (physiological) LSB with added heparin is dependent on its intended use. We prefer to store in high salt without heparin because it gives greater control over the relative effects of tryptase and heparin in various experiments, even if a direct consequence is that the stock solution must be diluted

13-fold prior to use in physiological conditions. Chymase tends to stick to surfaces, particularly plastic, and especially in a freeze-thaw cycle. One important consequence is that one must never freeze a dilute solution of chymase. It must always be concentrated to more than 1000 mU/mL before freezing. A concentration of 4000 mU/mL is best for the final purified product.

2. Materials

2.1. Tryptase Purification

1. LSB (4 L): 0.10 M NaCl, 0.05 M Mes (pH 6.1), 1 mM ethylenediaminetetraacetic acid (EDTA).
2. HSB (3 L): 2.0 M NaCl, 0.05 M Mes (pH 6.1), 1 mM EDTA.
3. Buffer A (1 L): 0.4 M NaCl, 10 mM Mes (pH 6.1), filtered (Millipore 0.45 µm) prior to use.
4. Buffer B (500 mL): 2.0 M NaCl, 10 mM Mes (pH 6.1), filtered (Millipore 0.45 µm) prior to use.
5. Buffer C (500 mL): 2.5 M NaCl, 20 mM Tris–HCl (pH 8.5).
6. 0.15 M benzamidine, 2.0 M NaCl, 10 mM Mes (pH 6.1) (20 mL).

2.2. Chymase Purification

1. LSB (4 L): 0.10 M NaCl, 0.05 M Mops (pH 6.8), 1 mM EDTA.
2. HSB (3 L): 2.0 M NaCl, 0.05 M Mops (pH 6.8), 1 mM EDTA.
3. Buffer D (1 L): 0.4 M NaCl, 10 mM Mops (pH 6.8), filtered (Millipore 0.45 µm) prior to use.
4. Buffer E (500 mL): 2.0 M NaCl, 10 mM Mops (pH 6.8), filtered (Millipore 0.45 µm) prior to use.
5. 3% (w/v) Triton X-100.

2.3. Activity Assays

2.3.1. Stock Solutions

1. Phosphate-buffered saline plus 0.2% (w/v) Tween-20 (PBST) (500 mL).
2. Blocking solution (100 mL): 3.0% (w/v) gelatin, 0.02% (w/v) sodium azide in 100 mL PBST. Warm to dissolve. This solution will gel on refrigeration. Heat to 35°C or higher to melt prior to use.
3. Standard Tryptase Assay Buffer (100 mL): 1.0 M glycerol, 0.1 M Tris–HCl (pH 8.0). Dispense in 20-mL aliquots and store at −20°C.
4. Standard Chymase Assay Buffer (100 mL): 0.3 M Tris–HCl (pH 8.0), 1.5 M NaCl. Store at 4°C.
5. 88.9 mM *N*-benzoyl-arginine *p*-nitroanilide (BAPNA) in dimethyl sulfoxide (DMSO) (38.66 mg/mL) (approximately 1 mL). Stable for several months at room temperature. Do not refrigerate – DMSO freezes at 18°C and BAPNA comes out of the solution irreversibly.
6. 88.9 mM pyroglutamyl-Pro-Arg-*p*-nitroanilide (S-2366, Chromogenix) in DMSO. Add 522 µL DMSO to a vial of 25 mg as supplied by manufacturer. Store at −20°C.

7. 88.9 mM *N*-methoxysuccinyl-Ala-Ala-Pro-Val-*p*-nitroanilide (AAPVpNA) in DMSO (52.50 mg/mL) (approximately 0.2 mL). Store at −20°C.
8. 88.9 mM *N*-succinyl-Ala-Ala-Pro-Phe-*p*-nitroanilide (AAPFpNA) in DMSO (55.54 mg/mL) (approximately 1 mL). Stable for several months at room temperature.

2.3.2. Working Solutions

1. 1.0 mM BAPNA (volume as required for number of samples): 11.25 µL 88.9 mM BAPNA for every 0.989 mL Standard Tryptase Assay Buffer. Stable at 4°C for 24 h. Do not freeze, as BAPNA will come out of solution irreversibly.
2. 0.555 mM S-2366 (volume as required for number of samples): 6.25 µL 88.9 mM S-2366 for every 0.994 mL Standard Tryptase Assay Buffer. What is left over after assay is stable in storage at −20°C.
3. 0.555 mM AAPVpNA (volume as required for number of samples): 6.25 µL 88.9 mM AAPVpNA for every 0.994 mL Standard Chymase Assay Buffer. Stable in storage at −20°C.
4. 0.777 mM AAPFpNA (volume as required for number of samples): 8.75 µL 88.9 mM AAPFpNA for every 0.991 mL Standard Chymase Assay Buffer. Stable in storage at −20°C.

2.4. Active Site Titration

2.4.1. Stock Solutions

1. 100 mM barbitone buffer, pH 8.3 (100 mL). Store at 4°C.
2. 10 mM 4-methylumbelliferone in dimethylformamide (1.98 mg/mL) (1.00 mL). Store at −20°C. Protect from light.
3. 10 mM 4-methylumbelliferyl *p*-guanidinobenzoate (MUGB) in dimethylformamide (3.74 mg/mL) (1 mL). Store at −20°C. Protect from light.

2.4.2. Working Solutions

4-Methylumbelliferone standard curve

(4-methylumbelliferone)	4-methylumbelliferone	Barbitone buffer
100 µM	10 µL 10 mM	990 µL
1 µM	30 µL 100 µM	2.970 mL
50 nM	25 µL 1 µM	475 µL
100 nM	50 µL 1 µM	450 µL
200 nM	100 µL 1 µM	400 µL
300 nM	150 µL 1 µM	350 µL
400 nM	200 µL 1 µM	300 µL
500 nM	250 µL 1 µM	250 µL
600 nM	300 µL 1 µM	200 µL
700 nM	350 µL 1 µM	150 µL
800 nM	400 µL 1 µM	100 µL
900 nM	450 µL 1 µM	50 µL

Substrate solution

20 µM MUGB (5 mL): made up fresh daily by mixing 10 µL 10 mM MUGB, 5 µL 1 M HCl, and 4.985 mL H_2O.

2.5. Equipment

2.5.1. Equipment for Extraction

1. Class I cabinet.
2. Waring Blendor, complete, with stainless steel bowl.
3. Preparative centrifuge with rotor for 6×250 mL bottles.
4. 6×250 mL centrifuge bottles with caps, inserts, and gaskets.
5. Plastic jug for pouring contents of blender into bottles.
6. Forceps, a pair of heavy duty kitchen scissors, scalpels, wooden chopping board.
7. 0.5-mm plastic gauze (tea strainer).
8. Standard size (20 cm) kitchen sieve.
9. Plastic spatulas.

2.5.2. Equipment for Purification

1. Low or medium-pressure protein purification system.
2. Selection of chromatographic columns.
3. Centrifuge with a fixed angle rotor suitable for centrifugal concentrators.

2.5.3. Equipment for Analysis

1. Microtiter plate reader with kinetics software.
2. UV spectrophotometer.
3. Fluorescence plate reader or fluorimeter.
4. Gel electrophoresis equipment.
5. Conductivity meter.

3. Methods

3.1. Regulations Concerning Work with Human Tissues

3.1.1. Ethical Approval

The use of clinical material for experimental purposes is subject to legal restrictions which vary with time and place. Workers are advised to consult with their local Ethics Committee on issues of informed consent (donor or next-of-kin), record-keeping, storage, and so on, and formal approval for the proposed work may be necessary.

3.1.2. Health and Safety Precautions

All processing of human tissue must be conducted inside a Class I safety cabinet, properly installed and routinely tested. Recommended protective clothing include a Howie-style lab coat, latex or nitrile gloves which overlap the cuffs of the lab coat, disposable plastic apron, surgical mask, and eye protection. These precautions are recommended for the chopping of lungs, the dissection of limbs, and all operations that might generate aerosols (use of blender, pouring of tissue extracts, filtration, etc.). Transport of extracts between rooms or across any public space should be done in sealed containers. Human tissues must be disposed of safely, following local guidelines. (In these laboratories, all materials are sent for incineration.) All work surfaces and all utensils must be properly cleaned and disinfected after use. Workers are advised to obtain vaccination against Hepatitis B.

These recommendations are subject to and may be superseded by any local Health and Safety regulations that may be in force. Workers are advised to consult with their local Safety Officer before proceeding.

3.2. Purification of Tryptase from Lung

*3.2.1. Tissue Preparation (see **Note 1**)*

1. *(Any time prior to extraction)* Lung tissue, obtained postmortem, is dissected clear of the major airways and roughly chopped into 2-cm cubes. For this procedure we tend to use a Chinese chopper and a wooden chopping board. Place pieces in tared storage containers (we use 150-mL pots), record the weight, and store at –20°C.
2. *(The evening before the extraction)* The desired amount of tissue (400–450 g) is placed at 4°C to thaw overnight. The storage jars should be placed in a tray so that if any of the containers crack during storage any leakage will be contained.

*3.2.2. Extraction (see **Note 1**)*

1. On the day of the extraction, place the centrifuge rotor (6 × 250 mL) in the cold room to chill, and place the lung samples in ice in the Class I cabinet.
2. Remove excess blood by washing the tissue pieces in ice-cold distilled water. Empty the contents of each pot into a standard size (20 cm) kitchen sieve, swirl around in a bucket of ice-cold distilled water, and drain before tipping into the blender.
3. Extract first in LSB and repeat until the supernatant is colorless. Then extract three times with HSB (*see* **Notes 2–4**).
4. The protocol for each extraction step is as follows (*see* **Notes 5** and **6**):
   a. Add 850 mL buffer to the lung tissue (or pellets for subsequent stages).
   b. Blend at low power for 30 s.
   c. Rest for 30 s.
   d. Blend at high power for 30 s.
   e. Rest for 1 min.
   f. Repeat steps 4 and 5 twice more.
   g. Pour the blender contents into a jug and use the jug to dispense the extract amongst the six 250-mL centrifuge bottles.
   h. Rinse the blender with approximately 100 mL buffer and top up the bottles.
   i. Balance the bottles pairwise using a pan balance and a Pasteur pipet or Pastette.
   j. Place the chilled rotor in the centrifuge, place the balanced bottles in it opposite each other, and replace the lid of the rotor.

    k. Centrifuge at 33,000g, 4°C, for 30 min.

    l. At the end of the run, remove bottles, place in ice, and return to Class I cabinet.

    m. Pour off the supernatant and keep.

    n. Transfer pellets to blender and repeat extraction.

5. Assay each extract for tryptic activity with BAPNA. What one normally sees at this stage is a small to moderate amount of activity in the first Low Salt Extract (LSE1), negligible amounts of activity in subsequent LSEs, a sizeable amount of activity in the first High Salt Extract (HSE1), and decreasing amounts of activity in HSE2 and HSE3. Discard all LSEs (the activity in LSE1 is not necessarily tryptase) and combine HSE1 and HSE2. Whether or not to combine HSE3 with the other two HSEs is a trade-off between the amount of additional enzyme gained and the extra volume to process and is decided on an individual basis for each extraction.

3.2.3. Treatment of Extract

1. Filter the pooled HSEs successively through (*see* **Note 7**)
Whatman 1 (pore size = 11 μm)
Whatman 50 (pore size = 2.7 μm)
Whatman GF/A (pore size = 1.6 μm)
Whatman GF/F (pore size = 0.7 μm)
Millipore HVLP (pore size = 0.45 μm)

2. Dialyze against a fourfold greater volume of 10 mM Mes, pH 6.1. It is better to use a long, moderate diameter tube than a shorter but fatter tube. (Optional – Change outer solution before going home for a buffer similar to Buffer A, but with slightly less NaCl (e.g., 0.36 M)). Leave to dialyze overnight.

3. Empty the dialysis sac into a measuring cylinder. Record volume.

4. Test the conductivity of the dialyzate and adjust to that of Buffer A (±5%), either by dilution with water or by addition of 4 M NaCl. (NB – Above 0.1 M, the relationship between conductivity and NaCl concentration is not linear.)

5. Filter through Millipore 0.45-μm membrane. The sample is now ready to load onto the heparin column.

3.2.4. Heparin Chromatography

A column with a bed volume of 20–30 mL of heparin agarose is recommended. We often use a syringe barrel with a centrally placed outlet which is loosely plugged with glass wool. Heparin agarose is available from a number of different suppliers – we would recommend one with a high heparin content, typically 5 mg/mL.

1. Put tubing in buffer bottles and flush through lines with the respective buffers.

2. Calibrate pump following manufacturer's instructions.

3. Plumb in column, set eluate to waste, and adjust pump speed to give a flux of 0.50 mL/min cm^2 through the column.

4. Wash column with three cycles of alternating Buffer B and Buffer A (2 bed volumes each).

5. Load sample at 0.50 mL/min cm^2. Run eluate to waste and collect the "run through" fraction in an appropriate container (*see* **Note 8**).

6. Wash the column with 200 mL Buffer A (approximately10 bed volumes).

7. Elute with a linear gradient of 0–69% Buffer B (0.4–1.5 M NaCl) in 300 mL, followed by 80 mL of 100% Buffer B. We begin fraction collection during the last 20 mL of the wash with Buffer A and adjust the fraction volume so that the entire gradient, including the final wash with Buffer B, is collected in 80 tubes. The elution program should be followed by three wash cycles (A/C/A/C/A/C) with a final wash of Buffer A containing 0.05% sodium azide as a column preservative.

8. Determine the tryptase activity and protein content (A_{280}) of each fraction, including the "run through". Calculate the specific activity of each fraction displaying significant activity and use that criterion, together with total activity, to decide which fractions to pool.

3.2.5. Benzamidine Chromatography (see **Notes 9 and 10**)

1. Equilibrate a column of *p*-benzamidine agarose (approximately 5 mL bed volume) with Buffer B.

2. Apply the pooled fractions from the heparin chromatography at a flux of 0.25 mL/min cm^2. Save and test the "run through" for tryptic activity.

3. Wash with 10 bed volumes of Buffer B.

4. Elute by pumping through 7 mL 0.1 M benzamidine whilst collecting fractions of 2.5 mL (recommended volume). Switch off the pump and leave the benzamidine to incubate with the column-bound tryptase for 30 min.

5. Resume flow (and fraction collection) and apply another bed volume of 0.1 M benzamidine. Switch off pump and leave the benzamidine to incubate with the column-bound tryptase for another 30 min.

6. Repeat step 5 once more.

7. Wash the column with 5 bed volumes of Buffer B and continue to collect fractions.

8. Identify the benzamidine-containing fractions by absorbance at 280 nm and pool them. (Because of the strong UV absorbance of benzamidine, it is not possible to identify the protein-containing fractions by this method.)

9. Concentrate by using centrifugal concentrators with a molecular weight cutoff (MWCO) of 30 kDa.

10. When down to approximately 0.5 mL in each concentrator, diafilter to remove excess benzamidine by topping up each concentrator with Buffer B and reconcentrating.

11. Combine concentrates, rinse each concentrator with 50 or 100 µL Buffer B, and combine. The final volume should be ~1 mL.

3.2.6. Gel Permeation Chromatography

1. Apply the concentrated benzamidine agarose eluate to a column of Sephacryl S-200 (approximately 70 ×2.6 cm) equilibrated with Buffer B (*see* **Notes 11–13**).

2. Elute at 0.40 mL/min. Collect a void volume of 120 mL, then fractions of 5.0 mL each.

3. Determine the tryptase activity and protein content (A_{280}) of each fraction. The two peaks should coincide exactly, and display a constant specific activity across the fractions containing tryptase activity.
4. Pool the peak fractions and determine protein content by absorbance at 280 nm, using the extinction coefficient for purified tryptase $E^{1\ mg/mL} = 2.81$ *(18)*. Also, determine the activity of the pooled fractions toward BAPNA and calculate the specific activity.
5. Concentrate in either an ultrafiltration cell or spin concentrators (30 kDa MWCO). Aliquot and store at −70°C.

3.2.7. Characterization of the Purified Protein

1. Determine the activity of the concentrated enzyme against BAPNA and test for contaminating chymase with suc-Ala-Ala-Pro-Phe-*p*-nitroanilide and for contaminating elastase with suc-Ala-Ala-Pro-Val-*p*-nitroanilide.
2. Determine the percentage of purified protein that is enzymatically active by titration of the active site with MUGB *(20)*. Use the previously determined specific activity to calculate the protein content of the concentrated sample.
3. Determine the homogeneity of the preparation by SDS-PAGE and Western blotting with antitryptase antibodies.

3.3. Purification of Chymase and Tryptase from Human Skin

3.3.1. Tissue Preparation

1. *(Any time prior to extraction)* Limbs obtained at amputation are stored at −20°C until dissection. The evening before the dissection is planned, transfer the limbs to the cold room. Skin removal is often easier if the underlying tissue is still partially frozen. Remove only normal looking skin. If in doubt, leave it. Remove any subcutaneous fat. This is best done by holding a piece of skin fat side up with a pair of forceps on a flat surface (we use a wooden chopping board) and scraping the fat off with a scalpel blade. Place pieces in tared storage containers (we use 150-mL pots), record the weight, and store at −70°C.
2. *(The evening before the extraction)* The desired amount of tissue (300–350 g) is placed in the cold room to thaw overnight. The storage jars should be placed in a tray so that if any of the containers cracked during storage any leakage will be contained.

On the day of the extraction:

1. Place the centrifuge rotor (6 × 250 mL) in the cold room to chill, and remove the skin samples and place, in ice, in the Class I cabinet.
2. Within the Class I cabinet, set up the Waring Blendor, a styrofoam box filled to a depth of 2–3 in. with liquid nitrogen, and the tray containing the thawed skin samples (*see* **Note 14**).
3. Remove pieces of skin from the storage container with forceps and while holding them over liquid N$_2$, cut into small pieces with the kitchen scissors. Pieces should be less than 0.5 cm^2. Top up liquid N$_2$ as necessary.

4. When finished, pour some liquid nitrogen into the blender, and when the boiling off has died down, add approximately one half of the tissue. Pour back into the styrofoam container any liquid N_2 remaining in the blender (*see* **Note 15**).

5. While pressing down firmly on the lid of the blender, switch it on to *high* power for approximately 1 min (*see* **Note 16**). Remove lid and using the plastic spatula, scrape down the sides. Add a small amount of liquid N_2, if necessary, to keep everything hard frozen (*see* **Note 17**). Mill at high speed for another minute, scrape down sides, and repeat again until all the skin is pulverized.

6. Add the remaining tissue (most easily done by tipping the contents of the styrofoam container into the blender, including liquid N_2). Once the boiling has died down, pour back liquid N_2 through the plastic gauze (tea strainer). Return any tissue caught in the strainer to the blender. Repeat the milling process as above. On the final milling, continue until the frost on the outside of the container melts.

3.3.2. Extraction

The procedure is the same as that described above (*see* **Section 3.2.2.**) for the extraction of tryptase from lung tissue, except that the buffers used contain Mops, pH 6.8, rather than Mes, pH 6.1.

3.3.3. Treatment of Extract

Method 1

1. While the combined HSE is stirring in the cold room, slowly add 3.0% solution of cetylpyridinium chloride (CPC) in proportions of 1 volume of CPC to 2 volumes of extract to give a final concentration of 1.0% CPC. Leave overnight. (The upper layer of solution may form a gel. Do not worry – by morning all will be stirring and mixing throughout.)

2. Centrifuge at 33,000g, 4°C, for 30 min.

3. Filter the supernatant successively through (*see* **Note 7**)
   Whatman 1 (pore size = 11 µm)
   Whatman 50 (pore size = 2.7 µm)
   Whatman GF/A (pore size = 1.6 µm)
   Whatman GF/F (pore size = 0.7 µm)
   Millipore HVLP (pore size = 0.45 µm)

4. Concentrate in a tangential flow ultrafiltration system (Pellicon, Millipore) to the minimum possible volume in the retentate vessel, drain system, measure volume of retentate, and calculate the amount of water and buffer to add to make the sample 0.4 M NaCl, 10 mM MOPS, pH 6.8, assuming that 10% of the sample is still trapped in the system.

5. Dilute sample as calculated and reconcentrate. When about 20–30 mL remains in retentate vessel, diafilter by adding Heparin Buffer A in small amounts (e.g., 30 mL), allowing the sample to concentrate down between each addition, until 300 mL has been added in total.

6. To finish and drain system, keep the return pipe from the manifold in the retentate vessel and put the intake pipe into 200 mL Heparin Buffer A. Switch on the pump to force the concentrated retentate out of the system with Buffer A, which will also serve to rinse out the system. When all has passed through, drain the system into the combined retentate and wash.

7. Test the conductivity of the filtered retentate with a conductivity meter. Adjust conductivity to that of Buffer A (±5%), either by dilution with water or by addition of 4 M NaCl.

8. Filter through Millipore 0.45-μm membrane. The sample is now ready to load onto the heparin column.

Method 2 – As **Section 3.2.3.** with the exception that all buffers are Mops, pH 6.8, rather than Mes, pH 6.1.

3.3.4. Heparin Chromatography

1. Set up the column as described in **Section 3.2.4.**, except use Buffer D to equilibrate the column.

2. Load the sample and wash with 10 bed volumes of Buffer D.

3. Elute with a linear gradient of 0–100% Buffer E (0.4–2.0 M NaCl) in 15 bed volumes, followed by 2 bed volumes of 100% Buffer E. We begin fraction collection during the last bed volume of the wash with Buffer D and adjust the fraction volume so that the entire gradient, including the final wash with Buffer E, is collected in 80 tubes. The elution program should be followed by three wash cycles (D/C/D/C/D/C) with a final wash of Buffer D containing 0.05% sodium azide as a column preservative.

4. Determine the chymase activity, the tryptase activity, and protein content (A_{280}) of each fraction. Calculate the specific activity of each fraction displaying enzymic activity and use that criterion, together with total activity, to decide on which fractions to pool. The chymase and tryptase elution peaks usually overlap, so the division between them tends to be rather subjective.

3.3.5. Benzamidine Chromatography

Follow the procedure described in **Section 3.2.5.**, except begin fraction collection as one starts to apply the sample.

1. Assay for chymase activity in the "run through" and wash fractions and pool the active samples.

2. Concentrate the chymase-containing samples in spin concentrators with a MWCO of 10 kDa. (Please note the use of a lower MWCO for chymase than for tryptase!)

3. Combine concentrates, rinse each concentrator with 50 or 100 μL Buffer B, and combine. The final volume should be ~1 mL.

4. Pool the benzamidine-containing fractions and process for gel filtration as described above (*see* **Section 3.2.5.**, steps 8–11).

3.3.6. Gel Permeation Chromatography

Purification of tryptase from benzamidine fractions – as **Section 3.2.6.**

Purification of chymase:

1. Apply the concentrated chymase-containing fractions to a column of Sephacryl S-200 (approximately 70×2.6 cm) equilibrated with Buffer B.
2. Elute at 4.0 mL/min (manufacturer's recommended flow rate). Collect a void volume of 120 mL, then fractions of 5.0 mL each.
3. Determine the chymase activity, tryptase activity, and protein content (A_{280}) of each fraction. If there is any tryptase present, reassay the fractions between the tryptase peak and the chymase peak, as well as the chymase-containing fractions, with the more sensitive tryptase substrate, S-2366.
4. Use the chymase and S-2366 activity data and the calculated specific activities for chymase to decide which fractions to pool.
5. Concentrate in either an ultrafiltration cell or in spin concentrators (10 kDa MWCO). Aliquot and store at $-70°C$.

3.3.7. Characterization of the Purified Protein

1. Determine the activity of the concentrated enzyme with suc-Ala-Ala-Pro-Phe-*p*-nitroanilide and test for contaminating tryptase with S-2366 and for contaminating elastase with suc-Ala-Ala-Pro-Val-*p*-nitroanilide.
2. Determine the protein content with Coomassie Protein Assay Reagent (Pierce), using bovine serum albumin as standard.
3. Determine the homogeneity of the preparation by SDS-PAGE and Western blotting with antichymase antibodies.

3.4. Activity Assays

3.4.1. Preparation of Microtiter Plates

Chymase adsorbs readily to plastic surfaces, so all plates used for assaying chymase must be coated. Trials have shown that gelatin is as good as any other agent tested and does not interfere with assays for tryptase. Adsorption to plastic does not appear to be a problem with tryptase, but we have found it convenient to use coated plates for all assays.

Plates: Greiner 96-well flat-bottomed plates (cat. no. 655101).

1. Add 110 µL blocking solution per well.
2. Incubate for 1 h at 37°C in shaking incubator.
3. Rinse three times with PBST (150 µL/well).
4. Rinse 2–3 times with distilled or RO water.
5. Leave to drain and dry completely (e.g., at a low heat in a glassware drying oven).
6. Seal in plastic bags and store at 4°C until ready for use.

3.4.2. Tryptase Assay (BAPNA)

1. Add 10 µL sample/well in the coated microtiter plate.
2. With a multichannel pipet, add 90 µL 1.0 mM BAPNA per well (final concentration of BAPNA = 0.90 mM).

3. Monitor change in absorbance at 410 nm in a microtiter plate reader fitted with a kinetics program.
4. The change in absorbance (mOD/min) can be converted to mU/mL (1 mU = 1 nmol substrate hydrolyzed/min) by multiplying by the factor 3.888. This is the enzyme activity in the 10 μL sample applied to the microtiter plate well. Any dilutions prior to this must be accounted for by multiplying by the appropriate dilution factor.

3.4.3. Tryptase Assay (S-2366)

As for BAPNA assay; except that for step 2, add 90 μL 0.555 mM S-2366 (final concentration of S-2366 = 0.50 mM).

3.4.4. Chymase Assay

As for BAPNA assay; except that for step 2, add 90 μL 0.777 mM AAPFpNA (final concentration of AAPFpNA = 0.70 mM).

3.4.5. Elastase Assay

As for BAPNA assay; except that for step 2, add 90 μL 0.555 mM AAPVpNA (final concentration of AAPVpNA = 0.50 mM).

3.5. Active Site Titration

1. On a fluorescence microtiter plate reader select the following filters:
   Excitation: 360 nm
   Emission: 460 nm

2. Choose a microtiter plate and take the fluorescence reading of the empty plate. If all wells to be used display a uniform, low background, then proceed. If not, then inspect for dirt, clean, try again, or try a different plate.
3. Dispense standards at 100 μL/well.

Suggested lay-out:

	1	2	3	4	5	6	7	8	9	10	11	12
A												
B	Buffer alone			500 nM								
C	50 nM			600 nM								
D	100 nM			700 nM								
E	200 nM			800 nM								
F	300 nM			900 nM								
G	400 nM			1 μM								
H												

4. Read plate testing several gain settings. Choose the best setting.
5. Dilute enzyme samples to fall within range of 100–400 nM active site (3.4–14 μg/mL). Dilute in barbitone buffer containing 100 μg/mL heparin.

6. Dispense samples and buffer controls 90 μL/well.

Suggested lay-out:

	1	2	3	4	5	6	7	8	9	10	11	12
A												
B	Buffer alone			500 nM			Buffer control					
C	50 nM			600 nM			Unknown 1					
D	100 nM			700 nM			Unknown 2					
E	200 nM			800 nM			Unknown 3					
F	300 nM			900 nM								
G	400 nM			1 μM								
H												

7. Add 10 μL/well of the MUGB substrate solution (20 μM) to the test samples. *Note the time at which you begin the addition.*

8. Read the plate at 1-min intervals (4 cycles, 1 scan each). *Note the time the first well is read.*

9. If the readings for your unknowns are between those for 50–400 nM 4-methylumbelliferone, export your data to a spreadsheet. If not, adjust your dilutions or sample volume and try again, ensuring that all reaction volumes are 100 μL.

10. From the standard curve for each time-point, determine the number of picomoles of 4-methylumbelliferone in each of the unknowns, and calculate the mean and SEM of replicate samples.

11. Subtract the value of the buffer-only control (spontaneous hydrolysis of MUGB) from each of the tryptase-containing samples.

12. Perform a linear regression of picomoles of substrate hydrolyzed versus time and extrapolate to time = 0. This value represents the amount of active tryptase in each well. Calculate the concentration in the original sample by using the appropriate values of volume and dilution factor.

4. Notes

1. For the purposes of planning, allow one and a half hours for each extraction, so although it is possible to complete the extractions in 1 d, most of us mortals like to pace ourselves. If at all possible, leave the tissues pellets suspended in high salt buffer overnight, i.e., complete all LSEs on Day 1, perform the first HSE in the blender, and then store the tissue suspension in the centrifuge bottles in ice in the cold room overnight. If you can push on to the second HSE and start the next stage of purification with the HSE1, you are well ahead of yourself.

2. There is often a fatty layer on top of the supernatant, especially for extracts from skin and heart. For LSEs, pour it off with the supernatant. For HSEs, strain it off with the tea strainer. If any remains in the bottle after removal of the pellet, rinse out the bottles with distilled water during the "rest" stages of the subsequent extraction.

3. For each extract, remove 0.5 mL of the supernatant and store in a labeled microcentrifuge tube.

4. Keep all extracts until they have been assayed for activity (usually midday on Day 2). LSEs can then be poured into a container of disinfectant, such as Virkon, left for half an hour, then tipped down the sink.

5. HSEs are saved, poured into a measuring cylinder, and the volume recorded.

6. Keep the tissue pellet from the third HSE in ice until the enzyme activity of HSE3 has been assayed. If it appears that no further extractions are needed, then dispose of the tissue according to the prevailing local Health and Safety regulations.

7. The supernatants from the HSEs contain particulate matter that will foul and block the heparin agarose column if not removed. We have found 0.45-μm pore-sized membranes to be adequate to prevent column blocking, but will themselves block very rapidly without prefiltration. A single prefiltration stage is not adequate, so we have developed a multistep filtration procedure.

8. Omission of a concentrating step between extraction and heparin chromatography has the disadvantage that it can take several days to load the sample onto the heparin column. This can be accommodated if the extraction is timed so that the sample is loaded over the weekend.

9. When this method works, it works very well with 95% of the applied tryptase binding to the column, and the eluted tryptase is 100% active by MUGB titration (after removal of the benzamidine by gel filtration). At other times, only a proportion of the tryptase binds, even with recycling the "run through" fraction through the column. There appear to be two factors at work here. One is batch-to-batch variation in the benzamidine agarose. The other appears to be partial degradation or inactivation of the tryptase, as what does not bind to the column has a lower specific activity after further purification than what does bind.

10. A very good alternative to benzamidine agarose affinity chromatography is a second chromatographic run on heparin agarose. A separate column is used so that one has a "dirty" column for treating the unfractionated HSE and a "clean" column for the partially purified tryptase. The efficacy of this method can usually be monitored in lung extracts in the presence of a yellow protein. This impurity tends to coelute with tryptase in the first heparin chromatographic run and be resolved from it in the second.

11. A longer or a narrower column may be used, but then void and fraction volumes would have to be adjusted accordingly. Sephacryl S-300 may be used as an alternative matrix for purifying tryptase from lung extracts, but S-200 should be used for skin extracts because it gives better separation between tryptase and chymase.

12. The manufacturer's recommended flow rate for this matrix and a column of these dimensions is 4.0 mL/min. The slower flow rate has been chosen to optimize the separation of bound benzamidine from the tryptase.

13. For purification from skin extracts, we initially ran the S-200 column in the same buffer as the final buffer in heparin chromatography, i.e., 2 M NaCl, 10 mM Mops, pH 6.8. However, we found that significant autolysis of chymase occurred under these conditions. Given that the enzymatic activity of chymase decreases dramatically over the pH range from 7.0 to 5.5 *(9)*, we have tried elution at lower pH values. At pH 5.5 there was very little autolysis, but there was significant

contamination with inactive monomeric tryptase. The use of pH 6.1 seems to be a suitable compromise.

14. We have only used this liquid nitrogen extraction in a stainless steel blender bowl. We would not wish to comment on the safety or suitability of using a Pyrex bowl.

15. Switching the motor on while liquid N_2 is still in the chamber will cause a rapid boiling off of N_2 gas which will blow off the lid and scatter the contents of the blender.

16. If the motor is labored, use shorter bursts, and, if necessary, tip out some of the material.

17. If the frost on the outside of the blender starts to melt before the final milling, stop and refreeze with liquid N_2.

References

1. Walls, A. F. (2000) The roles of neutral proteases in asthma and rhinitis. In *Asthma and Rhinitis* (Busse, W. W. and Holgate, S. T., eds), Blackwell, Boston, pp. 968–998.
2. Beil, W. J., Schulz, M., McEuen, A. R., Buckley, M. G., and Walls, A. F. (1997) Number, fixation properties, dye-binding and protease expression of duodenal mast cells: comparisons between healthy subjects and patients with gastritis or Crohn's disease. *Histochem. J.* **29,** 759–773.
3. Beil, W. J., McEuen, A. R., Schulz, M., et al. (2003) Selective alterations in mast cell subsets and eosinophil infiltration in two complementary types of intestinal inflammation: ascariasis and Crohn's disease. *Pathobiology* **70,** 303–313.
4. Walls, A. F. (2000) Structure and function of human mast cell tryptase. In *Mast Cells and Basophils* (Marone, G., Lichtenstein, L. M., and Galli, S. J., eds), Academic Press, New York, pp. 291–309.
5. Walls, A. F. (2001) Tryptase inhibitors. In *Therapeutic Immunology* (Austen, K. F., Burakoff, S. J., Rosen, F. S., and Strom, T. B., eds), 2nd edition, Blackwell, Boston, pp. 150–158.
6. Krishna, M. T., Chauhan, A., Little, L., et al. (2001) Inhibition of mast cell tryptase by inhaled APC 366 attenuates allergen-induced late-phase airway obstruction in asthma. *J. Allergy Clin. Immunol.* **107,** 1039–1045.
7. Peng, Q., McEuen, A. R., Benyon, R. C., and Walls, A. F. (2003) The heterogeneity of mast cell tryptase from human lung and skin – differences in size, charge and substrate affinity. *Eur. J. Biochem.* **270,** 270–283.
8. McEuen, A. R., GaÇa, M. D. A., Buckley, M. G., et al. (1998) Two distinct forms of human mast cell chymase. Differences in affinity for heparin and in distribution in skin, heart, and other tissues. *Eur. J. Biochem.* **256,** 461–470.
9. Schechter, N. M., Fräki, J. E., Geesin, J. C., and Lazarus, G. S. (1983) Human skin chymotryptic proteinase. Isolation and relation to cathepsin G and rat mast cell proteinase I. *J. Biol. Chem.* **258,** 2973–2978.
10. Schechter, N. M., Choi, J. K., Slavin, D. A., et al. (1986) Identification of a chymotrypsin-like proteinase in human mast cells. *J. Immunol.* **137,** 962–970.
11. McEuen, A. R., Sharma, B., and Walls, A. F. (1995) Regulation of the activity of human chymase during storage and release from mast cells: the contributions

of inorganic cations, pH, heparin and histamine. *Biochem. Biophys. Acta* **1267,** 115–121.

12. He, S. and Walls, A. F. (1998) The induction of a prolonged increase in microvascular permeability by human mast cell chymase. *Eur. J. Pharmacol.* **352,** 91–98.
13. He, S. and Walls, A. F. (1998) Human mast cell chymase induces the accumulation of neutrophils, eosinophils and other inflammatory cells *in vivo. Br. J. Pharmacol.* **125,** 1491–1500.
14. Schwartz, L. B., Bradford, T. R., Lee, D. C., and Chlebowski, J. F. (1990) Immunologic and physicochemical evidence for conformational changes occurring on conversion of human mast cell tryptase from active tetramer to inactive monomer. *J. Immunol.* **144,** 2304–3211.
15. He, S., Peng, Q., and Walls, A. F. (1997) Potent induction of a neutrophil and eosinophil-rich infiltrate in vivo by human mast cell tryptase. Selective enhancement of eosinophil recruitment by histamine. *J. Immunol.* **159,** 6216–6225.
16. Stack, M. S. and Johnson, D. A. (1994) Human mast cell tryptase activates single-chain urinary-type plasminogen activator (pro-urokinase). *J. Biol. Chem.* **269,** 9416–9419.
17. Walls, A. F., Bennett, A. R., McBride, H. M., et al. (1990) Production and characterisation of monoclonal antibodies specific for human mast cell tryptase. *Clin. Exp. Allergy* **20,** 581–589.
18. Schechter, N. M., Jordan, L. M., James, A. M., et al. (1993) Reaction of human chymase with reactive site variants of α_1-antichymotrypsin. Modulation of inhibitor *versus* substrate properties. *J. Biol. Chem.* **268,** 23,626–23,633.
19. Smith, T. H., Hougland, M. W., and Johnson, D. A. (1984) Human lung tryptase. Purification and characterization. *J Biol. Chem.* **259,** 11,046–11,051.
20. McEuen, A. R., He, S., Brander, M. L., and Walls, A. F. (1996) Guinea pig lung tryptase: localisation to mast cells and characterisation of the partially purified enzyme. *Biochem. Pharmacol.* **52,** 331–340.
21. Compton, S. J., Cairns, J. A., Holgate, S. T., and Walls, A. F. (1998) The role of mast cell tryptase in regulating endothelial cell proliferation, cytokine release and adhesion molecule expression. Tryptase induces expression of mRNA for IL-1ß and IL-8 and stimulates the selective release of IL-8 from human umbilical vein endothelial cells. *J. Immunol.* **161,** 1939–1946.
22. Berger, P., Perng, D.-W., Thabrew, H., et al. (2001) Tryptase and agonists of PAR-2 induce the proliferation of human airway smooth muscle cells. *J. Appl. Physiol.* **91,** 1372–1379.

26

Experimental Activation of Mast Cells and Their Pharmacological Modulation

Shaoheng He and Andrew F. Walls

Abstract

The activation of mast cells is of pivotal importance in the pathogenesis of allergic conditions. Mast cell activation can provoke rapid increases in microvascular permeability, induce bronchoconstriction after blood flow, stimulate the recruitment and activation of other inflammatory cells, and has come to be associated with the processes of tissue remodeling and fibrosis. Such changes may be mediated by the release of a range of potent mediators of inflammation: preformed in secretory granules, or newly generated, or both.

There are major differences in the responsiveness to various stimuli and to pharmacological agents for mast cells from different body compartments. A method is presented here for the purification of mast cells from enzymatically dispersed human tissues. The methods described for the experimental activation of mast cells can be readily adapted to studies with cell lines or mast cells obtained through long-term culture.

Key Words: Mast cell; activation; modulation of mast cells.

1. Introduction

Mast cell activation is of pivotal importance in the pathogenesis of allergic conditions. Histological evidence for mast cell activation in bronchial tissues and the presence of increased concentrations of mast cell products, including histamine, tryptase, and prostaglandin D_2 (PGD_2), have been noted in bronchoalveolar lavage fluid and sputum from asthmatics [1,2]. Even during relatively asymptomatic periods, there is an increased degree of mast cell activation in asthma, and levels may be dramatically increased following exposure to allergen [3,4]. Similarly, allergen challenge of rhinitis results in increased release of mast cell products into nasal lavage fluid [5,6], and allergen challenge in the skin of sensitized subjects is associated with the secretion of these mediators in skin blister fluid [7].

From: *Methods in Molecular Medicine: Allergy Methods and Protocols*
Edited by: M. G. Jones and P. Lympany © Humana Press Inc., Totowa, NJ

Mast cell activation can provoke rapid increases in microvascular permeability, induce bronchoconstriction after blood flow, stimulate the recruitment and activation of other inflammatory cells, and has come to be associated with the processes of tissue remodeling and fibrosis (reviewed in **Ref.** *[8]*). Such changes may be mediated by the release of a range of potent mediators of inflammation *(9,10)*. These have been divided into two main classes: those which are preformed and released from secretory granules and those which are newly generated following mast cell activation. Prominent among the former group are histamine, proteases (including tryptase, chymase, and carboxypeptidase), and proteoglycans. Products of arachidonic acid metabolism and particularly PGD_2 and leukotriene C_4 (LTC_4) constitute the newly generated mediators. Mast cell cytokines may constitute a third category, in that they may be both preformed and newly synthesized. Those produced by human mast cells include IL-4, IL-5, IL-6, and TNFα.

Investigation of the stimuli, mechanisms of mast cell activation, and the means for pharmacological modulation have become important areas in the study of allergic disease. The activation of mast cells by allergen binding to specific IgE on high-affinity receptors (FCεR1) is the best understood mechanism of mast cell activation. This process of 'immunological activation' may be mimicked experimentally using antiserum specific for IgE which can crosslink membrane-bound IgE. Calcium ionophores can also prove useful as experimental stimuli, and like anti-IgE, can induce the activation of all populations of mast cells. Other 'nonimmunonological' stimuli ('secretagogues') for mast cell activation include substance P, vasoactive intestinal peptide (VIP), C5a and C3a, somatostatin, compound 48/80, morphine, pepstatin, eosinophil major basic protein (MBP), platelet activating factor, platelet factor 4, and very low density lipoproteins (reviewed in **Ref.** *[11,12]*); all these have differential effects on mast cells from different sources of tissue. The mast cell product tryptase can also stimulate the activation of human tonsil mast cells and perhaps act as an amplification signal with other stimuli *(13)*. In contrast, substance P, a stimulus for human skin mast cell activation, fails to activate mast cells of tonsil, lung, or gut tissue *(12)*.

Selecting an appropriate model system for the investigation of mast cell activation can present a challenge, given the extent of mast cell heterogeneity. There are major differences in responsiveness to various stimuli and to pharmacological agents for mast cells from different body compartments. Ideally, in seeking to investigate the behavior of mast cells in a particular site, the cells should be derived from tissues from that site. Various human tissues may be obtained from operating theatres (with appropriate local research ethics committee approval; *vide infra*), although it should be borne in mind that such tissues are generally from diseased subjects and may not be typical. It may be possible to obtain 'normal' tissue that has proven unsuitable for transplant surgery or nondiseased skin which is removed at circumcision, but otherwise tissues will be inflamed, damaged, or cancerous, or adjacent to such tissues. Cells and tissues from rodents have been widely employed in investigations of mast cell degranulation in vitro, with mast cells recovered from the peritoneum or from chopped lung tissue *(14)*. However, important differences in mast cell behavior have emerged from studies with different species, and caution is required in extrapolating from findings with rodent mast cells to the situation in man.

Early investigations of the activation of tissue mast cell in vitro relied on mechanical processes of tissue dispersion. Better standardization of the technique may be achieved by incubating chopped tissues with proteases to generate a homogeneous cell suspension. A mixture of pronase, chymopapain, elastase, and collagenase has been employed *(15)*, although a mixture of collagenase and hyaluronidase alone may be more effective *(16)*. The proportion of mast cells within dispersed tissue preparations ranges from 0.5–10% depending on the tissues. Such preparations may be suitable for the study of mast cells where the product of activation is produced mainly by this cell type. Histamine has been widely employed as a marker for mast cell activation, and a method for its measurement is provided here. Mast cell tryptase or chymase could also be employed, or PGD_2. It is important to realize, however, that there may be differential release of mast cell products with different stimuli. Thus, whereas anti-IgE can induce the release of histamine, PGD_2, and LTC_4 from human skin mast cells, substance P can stimulate the secretion of histamine from these cells without apparent release of PGD_2 and LTC_4 *(12)*.

It could be argued that the activation of mast cells in vivo occurs in the presence of other cell types, and that it may thus be appropriate to employ mixed cell preparations to study the process. In some circumstances, however, there are advantages to using a pure preparation of mast cells, e.g., where a mediator to be analyzed is also produced by other cell types. A method is presented here for the purification of mast cells from enzymatically dispersed human tissues that involves isolation by density sedimentation with Percoll, followed by a positive selection procedure with an anti-c.*kit* monoclonal antibody and Dynabeads *(17)*. The long-term culture of mast cells from precursors in bone marrow, fetal liver, or blood does offer a means of obtaining preparations of mature mast cells of high purity, although the purchase of the growth factors may be expensive. Another approach could involve the use of a cell line with mast cell-like features. Some lines (e.g., HMC1) have proved of limited value on account of their immature phenotype. The stem cell factor-dependent LAD1 and LAD2 cell lines derived from a patient with mast cell sarcoma/leukemia have many of the characteristics of mature tissue mast cells *(18)* and can offer a useful model for studies with mast cells. The methods described here for the experimental activation of mast cells can be readily adapted to studies with cell lines or mast cells obtained through long-term culture.

Various antiallergic drugs have been found to possess mast cell-stabilizing properties. These include ketotifen, sodium cromoglycate, salbutamol *(16)*, some histamine H$_1$ receptor antagonists *(12)*, and certain inhibitors of mast cell tryptase *(13,19)* and chymase *(20)*. Major differences in responsiveness have been found for mast cells from different sources and from different species. The extent of mast cell heterogeneity calls for the use of several different mast cell models when investigating mast cell function and pharmacological control.

2. Materials
2.1. Equipment
1. Class I cabinet.
2. Forceps and scissors.
3. Centrifuge.
4. Shaking water bath.
5. Water bath.
6. Hot plate.
7. Spiramix.
8. Magnetic cell sorter (MACS) (Miltenyi Biotec, Bergisch Gladbach, Germany).
9. Histamine analyzer (The Reference Library, Copenhagen, Denmark) with glass fiber-coated plates (Lundbeck Diagnostics, Copenhagen, Denmark).
10. Plate washing apparatus.
11. Dry incubator.

2.2. Media and Buffers
1. Hank's balanced salt solution (HBSS):
   4 g NaCl.
   2.4 g Hepes.
   0.5 g glucose.
   500 mL distilled water.
   0.5 mL 0.2 g/mL KCl.
   0.5 mL 0.06 g/mL NaH$_2$PO$_4$.
2. Complete HBSS:
   100 mL HBSS.
   100 μL 0.265 g/mL CaCl$_2$.
   100 μL 0.102 g/mL MgCl$_2$.
3. HBSS culture medium:
   500 mL HBSS.
   2% FCS.
   1% (v/v) streptomycin and penicillin.
   1% fungizone.

4. Minimal essential medium (MEM) culture medium:
   500 mL Eagle's MEM.
   2% (v/v) fetal calf serum (FCS).
   2% (v/v) streptomycin and penicillin.
   1% (v/v) fungizone.

5. DMEM culture medium:
   500 mL Dulbecco's modification of Eagle's medium.
   2% (v/v) FCS.
   1% (v/v) streptomycin and penicillin.
   10% MEM nonessential amino acid solution.
   1% (v/v) L-glutamine.

6. Phosphate-buffered saline (PBS) culture medium:
   500 mL PBS.
   2% (v/v) FCS.
   1% (v/v) streptomycin and penicillin.
   0.3 mg/mL deoxyribonuclease (DNase).

7. Digestion solution:
   Tonsil:
   10 mL MEM culture medium for every gram of tissue.
   1.5 mg/mL collagenase.
   0.75 mg/mL hyaluronidase.
   10% FCS.

   Lung*:
   10 mL MEM culture medium for every gram of tissue.
   2 mg/mL collagenase.
   1 mg/mL hyaluronidase.
   10% FCS.

   Skin or synovium:
   10 mL MEM culture medium for every gram of tissue.
   2.5 mg/mL collagenase.
   1.5 mg/mL hyaluronidase.
   10% FCS.
   25 mg/mL bovine serum albumin (BSA).

8. 0.5% (w/v) Alcian blue dye in saline.
9. 65% continuous Percoll gradient:
   2.16 mL 10× conc. HBSS without Ca or Mg.
   19.5 mL N Percoll (Sigma, St Louis, MO).
   3.4 mL HBSS.
   0.3 mg/mL DNase.

---

*For purification of lung mast cells (Methods 3.2), the digestion solution should contain 15 mg/mL DNAse and 1 mM dithioerythritol.

10. Blocking buffer:
    90 mL PBS.
    10 mL FCS.
    1 g BSA.
11. 0.4% (w/v) SDS (sodium dodecyl sulfate or lauryl sulfate) solution.
12. Coupling reagent:
    0.5 mg/mL O-phthaldialdehyde.
    5% (v/v) methanol.
    2 mg/mL NaOH.
13. 58 mM $HClO_4$.

3. Methods

3.1. Regulations, Safety, and Ethical Considerations

3.1.1. Ethical Issues

Whereas in the past surgically removed tissues have been treated as 'clinical waste' from operating theaters and used with relatively few restrictions in research, such studies may now require the specific approval of the Local Research Ethics Committee. Issues of informed consent (donor or next of kin), record keeping, and tissue storage require consideration. In many cases an 'unlinked, anonymized' study design will be adequate, where findings are not linked to the identity of a given patient.

3.1.2. Health and Safety Precautions

Workers are advised to consult their Local Safety Office before proceeding. Processing of tissues should be carried out in a Class I safety cabinet. It is recommended that protective clothing for the chopping of tissues should include a Howie-style lab coat, latex or nitrile gloves which overlap the cuffs of the lab coat, a disposable plastic apron, surgical mask, and eye protection. Tissues should be transported in sealed containers. Human tissues should be disposed of safely (e.g., by incineration) according to local guidelines. All work surfaces and utensils should be cleaned thoroughly and disinfected after use. Vaccination of workers against Hepatitis B is advised.

3.2. Mast Cell Dispersion and Challenge (see Notes 1 and 2)

1. Collect fresh lung (at lung resection; >3 g), tonsil (at tonsillectomy; >3 g), skin (at circumcision; >1 g), and synovial tissue (at knee replacement operations; >3 g) in MEM.
2. Weigh tissue.
3. Remove blood vessels and keep only macroscopically normal tissue for experiment.
4. Cut tissue into a few pieces and squeeze blood out from lung tissue in a 100 mm × 20 mm Petri dish.

5. Wash twice with ~15 mL MEM culture medium.
6. Decant off the supernatant and add ~3 mL MEM culture medium to tissue and chop finely (approx. $0.5 \times 1 \times 2$ mm^3) with a pair of scissors.
7. Collect tissue fragments in 50-mL centrifuge tubes (approx. 2.5 g tissue per tube).
8. Top up tubes to 50 mL with MEM culture medium and centrifuge at 500g for 6 min at 4°C.
9. Discharge supernatant and resuspend tissue pellet in about 10 mL MEM culture medium and top up tube with MEM culture medium and centrifuge as above.
10. Repeat step 9 twice more.
11. Resuspend tissue pellet in the digestion solution and incubate at 37°C in a shaking water bath for 65 min for tonsil, 70 min for lung, and 80 min for skin and synovial tissue.
12. Separate cells from undigested tissue debris by passing through two sets of nylon mesh filters of pore size 100 μM (nylon tea strainers are ideal).
13. Continue to digest the undigested tissue as before in order to obtain more cells if required.
14. Centrifuge the filtrate at 500g for 6 min at 4°C.
15. Aspirate supernatant, resuspend cells in about 10 mL MEM culture medium, top up tubes to 50 mL, and centrifuge as above.
16. Repeat the above washing procedure.
17. Resuspend the cells in about 10 mL MEM culture medium with 10% FCS and adjust the volume to 50 mL.
18. Leave the cells on a roller overnight at room temperature.
19. Centrifuge the tubes at 500g for 6 min at room temperature.
20. Resuspend the cells in 10 mL MEM culture medium.
21. To estimate the cell numbers, mix 10 μL of the cell suspension with 10 μL 0.5% Alcian blue dye in saline for 20 min at room temperature. Count total and positive stained cells with a hemocytometer. With an improved Neubauer hemocytometer, counting the middle large triple-ruled square, cells/mL = cell numbers counted $\times$ $10^4 \times 2$ (dilution factor). Add 40 mL more MEM culture medium to the cell suspension and leave on roller at room temperature until use.
22. Add 25 μL secretagogue and 25 μL pharmacological agonist (or complete HBSS) in 4-mL polypropylene tubes on ice (for spontaneous and total histamine release, add 50 μL complete HBSS into each tube).
23. Centrifuge the cell suspension at 500g for 6 min at 25°C.
24. Aspirate the supernatant, resuspend cells in about 10 mL HBSS + 2% FCS, top up tubes to 50 mL, and centrifuge as above.
25. Repeat above.
26. Aspirate the supernatant, resuspend cells in about 10 mL HBSS, top up tubes to 50 mL, and centrifuge at 500g for 6 min at 25°C.
27. Resuspend cells in complete HBSS to the desired volume (so that 100 μL of cell suspension contains 2500–5000 mast cells).
28. Prewarm mast cell suspension and tubes in 37°C water bath for approx. 5 min.
29. Add 100 μL cell suspension into each tube and mix them carefully.

30. Incubate tubes for 15 min.
31. Place tubes on ice and immediately add 150 µL cold HBSS in each tube.
32. Boil the tubes for total histamine release for 6 min, then put them on ice.
33. Centrifuge all tubes at 900g for 10 min at 4°C.
34. Transfer the supernatants into capped 1.5-mL tubes and store at −20°C until assaying for histamine.

3.3. Purification of Lung Mast Cells (see Note 3)

The whole procedure should be carried out under sterile conditions:

1. Collect fresh lung tissue (>15 g) and maintain in HBSS.
2. Weigh tissue in tared 50-mL container.
3. Remove blood vessels and bronchi from tissue.
4. Cut lung tissue into a few pieces and gently squeeze blood out from tissue in a 100 mm × 20 mm Petri dish.
5. Wash tissue twice with about 15 mL of HBSS culture medium.
6. Add approx. 3 mL HBSS culture medium to lung tissue and chop finely (to pieces approx. $0.5 \times 1 \times 2$ mm^3) with a pair of scissors.
7. Collect tissue fragments in 50-mL centrifuge tubes (approx. 2.5 g tissue per tube).
8. Top up tubes to 50 mL with HBSS culture medium and centrifuge at 500g for 6 min at 4°C.
9. Discharge supernatant and resuspend tissue pellet in about 15 mL HBSS culture medium and top up tube to 50 mL with HBSS culture medium and centrifuge as above.
10. Wash tissue twice with 50 mL HBSS culture medium.
11. Resuspend tissue pellet in 50 mL DMEM culture medium and leave on roller overnight at 4°C.
12. Centrifuge at 500g for 6 min at 4°C.
13. Resuspend tissue pellet in lung digestion solution (containing 15 mg/mL DNAse and 1 mM dithioerythritol). Incubate at 37°C in a shaking water bath for 90 min.
14. Separate cells from undigested tissue debris by passing through two sets of nylon mesh filter of pore size 100 µM (nylon tea strainers are ideal).
15. Redigest the undigested tissue as before in order to obtain more cells if required.
16. Centrifuge the filtrate at 500g for 6 min at 4°C.
17. Resuspend cells in about 10 mL MEM culture medium, and divide into two 50 mL centrifuge tubes. Top up tubes to 50 mL and centrifuge as above.
18. Combine all the cells in a single 50-mL tube and wash twice with 50 mL MEM culture medium.
19. Resuspend the cells gently in a small volume of DMEM and adjust to 5 mL.
20. Mix 5 mL cell suspension with 25 mL Percoll and centrifuge at 1400g for 20 min at 4°C (if cells from more than 15 g tissue used, then increase the quantity of Percoll).
21. Remove supernatant and transfer into a number of 50-mL tubes −5 mL per tube.
22. Aspirate red blood cells and wash tube with small volume of PBS culture medium in order to recover more mast cells.

23. Add 30 mL PBS culture medium to each tube, mix gently, and centrifuge at 500g for 10 min at 4°C.
24. Combine all cells and wash twice more with 30 mL PBS culture medium.
25. Resuspend cells in 1 mL PBS culture medium and mix 10 µL of it with 0.5% Alcian blue solution for 20 min at room temperature.
26. Count total and positive stained cells with a hemocytometer (as in **Section 3.1.**).
27. Add 2 mL blocking buffer to 1 mL of cell suspension, then add 30 µL 5 mg/mL IgG (final concentration 50 µg/mL).
28. Incubate the mixture for 30 min on ice on a roller.
29. Top up the mixture with 30–40 mL PBS culture medium and centrifuge at 500g for 10 min at 4°C.
30. Aspirate the supernatant and resuspend cells in 600 µL blocking buffer.
31. Add 15 µL of 5 µg/mL monoclonal antibody YB5B8 (specific for c.*kit*; Pharmingen, San Diego, CA) to the cells dispersed from 15 g tissue and mix carefully, ensuring the cells do not clump.
32. Incubate the mixture for 30 min on ice on a roller.
33. Disperse the clumps with a pipet and incubate for a further 30 min.
34. Meanwhile:
    a. Add 30 µL of Dynabeads to 20 mL PBS culture medium in a universal container and expose the container to a magnetic field for 3 min.
    b. Aspirate the supernatant and resuspend the Dynabeads in 20 mL PBS culture medium and expose to a magnetic field for a further 3 min. Repeat twice more.
    c. Resuspend Dynabeads in 500 µL blocking buffer.

35. Centrifuge the cells at 1000 rpm, 4°C for 10 min in a microcentrifuge.
36. Resuspend cells with Dynabeads solution at a ratio of 5–8 beads per mast cell, mix well with a pipet, and incubate the mixture for 90 min on ice on a roller (disperse cells every 30 min).
37. Dilute the mixture to 20 mL with PBS culture medium and expose to magnetic field for 3 min.
38. Aspirate the supernatant and repeat step 37 above thrice more.
39. Resuspend the cells in DMEM for culture or HBSS culture medium for challenge.
40. Stain cells with 0.5% Alcian blue solution in saline for 20 min at room temperature. Count the total and positive stained cells with a hemocytometer.

3.4. Histamine Measurement (see Note 4)

1. Add 50 µL sample, 50 ng/mL histamine standard, or HBSS to each well of 96-well glass fiber coated plate.
2. Incubate in dry incubator for 60 min at 37°C.
3. Wash plate with distilled water using plate washing apparatus for 2 min.
4. Add 150 µL 0.4% SDS solution to each well.
5. Incubate in dry incubator for 30 min at 37°C.
6. Wash plate as above.
7. Add 75 µL coupling reagent to each well.

8. Incubate in dark for 10 min at room temperature.
9. Add 75 µL 58 mM $HClO_4$ to each well to stop reaction.
10. Read plate on a histamine analyzer.

Histamine release should be expressed as a percentage of total cellular histamine levels and corrected for the spontaneous release measured in tubes in which cells had been incubated with the HBSS diluent alone (i.e., percentage net histamine release = [(histamine release with stimulus – spontaneous histamine release)/total histamine content] × 100.

4. Notes

1. The procedure for tissue chopping and mast cell dispersion and challenge is here described as a continuous procedure that may be carried out in a single working day. However, chopped tissues (step 7) may be maintained overnight at 4°C on a mechanical roller, and the cell dispersion and challenge can take place the following day. This has advantages to the worker when large numbers of experiments are to be performed or when tissues are received late in the day. Incubating the tissue overnight may also lead to lower spontaneous histamine release in subsequent mast cell challenge experiments.

2. The number of experiments that may be carried out at one time can depend on the skill and the experience of the worker. The novice may prefer to restrict themselves to some 20–30 tubes, but several hundred are possible (in which case it is essential that tubes for estimation of spontaneous or total histamine are included at regular points throughout and the potential for a drift in values assessed).

3. The yield and purity of the mast cells are generally difficult to predict at the outset of such experiments, and there may be a trade-off between the two. Whereas it is possible to obtain mast cells more than 95% pure, the proportion of contaminating cells may be much greater in some cases. Differences can reflect differences between lung tissues and the skill of the worker.

4. Other methods for the measurement of histamine may be considered, such as specific enzyme immunoassay (Beckman Coulter, Fullerton, CA) which is more sensitive but expensive if many experiments are planned. The measurement of other specific mast cell products (e.g., tryptase, chymase, PGD_2) may also be considered, and there are commercially available assays. For certain products of mast cell activation produced by other cell types also (e.g., LTC_4, cytokines), it may be necessary to restrict studies to purified cells. Cytokine release from activated mast cells may be increased many hours following addition of the stimulus, and so longer incubation periods should be employed when cytokine release is to be measured (ideally several time-points).

References

1. Broide, D. H., Gleich, G. J., Cuomo, A. J., et al. (1991) Evidence of ongoing mast cell and eosinophil degranulation in symptomatic asthma airway. *J. Allergy Clin. Immunol.* **88,** 637–648.

2. Jarjour, N. N., Calhoun, W. J., Schwartz, L. B., and Busse, W. W. (1991) Elevated bronchoalveolar lavage fluid histamine levels in allergic asthmatics are associated with increasing airway obstruction. *Am. Rev. Respir. Dis.* **144,** 83–87.

3. Wenzel, S. E., Fowler, A. A., and Schwartz, L. B. (1988) Activation of pulmonary mast cells by bronchoalveolar allergen challenge. *In vivo* release of histamine and tryptase in atopic subjects with and without asthma. *Am. Rev. Respir. Dis.* **137,** 1002–1008.

4. Salomonsson, P., Gronneberg, R., Gilljam, H., et al. (1992) Bronchial exudation of bulk plasma at allergen challenge in allergic asthma. *Am. Rev. Respir. Dis.* **146,** 1535–1542.

5. Castells, M. and Schwartz, L. B. (1988) Tryptase levels in nasal lavage fluid as an indicator of the immediate allergic response. *J. Allergy Clin. Immunol.* **82,** 348–355.

6. Proud, D., Bailey, G. S., Naclerio, R. M., et al. (1992) Tryptase and histamine as markers to evaluate mast cell activation during the responses to nasal challenge with allergen, cold, dry air, and hyperosmolar solutions. *J. Allergy Clin. Immunol.* **89,** 1098–1110.

7. Shalit, M., Schwartz, L. B., Golzar, N., et al. (1988) Release of histamine and tryptase *in vivo* after prolonged cutaneous challenge with allergen in humans. *J. Immunol.* **141,** 821–826.

8. Bradding, P., Walls, A. F., and Church, M. K. (1995) Mast cells and basophils: their role in initiating and maintaining inflammatory responses. In *Immunology of the Respiratory System* (Holgate, S. T., ed.), Academic Press, London, pp. 53–84.

9. Church, M. K., Holgate, S. T., Shute, J. K., Walls, A. F., and Sampson, A. P. (1998) Mast cell derived mediators. In *Allergy: Principles and Practise*(Middleton, E., Reed, C. E., Ellis, E., Adkinson, N. F., Yunginger, J. W., and Busse, W. W., eds.), 5th Ed., Mosby, St Louis, pp. 146–167.

10. Walls, A. F. (2000) The roles of neutral proteases in asthma and rhinitis. In *Asthma and Rhinitis* (Busse, W. W. and Holgate, S. T. eds.), 2nd Ed., Blackwell, Boston, pp. 968–998.

11. Peters, S. P. (1995) Mechanism of mast cell activation. In *Asthma and Rhinitis* (Busse, W. W. and Holgate, S. T. eds.), Blackwell, Boston, pp. 221–230.

12. Church, M. K. and Caulfield, J. P. (1993) Mast cell and basophil functions. In *Allergy* (Holgate, S. T. and Church, M. K. eds.), Gower Medical Publishing, London, pp. 5–12.

13. He, S., Gaça, M. D. A., and Walls, A. F. (1998) A role for tryptase in the activation of human mast cells: modulation of histamine release by tryptase and inhibitors of tryptase. *J. Pharmacol. Exp. Ther.* **286,** 289–297.

14. He, S. and Walls, A. F. (1997) Human mast cell tryptase: a stimulus of microvascular leakage and mast cell activation. *Eur. J. Pharmacol.* **328,** 89–97.

15. Caulfield, J. P., Lewis, R.A., Hein, A., and Austin, K. F. (1980) Secretion in dissociated human pulmonary mast cells. Evidence of solubilisation of granule contents before discharge. *J. Cell Biol.* **85,** 299–311.

16. Okayama, Y. and Church, M. K. (1992) Comparison of the modulatory effect of ketotifen, sodium cromoglycate, procaterol and salbutamol in human skin, lung and tonsil mast cells. *Int. Arch. Allergy Appl. Immunol.* **97,** 216–222.

17. Okayama, Y., Benyon, R. C., Lowman, M. A., and Church, M. K. (1994) *In vitro* effects of H1-antihistamine and PGD2 release from mast cells of human lung, tonsil and skin. *Allergy* **49,** 246–253.
18. Kirshenbaum, A. S., Akin, C., Wu, Y. L., et al. (2003) Characterization of novel stem cell factor responsive human mast cell lines LAD 1 and 2 established from a patient with mast cell sarcoma/leukemia; activation following aggregation of Fc epsilon RI or Fc gamma RI. *Leukemia Res.* **27,** 677–682. Erratum published *Leukemia Res.* **27,** 1171.
19. He, S., Aslam, A., Gaça, M. D. A., et al. (2004) Inhibitors of tryptase as mast cell-stabilizing agents in the human airways: effects of tryptase and other agonists of proteinase-activated receptor 2 on histamine release. *J. Pharmacol. Exp. Ther.* **309,** 119–126.
20. He, S., Gaça, M. D. A., McEuen, A. R., and Walls, A. F. (1999) Inhibitors of chymase as mast cell-stabilising agents: contribution of chymase in the activation of human mast cells. *J. Pharmacol. Exp. Ther.* **291,** 517–523.

27

In situ Hybridization

Kayhan T. Nouri-Aria

Abstract

Hybridization is the formation of hybrid nucleic acid molecules with complementary nucleotide sequences in DNA:DNA, DNA:RNA, or RNA:RNA forms. In situ hybridization is a highly sensitive technique that allows detection and localization of specific DNA or RNA molecules in morphologically preserved isolated cells, histological tissue sections, or chromosome preparations. In situ hybridization has broad range of applications and has been used to (a) localize viral infection, (b) identify sites of gene expression, (c) analyze mRNA transcription and tissue distribution, and (d) map gene sequences in chromosomes. There are several advantages of the use of in situ hybridization including the fact that it can be applied to archival materials and frozen tissues and can be combined with immunohistochemistry to detect protein as well as mRNA of interest or phenotype of cells expressing the target genome, detecting more than one nucleic acid sequences using different labeling methods.

The major steps involved in in situ hybridization are as follows: probe preparation and labeling, tissue fixation, permeabilization, hybridization, and signal detection and these are described in detail in this chapter.

Key Words: In situ hybridization; DNA; RNA; blotting.

1. Introduction
1.1. Background

Hybridization is the formation of hybrid nucleic acid molecules with complementary nucleotide sequences in DNA:DNA, DNA:RNA, or RNA:RNA forms. In situ hybridization is a highly sensitive technique that allows detection and localization of specific DNA or RNA molecules in morphologically preserved isolated cells, histological tissue sections, or chromosome preparations (1). The technique was first described by Gall and Pardue (2) and independently by John et al. (3) in 1969. In situ hybridization is believed to have higher sensitivity than filter hybridization (Northern or Southern) where the nucleic acid sequence of interest is

From: *Methods in Molecular Medicine: Allergy Methods and Protocols*
Edited by: M. G. Jones and P. Lympany © Humana Press Inc., Totowa, NJ

present in low copies or in a small proportion of cells within tissue. The concept behind the in situ hybridization of nuclear DNA or cytoplasmic RNA is similar, although the techniques used in practice vary considerably. The hybridized sequences can subsequently be detected using autoradiography *(4)* or immunohistochemistry *(5)* depending on whether radiolabeled or chromogenic labeled probes have been used.

In situ hybridization has broad range of applications and has been used to (a) localize viral infection, (b) identify sites of gene expression, (c) analyze mRNA transcription and tissue distribution, and (d) map gene sequences in chromosomes.

Advantages of in situ hybridization include: (1) greater sensitivity than Northern blotting, (2) precise cellular or subcellular localization of DNA or RNA, (3) application to archival materials (formalin-fixed paraffin embedded tissues) as well as frozen tissues, (4) combination with immunohistochemistry to detect protein as well as mRNA of interest or (5) phenotype of cells expressing the target genome, (6) detecting more than one nucleic acid sequences using different labeling methods *(5–9)*.

However, in situ hybridization is cumbersome, expensive, and time consuming. The major steps involved in in situ hybridization are as follows: *probe preparation and labeling* (*see* **Fig. 1**), *tissue fixation, permeabilization, hybridization,* and *signal detection* (*see* **Fig. 2**).

Probe preparation: Different types of probes (double-stranded DNA, single-stranded DNA, single-stranded RNA, and oligonucleotide) can be used for in situ hybridization *(6,10–13)*. Oligonucleotides represent the least sensitive probes and can also bind electrostatically (nonspecifically) to genomic components of cells owing to their small size. In contrast, ribo-probes (RNA probes) are the most sensitive probes, binding specifically to the target mRNA using hydrogen bonds.

Probe labeling: A number of methods are available to label probes. These include nick translation and random primer labeling which is applied in labeling of cDNA probes; 3′ or 5′ end labeling for labeling oligonucleotides; and in vitro transcription to synthesize RNA probes *(14–17)*.

Radioisotope and *nonradioisotope labeling* are used for probe labeling in in situ hybridization.

(a) *Radioactive labels:* Tritium (^{3}H), sulfur (^{35}S), and phosphorus (^{32}P) have been widely used to label probes *(18,19)*. ^{3}H has the lowest energy emission and gives the finest resolution. However, using ^{3}H requires the longest exposure time and in some studies several months of exposure have been reported. Therefore, despite high resolution (localizing signals at subcellular levels), ^{3}H is not commonly used in in situ hybridization. In contrast, ^{32}P, a highly energetic nuclide requires a very short exposure time (3–5 d), but provides poor resolution. Amongst radioisotopes, ^{35}S has been widely applied because of its relatively short exposure time (10–20 d) and good resolution. Radioisotope labels are highly sensitive, provide reproducible

Probe preparation

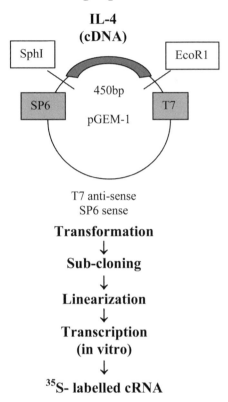

Fig. 1. Schematic representation of probe preparation and labelling. pGEM vector expressing human IL-4 genome cDNA is shown. RNA promoter sites and restriction enzyme sites for sense and anti senses are also illustrated.

results, and are easily incorporated into newly synthesized DNA or RNA. However, these labels are expensive, require long exposure, and their safety measures and waste disposal should all be taken into consideration before application.

(b) *Nonradioactive labels:* A number of nonisotopic labels have been used in in situ hybridization. These include digoxigenin, biotin, and fluorescein. In contrast to radiolabeled probes with limited half-life (with the exception of ^{3}H), chromogenic labeled probes are stable, economical, and do not require long exposure. Furthermore, they provide excellent resolution and are safe to handle. However, because of their relatively low sensitivity they are not applicable where low copies of the target genome are present in a small proportion of cells within tissues *(20–22)*.

This chapter focuses on in situ hybridization to detect mRNA using radio-labeled ribo-probes.

In situ hybridisation

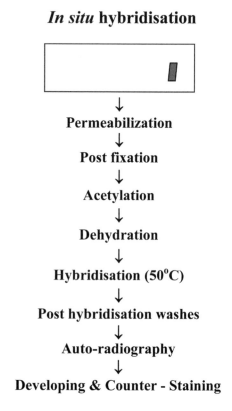

↓
Permeabilization
↓
Post fixation
↓
Acetylation
↓
Dehydration
↓
Hybridisation (50°C)
↓
Post hybridisation washes
↓
Auto-radiography
↓
Developing & Counter - Staining

Fig. 2. Schematic representation and steps involved in in situ hybridization are illustrated.

Fixation: Tissue fixation is one of the most critical steps in in situ hybridization. This is used to maintain tissue architecture as well as to ensure the retention of the target RNA or DNA within the specimens. Fixation should be carried out with minimal delay from tissue separation particularly when the target nucleic acid is RNA. Tissue fixation also influences probe penetration to the target genome. A variety of fixatives have successfully been used for tissue fixation in in situ hybridization. These include acetone, ethanol, formalin, paraformaldehyde, and gluteraldehyde. The crosslinking fixatives such as formalin, paraformaldehyde, and gluteraldehyde are the most appropriate fixatives when RNA transcripts are the target genome, whereas precipitating fixatives such as acetone and ethanol are often used for cytospin preparations *(23)*.

Permeabilization: This step is intended to remove proteins that surround nucleic acids, involves protease digestion, and increases signal intensity. Weak acid or detergent (Triton) treatment of sections prior to hybridization would also amplify signals by removing lipids within tissues.

Hybridization: Hybridization buffer consists of a number of high molecular weight chemicals such as dextran sulfate and Denhardt's solution which maintains a close contact between the labeled probe and target nucleic acid sequence of interest, hence formation of hybrid molecules. The use of formamide in hybridization buffer assists the formation of hybrids at lower temperature resulting in better specimen morphology (i.e., 1% formamide reduces hybridization temperature by 0.61°C for DNA:DNA and 0.35°C for RNA:RNA).The salt concentration and pH of the buffer determine the stringency conditions during hybridization. Hybridization temperatures of ~37°C for oligonucleotide, 40°C for cDNA, and 50°C for RNA probes are used and the procedure is normally carried out overnight *(24)*.

Detection of hybridized signals: Autoradiography is the only means of detecting signals when radioactive probes are applied. Immunohistochemistry is the method of detecting hybridized signals when nonradioactive probes are used. Radioactive detection is more robust, sensitive, and reproducible, whereas nonradioactive probes provide more rapid results.

Controls for in situ hybridization: As many factors influence the outcome of in situ hybridization, several controls should be included in each run to ensure that the results are not because of experimental artifacts. The technique is controlled by including negative and positive control sections for each probe, RNase treatment of sections prior to hybridization (which should remove hybridization signals), and inclusion of a sense probe which should result in no hybridization signals. Similarly sections hybridized in the absence of the probe, but which have gone through all other steps including autoradiography serve as a further negative control.

1.2. Ribo-Probes and Their Application

Ribo-probes are also called cRNA (complementary RNA) or antisense probes which have sequences complementary to that of target mRNA. The binding between these probes and target mRNA are specific (hydrogen bonds) and not easily dissociated *(25–26)*. To generate ribo-probes, the cDNA of interest must be inserted into specific vectors expressing RNA polymerase sites and restriction enzyme sites to allow synthesis of a sense (with a sequence identical to mRNA) and an antisense (with a sequence complementary to mRNA) probe (*see* **Fig. 1**).

Several RNA expressing vectors such as pGEM and Bluescript are commercially available. Ribo-probes have several advantages: (a) they have high affinity and thermal stability which are greater for RNA:RNA than DNA:DNA or DNA:RNA hybrids, (b) they have constant and defined size following labeling (directly) or indirectly can be made to a smaller size by alkaline hydrolysis following labeling, (c) they are produced without vector sequences, (d) they have higher specificity compared to oligoprobes, (e) unbound probe can be removed using RNase treatment post hybridization, (f) using a sense probe (with identical sequence homology with the RNA of interest), hybridization signals can be controlled.

2. Materials

All reagents should be of molecular biology grade.

2.1. Specimen Preparation

1. 0.1 M phosphate-buffered saline (PBS) (NaCl, KH_2PO_4, Na_2HPO_4).
2. 4% paraformaldehyde/PBS.
3. 15% sucrose/PBS.
4. OCT (BDH, Lutterworth, Leicestershire, UK).
5. Isopentane (BDH).
6. Liquid nitrogen.
7. Polysine™ microscopic slides (BDH).

2.2. Probe Preparation

2.2.1. Transformation

1. Polypropylene test tube (10 mL).
2. Maxi Efficiency DH5α™ Competent cells (Life Technologies, Paisley, Scotland, UK).
3. LB broth base medium (Sigma, Dorset, UK).
4. LB agar medium (Sigma).
5. Ampicillin (Sigma).

2.2.2. Mini-Preparation

1. LB broth base medium (Sigma).
2. Ampicillin (Sigma).
3. Eppendorf tubes (1.5 mL).
4. Denaturing buffer: 0.1 M NaCl, 10 mM Tris–HCl (pH 8.0), 1 mM EDTA (pH 8.0), 5% Triton X-100.
5. 10 mg/mL lysozyme (Roche, Sussex, UK).
6. 10 mM Tris–HCl (pH 8.0).
7. Gene Clean II Kit (Stratech Scientific Ltd, Luton, Bedfordshire, UK).
8. Restriction enzymes (as required) (Life Technologies).
9. Reagents for gel electrophoresis.
   a. Agarose (Sigma).
   b. Ethidium bromide (10 mg/mL) (Promega, Southampton, UK).
   c. TBE buffer: 45 mM Tris–borate, 10 mM EDTA.
   d. Gel loading solution (6× concentrate) (Sigma).
   e. Molecular weight marker (100 bp and λ DNA Hind III) (Promega).

2.2.3. Maxi-Preparation

1. LB broth base (Sigma).
2. Ampicillin (Sigma).
3. Plasmid Maxi kit (Qiagen Ltd, Dorking, Surrey, UK).
4. Restriction enzymes (as required) (Life Technologies or Promega).
5. Reagents for gel electrophoresis (*see* **Section 2.2., 2.9.**).

2.2.4. Linearization

1. DNA template, e.g., human IL-4 plasmid (hIL-4).
2. Restriction enzyme (as required) (Life Technologies or Promega).
3. Phenol (pH 6.7) (Sigma).
4. Chloroform (BDH).
5. Isoamyl alcohol (BDH).
6. Reagents for electrophoresis (*see* **Section 2.2., 2.9.**).

2.3. In Vitro Transcription

1. 5X transcription buffer (Promega).
2. 100 mM DTT (Promega).
3. RNasin 20 U/µL (Promega).
4. ^{35}S – UTP 20 mCi/mL (Amersham, Buckinghamshire, UK).
5. cDNA template (1 µg/µL).
6. ATP, GTP, CTP (7.25 mM each) (Promega).
7. RNA polymerase (SP6 or T7 or T3) (10 U/µL) (Promega).
8. 4 M NaCl.
9. RNase-free DNase (1 µg/µL) (Promega).
10. tRNA (20 µg/µL) (Sigma).
11. 7 M ammonium acetate.
12. Phenol:chloroform:isoamyl alcohol (25:24:1) (pH = 5.2) (BDH, UK).
13. Chloroform:isoamyl alcohol (24:1) (BDH).
14. Ethanol (70 and 100%).
15. Diethyl pyrocarbonate treated H_2O (DEPC, Sigma).
16. Filter paper #1 (Whatman).

2.4. Pretreatment of Specimen Prior to Hybridization

1. 0.1 M PBS (as previously described).
2. 0.75% glycine in 0.1 M PBS.
3. 0.3% Triton-X 100 in 0.1 M PBS.
4. 4% paraformaldehyde in 0.1 M PBS.
5. 100 mM Tris–HCl, 50 mM EDTA buffer.
6. Proteinase K (1 µg/µL) in Tris–EDTA (pH 8.0) (Sigma).
7. 0.25% acetic anhydride in 0.1 M triethanolamine (pH 8.0).
8. 50% formamide in 2× saline sodium citrate (2× SSC; 0.3 M NaCl, 0.03 M NaCitrate).
9. Ethanol (70, 90, and 100%).

2.5. Hybridization Mixture

1. 10% dextran sulfate (Sigma).
2. 5× Denhardt's solution (Sigma).
3. 50% formamide.
4. 0.5% sodium dodecyl sulfate (SDS) (Promega).
5. 0.5% sodium pyrophosphate (Sigma).
6. 100 mM dithiothreitol (DTT) (Promega).

2.6. Post Hybridization

1. 20× SSC (3 M NaCl, 0.3 M NaCitrate, pH 7.0).
2. RNase-A (20 µg/µL) (Sigma).
3. 0.3 M ammonium acetate in 70% ethanol.
4. 0.3 M ammonium acetate in 90% ethanol.
5. 0.3 M ammonium acetate in 100% ethanol.

2.7. Autoradiography

1. Photography emulsion – Hypercoat (Amersham).
2. Dipping chamber (Amersham).
3. Kodak Safelight filter (Type GBX-2) (Sigma).
4. Slide rack (RA Lamb, London, UK).
5. Black box and black rack (RA Lamb).

2.8. Developing and Detection

1. Developer (Kodak D-19) (Sigma).
2. Rapid fixer (Sigma).
3. Hematoxylin (mercury free) (BDH).
4. Ethanol (90, 100, and 100%).
5. Xylene (BDH).
6. DPX mountant for microscopy (BDH).

3. Methods (see Notes 1–3)

3.1. Specimen Preparation

1. Place biopsy in 4% paraformaldehyde for 2 h at 4°C (*see* **Notes 4** and **5**).
2. Transfer the biopsy into 15% sucrose for 1 h at 4°C.
3. Transfer the biopsy into fresh 15% sucrose overnight at 4°C.
4. Embed the biopsy in OCT, mount on a piece of cork, snap freeze in isopentane precooled in liquid nitrogen, and store at −80°C.
5. Cut 6-µm sections and place on polysine™ microscope slides, dry overnight at 37°C, and store at −80°C.

3.2. Probe Preparation

3.2.1. Transformation

1. Make up LB medium agar plates in advance. Add 30.5 g LB agar base to 1 L distilled water or according to the manufacturer's instructions. Autoclave for 15 min at 121°C. Allow to cool to 55°C before adding 50 µg/mL ampicillin. Under sterile conditions, pour into plates (30–35 mL per 85-mm sterile Petri dish) and allow to solidify. Plates can be stored, covered by a lid, sealed, and inverted at 4°C prior to use.
2. Place 100 µL DH5α competent cells into a 10-mL polypropylene tube (*see* **Note 6**).
3. Add 10 ng plasmid (e.g., hIL-4) DNA to the above cells.

4. Place on ice for 30 min.
5. Incubate at 42°C for 45 s.
6. Place on ice for 2 min.
7. Add 900 μL LB broth medium and incubate at 37°C for 1 h in an orbital shaker (shake vigorously).
8. Plate 100 μL of the above mixture onto LB agar plates containing 50 μg/ml ampicillin and incubate at 37°C for 16 h.

3.2.2. Mini-Preparation (see **Note 7**)

1. Select one single bacteria colony and resuspend in 5 mL LB medium (*see* **Note 8**) containing 50 μg/mL ampicillin. Repeat this for two more colonies. Incubate at 37°C overnight in an orbital shaker with vigorous shaking.
2. Take 1.5 mL of bacteria cell suspension and spin at 12,000g for 30 s.
3. Resuspend the pellet in 350 μL of denaturing buffer and add 25 μL lysozyme.
4. Place the tube in boiling water for 40 s. Spin the bacteria lysate at 12,000g for 10 min.
5. Transfer supernatant to a new 1.5-mL tube and proceed using a Gene Clean Kit to isolate DNA.
6. Digest DNA using appropriate restriction enzymes. This is most commonly at 37°C for ~3 h but consult the manufacturer's instructions.
7. Prepare 1.5% agarose gel containing 0.5 μg/mL ethidium bromide (*see* **Note 9**).
8. Run the digested DNA and M.W. markers in the agarose gel for 1 h at 80 mA.
9. Visualize bands under the UV light (*see* **Fig. 3**). Check the digested DNA has the correct size (*see* **Fig. 3b**) (*see* **Note 10**).

3.2.3. Maxi-Preparation

1. Prepare 250 mL LB broth medium in a conical flask. Autoclave the medium for 20 min at 121°C.
2. Allow to cool to 55°C, then add ampicillin at 50 μg/mL.
3. Add 3 mL of bacteria from the mini-prep tube with confirmed insert size.
4. Incubate at 37°C overnight in an orbital shaker with vigorous shaking.
5. Perform DNA extraction using plasmid maxi kit according to the manufacturer's instruction. At the final step of the procedure check the purity of and quantify the DNA obtained:

    Dilute plasmid DNA in H_2O (~500 μL). Measure OD at 260 and 280 nm using spectrophotometry. The ratio 260:280 must be ≥1.8 (*see* **Note 11**). If the ratio is less than 1.6, discard the preparation.

    Calculate the amount of DNA; e.g., OD reading at 260 nm × 50 × volume of solution = Concentration of DNA/μL.
6. Digest the DNA (~2μg) with appropriate restriction enzymes (i.e., those which will excise the probe from the plasmid) for about 3 h at 37°C or according to the manufacturer's instructions.
7. Run the digested DNA in agarose gel to confirm the correct size of the probe. Store at −20°C (*see* **Fig. 3b**).

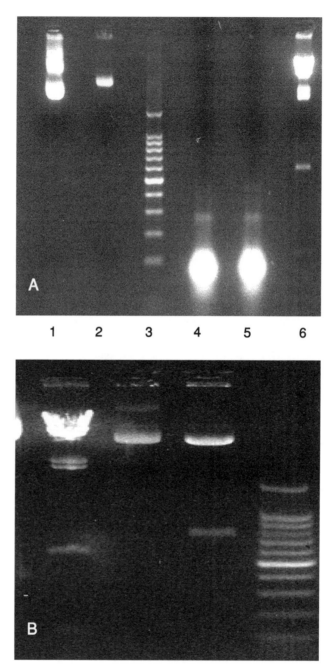

3.2.4. Linearization

The plasmid DNA at this stage is in a circular form. To linearize the probe, plasmid DNA should be digested using appropriate enzymes to allow RNA polymerases to initiate at appropriate promoter sites.

1. Digest DNA (~10 µg) with an appropriate restriction enzyme for sense and another restriction enzyme for antisense probe labeling.
2. Incubate at 37°C for ~3 h.
3. Extract linearized DNA with equal volume phenol:chloroform:isoamyl alcohol (25:24:1).
4. Repeat step 3 using an equal volume of chloroform:isoamyl alcohol (24:1).
5. Remove the upper phase containing the DNA and precipitate it with 0.5 volumes 7 M ammonium acetate and 2.5 volumes of chilled ethanol.
6. Incubate at −20°C for a minimum of 3 h. Centrifuge at 13,000g for 10 min.
7. Wash the pellet with 70% ethanol. Dry the pellet and dissolve in ~10 µL of autoclaved H_2O.
8. Take 1 µL for electrophoresis (to confirm the linearization is complete) (*see* **Fig. 3a**).

3.3. In Vitro Transcription

Add the following to 1.5-mL Eppendorf tube:

1. 2 µL transcription buffer (5×).
2. 1 µL 100 mM DTT.
3. 0.5 µL RNasin.
4. 2 µL ATP, GTP, and CTP.
5. 1 µL linearized DNA template.
6. 2.5 µL ^{35}S UTP (*see* **Note 13**).
7. 1 µL SP6 or T7 or T3 RNA polymerases (as required). Incubate at 37°C for 1 h.
8. Add 1 µL of RNase-free DNase and incubate the mixture at 37°C for 10 min to digest template DNA.
9. Add 1 µL yeast tRNA, 5 µL 4 M NaCl, 175 µL DEPC-H_2O and equal volume (200 µL) of phenol:chloroform:isoamyl alcohol, vortex for 1 min. Centrifuge at 13,000g for 5 min.
10. Collect the upper phase and transfer to a new Eppendorf tube.
11. Add 0.5 volumes ammonium acetate and 2.5 volumes cooled ethanol. Incubate the mixture at −20°C for overnight or −80°C for at least 2 h.
12. Centrifuge at 12,000g at 4°C for 20 min.

Fig. 3. Agarose gel electrophoresis under UV light demonstrating (A) lane 1, plasmid DNA before linearization; lane 2, plasmid DNA after linearization. Lane 3, 100 bp molecular weight markers; lane 4, a ribo-probe sense (~300 bp); lane 5, a ribo-probe antisense (~300 bp); lane 6, Lambda DNA *Hin*dIII digested (B) lane 1, Lambda DNA *Hin*dIII digested; lane 2, plasmid DNA before digestion; lane 3, plasmid DNA after digestion with an insert of ~800 bp; lane 4, 100 bp molecular weight markers are shown.

13. Remove the supernatant and wash the pellet with 70% cold ethanol.
14. Dry the pellet for 3–5 min at room temperature. Resuspend the pellet in 20 µL H_2O (*see* **Fig. 3a**).
15. Take 1 µL and apply to a filter paper to determine ^{35}S incorporation. Place filter paper in scintillation fluid and count on β-counter.
16. Take 1 µL for gel electrophoresis to confirm the correct size of the newly synthesized radiolabeled ribo-probe (*see* **Fig. 3a**). Store the remaining at −80°C.

3.4. Pretreatment of Sections Prior to Hybridization

1. Rehydrate in PBS for 5 min at room temperature.
2. 0.75% glycine in PBS, for 5 min at room temperature.
3. Wash in 1× PBS.
4. 0.3% Triton X-100 in PBS for 5 min at room temperature.
5. Wash in PBS.
6. Proteinase K in Tris buffer for 20 min at 37°C.
7. Postfix sections in 4% paraformaldehyde for 5 min at room temperature.
8. Wash 2× in PBS at room temperature.
9. Block nonspecific binding using triethanolamine and acetic anhydride for 10 min at 37°C.
10. Prehybridize in 50% formamide in 2× SSC for 15 min at 37°C.
11. Dehydrate for 5 min each in 70, 90, and 100% ethanol. Allow slides to dry at room temperature.

3.5. Hybridization (see Note 14)

1. Prepare a mixture of hybridization buffer and the probe (allow 1×10^6 cpm of ^{35}S-labeled probe per section and 14–20 µL buffer per slide) (*see* **Notes 15–18**).
2. Incubate the mixture at 60°C for 30 min in a shaking water bath (*see* **Note 19**).
3. Place the mixture on ice for 5 min.
4. Place slides on a staining rack. Apply 14–20 µL hybridization buffer containing the labeled probe onto each slide.
5. Cover the section with an appropriate size coverslip and incubate at 50°C for ~16 h.

3.6. Post Hybridization

Post hybridization washes are carried out as follows for 20 min at 42°C in shaking water bath (*see* **Note 21**):

1. 3 times in 4× SSC.
2. Once in RNase in 2× SSC at 37°C.
3. Once in 2× SSC.
4. Once in 1× SSC.
5. Once in 0.5× SSC.
6. Once in 0.1× SSC.

The following steps are performed at room temperature for 10 min:

1. 70% ethanol in 0.3 M ammonium acetate.

2. 90% ethanol in 0.3 M ammonium acetate.
3. 100% ethanol in 0.3 M ammonium acetate.

Allow slides to dry at room temperature.

3.7. Autoradiography

Perform the following in the dark room under safelight:

1. Melt emulsion in water bath at 42°C for ~30 min (*see* **Note 21**).
2. Pour some into a dipping chamber. Dip slides and allow to dry for at least 3 h at room temperature.
3. Place slides in a black box, seal, and store at 4°C for ~2–3 wk.

3.8. Developing and Detection

Prepare the fixer and the developer according to the manufacturer's instructions. Perform the following in the dark room under safelight:

1. Allow boxes containing slides to warm up to room temperature for ~30 min.
2. Place the rack containing slides in the developer's trough for 3.5 min.
3. Transfer the rack in a trough containing H_2O for 30 s.
4. Transfer the rack to a trough containing the fixer for 5 min.
5. Place the rack under running tap H_2O for ~20 min.

The remaining of experiment can be carried out in the laboratory under the normal light:

1. Scrape the excess of emulsion surrounding the section(s) from slides.
2. Counterstain with hematoxylin for 2 min. Wash slides thoroughly.
3. Dehydrate slides in 90, 100, and 100% ethanol for 2 min each.
4. Immerse slides in xylene 2×2 min (*see* **Note 22**).
5. Mount in DPX and cover section(s) with coverslip.
6. Observe signals using light or dark field microscopy (*see* **Fig. 4**).

4. Notes

All reagents should be molecular biology grade materials.

1. Gloves must be worn throughout the experiment and changed frequently to avoid RNase contamination.
2. Glassware must be baked at 220°C overnight.
3. All buffers must be treated with 0.1% DEPC, then autoclaved to ensure no traces of DEPC remain. Tris buffer is an exception, it should be prepared with autoclaved DEPC-treated H_2O.
4. Biopsies must be fixed immediately in freshly prepared 4% paraformaldehyde to prevent RNA degradation and to retain the tissue architecture. The length of fixation depends on the size of the biopsy, i.e., larger biopsies require longer fixation. In contrast, cytospin preparations do not require more than 20 min of fixation.

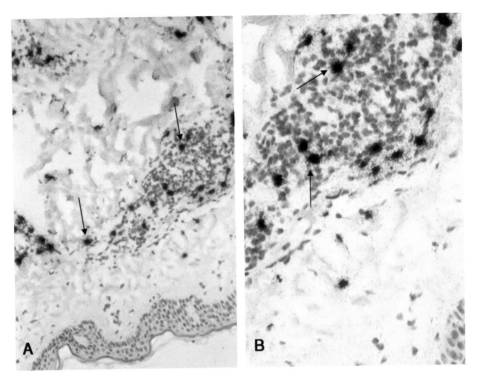

Fig. 4. Light microscopic examination of in situ hybridization performed on a skin biopsy (obtained 24 h after challenge with grass pollen extract) using ^{35}S-labelled IL-13 ribo-probe. Hybridization signals are shown as clusters of silver grains over nuclei of mononuclear cells *(a)* 20× and *(b)* 40× magnification.

5. Paraformaldehye should be prepared in fume hood. Preheat PBS to 60°C. Add paraformaldehyde and monitor the temperature. Do not allow the temperature to exceed 60°C.
6. Extra care should be taken when handling DH5α™ Competent cells (*E. Coli*).
7. Mini-preparation can also be performed using Plasmid Mini Kit (Qiagen).
8. LB broth and LB agar are prepared according to the manufacturer's instructions.
9. Ethidium bromide is believed to be carcinogen and should not be discarded in the waste sink. It should be inactivated before discarding.
10. Protect eyes when analyzing gels under the UV light by viewing under perspex screen and/or wearing eye goggles.
11. Ratios below 1.8 for 260/280 nm indicate impurity of DNA preparation.
12. Phenol should be handled with care and not discarded in the waste sink.
13. When using ^{35}S, the procedure should be carried out behind the perspex screen.
14. All steps used in any in situ hybridization should be empirically determined as type of tissue, method of fixation used, choice of probe, type of and method of labeling,

concentration of the probe, the stringency of hybridization and post hybridization conditions, and type and level of expression of the target nucleic acid sequence of interest all influence the outcome of the results.

15. Formamide used in hybridization buffer should be deionized before use (using 10% (w:v) Mixed Bed Resin M-8032, Sigma).
16. Formamide can methylate DNA and is harmful to unborn babies and should therefore be handled with extreme care in the fume hood.
17. Acetylation of amino groups reduces nonspecific electrostatic binding of probes, particularly when ^{35}S-labeled probe is used.
18. Acetic anhydride should be used in the fume hood.
19. Heating the probe at 60°C is intended to unfold tertiary structure of ribo-probe and facilitate hybridization.
20. 20× SSC is prepared by 175.3 g sodium chloride and 88.2 g sodium citrate in 1.0 liter (pH = 7.0).
21. The stringency of post hybridization washes is critical for specific hybridization signals. Therefore high temperature and low salt concentration should be included in post hybridization washes to ensure hybridized signals are not artifacts.
22. Emulsion should not be stored in the same fridge as radioisotopes.
23. Xylene must be handled in the fume hood wearing nitrile gloves.

Acknowledgment

The author is grateful to Professor SR Durham and Dr MR Jacobson for their helpful comments on this chapter.

References

1. Pardue, M. L. and Gall, J. G. (1969) Molecular hybridisation of radioactive DNA to the DNA of cytological preparations. *Proc. Natl Acad. Sci. USA* **64,** 600–604.
2. Gall, J. G. and Pardue, M. L. (1969) Formation and detetion of RNA-DNA hybrid molecules in cytological preparations. *Proc. Natl Acad. Sci. USA* **63,** 378–383.
3. John, H., Birnstiel, M., and Jones, K. (1969) RNA:DNA hybrids at the cytological level. *Nature* **223,** 582–587.
4. Nouri-Aria, K. T., Arnold, J., Davison, F., et al. (1991) Hepatic IFN-α gene transcripts and products in liver specimens from acute and chronic hepatitis B virus infection. *Hepatology* **13,** 1029–1034.
5. Nouri-Aria, K. T., Sallie, R., Sanger, D., et al. (1993) Detection of genomic and intermediate replicative strands of hepatitis C virus in liver tissue by *in situ* hybridisation. *J. Clin. Invest.* **91,** 2226–2234.
6. Naoumou, N. V., Alexander, G. J. M., Eddleston, A. L. W. F., and Williams, R. (1988) *In situ* hybridisation in formalin fixed paraffin wax embedded liver specimens: method for detecting human and viral DNA using biotinylated probes. *J. Clin. Pathol.* **158,** 279–286.
7. Porter, H. J., Heryet, A., Quantrill, A. M., and Fleming, K. A. (1990) Combined non-isotopic *in situ* hybridization and immunohistochemistry on routine paraffin wax embedded tissue: identification of cell type infected by human parvovirus and

demonstration of cytomegalovirus DNA and antigen in renal infection. *J. Clin. Pathol.* **43**, 129–132.

8. Bakkus, M. H. C., Brakel-Van Peer, K. M. J., Adriaansen, H. J., et al. (1989) Detection of oncogene expression by fluorescent in situ hybridisation in combination with immunofluorescent staining of cell surface markers. *Oncogene* **4**, 1255–1262.

9. Nouri-Aria, K. T., Masuyama, K., Jacobson, M. R., et al. (1998) Granulocyte/macrophage-colony stimulating factor in allergen-induced rhinitis: cellular localization, relation to tissue eosinophilia and influence of topical corticosteroid. *Int. Arch. Allergy Immunol.* **117**, 248–254.

10. van Dekken, H. (1988) Enzymatic production of single-stranded DNA as a target for fluorescence *in situ* hybridisation. *Chromosoma* **97**, 1–5.

11. d'Arville, C. N., Nouri-Aria, K. T., Johnson, P., and Williams, R. (1991) Regulation of insulin-like growth factor II gene expression by hepatitis B virus in hepatocellular carcinoma. *Hepatology* **13**, 310–315.

12. Denny, P., Hamid, Q., Krause, J. E., Polak, J. M., and Legon, S. (1988) Oligoriboprobes: Tools for *in situ* hybridisation. *Histochemistry* **89**, 481–483.

13. Giaid, A., Hamid, Q., Adams, C., et al. (1989) Non-isotopic RNA probes: comparison between different labels and detection systems. *Histochemistry* **93**, 191–196.

14. Farquharson, M., Harvie, R., and McNicol, A. M. (1990) Detection of mRNA using a digoxigenin end labelled oligodeoxynucleotide probe. *J. Clin. Pathol.* **43**, 424–428.

15. Singler, R. H., Lawrence, J. B., and Villnave, C. (1986) Optimization of *in situ* hybridisation using isotopic and non-isotopic detection methods. *BioTechniques* **4**, 230–250.

16. Niedobitek, G. (1989) In situ hybridisation using biotinylated probes. An evaluation of different detection systems. *Path. Res. Pract.* **184**, 343–348.

17. Baldino, F. Jr. and Lewis, M. E. (1989) Nonradioactive *in situ* hybridization histochemistry with digoxigenin-deoxyuridine 5′-triphosphate-labeled oligonucleotides. In: Conn. P. M. (ed.) Gene probes. *Methods in Neuroscience.* Academic Press, San Diego, pp. 282–292.

18. Nouri-Aria, K. T., O'Brien, F., Noble, W., et al. (2000) Cytokine expression during allergen-induced late nasal responses: IL-4 and IL-5 mRNA is expressed early (at 6 h) predominantly by eosinophils. *Clin. Exp. Allergy* **30**, 1709–1716.

19. Maitland, N. J., Cox, M. F., Lynas, C., et al. (1987) Nucleic acid probes in the study of latent viral disease. *J. Oral Pathology* **16**, 199–211.

20. Clavel, C., Binninger, I., Boutterin, M-C., Polette, M., Birembaut, P. (1991) Comparison of four non-radioactive and ^{35}S-based methods for the detection of human papillomavirus DNA by in situ hybridization. *J. Virol. Methods.* **33**, 253–266.

21. Crum, C. P., Nuovo, G., Friedman, D., Silverstein, S. J. (1988) A comparison of biotin and isotope-labelled ribonucleic acid probes for in situ detection of HPV-16 ribonucleic acid in genital pre-cancers. *Lab Invest.* **8**, 354–359.

22. Nuovo, G. L. and Richart, R. M. (1989) A comparison of biotin- and ^{35}S-based in situ hybridization methodologies for detection of human papillomavirus DNA. *Lab. Invest.* **61**, 471–476.

23. Roch Molecular Biochemicals: Nonradioactive in situ hybridisation – Application Manual. 2nd Ed. Combined DNA in situ hybridiation and IMH for the simultaneous detection of nucleic acod sequences, protein and incorporated BrdU in cell preparation. Speel EJM, Ramaekers FCS, HopmanAHN, pp. 111.
24. Isotopic *in situ* hybridisation (Handbook). Methods and Reagents, pp. 17. Amersham International plc (UK).
25. Cox, K. H., Deleon, D. V., Angerer, L. M., and Angerer, R. C. (1984) Detection of mRNAs in sea urchin embryos by *in situ* hybridization using asymmetric RNA probes. *Dev. Biol.* **101,** 485–502.
25. Durham, S. R., Walker, S., Varga, E. M., et al. (1999) Long term clinical efficacy of grass-pollen immunotherapy. *New Engl. J. Med.* **341,** 468–475.

Index

Printed in The United States of America